MCQs in Medical Surgical Nursing

(With Explanatory Answers)

MCQs in Medical Surgical Nursing
(With Explanatory Answers)

Second Edition

Srinanda Ghosh MN
Formerly, Principal
Woodlands College of Nursing
Kolkata, West Bengal, India

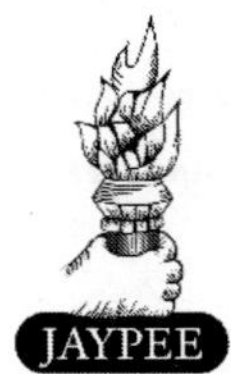

JAYPEE BROTHERS MEDICAL PUBLISHERS
The Health Sciences Publisher
New Delhi | London

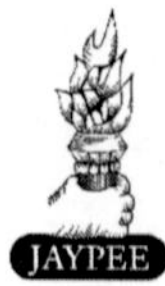

Jaypee Brothers Medical Publishers (P) Ltd

Headquarters
Jaypee Brothers Medical Publishers (P) Ltd
23/23-B, Ansari Road, Daryaganj
New Delhi 110 002, India
Phone: +91-11-23272143, +91-11-23272703
+91-11-23282021, +91-11-23245672
E-mail: jaypee@jaypeebrothers.com

Corporate Office
Jaypee Brothers Medical Publishers (P) Ltd.
4838/24, Ansari Road, Daryaganj
New Delhi 110 002, India
Phone: +91-11-43574357
Fax: +91-11-43574314
E-mail: jaypee@jaypeebrothers.com

Overseas Offices
J.P. Medical Ltd
83 Victoria Street, London
SW1H 0HW (UK)
Phone: +44 20 3170 8910
Email: info@jpmedpub.com

EU GPSR Authorised Representative
Logos Europe, 9 rue Nicolas Poussin
17000, La Rochelle, France
Phone: +33 (0) 6 67 93 73 78
E-mail: Contact@logoseurope.eu

Website: www.jaypeebrothers.com
Website: www.jaypeedigital.com

© 2019, Jaypee Brothers Medical Publishers

The views and opinions expressed in this book are solely those of the original contributor(s)/author(s) and do not necessarily represent those of editor(s) of the book.

All rights reserved. No part of this publication may be reproduced, stored or transmitted in any form or by any means, electronic, mechanical, photocopying, recording or otherwise, without the prior permission in writing of the publishers.

All brand names and product names used in this book are trade names, service marks, trademarks or registered trademarks of their respective owners. The publisher is not associated with any product or vendor mentioned in this book.

Medical knowledge and practice change constantly. This book is designed to provide accurate, authoritative information about the subject matter in question. However, readers are advised to check the most current information available on procedures included and check information from the manufacturer of each product to be administered, to verify the recommended dose, formula, method and duration of administration, adverse effects and contraindications. It is the responsibility of the practitioner to take all appropriate safety precautions. Neither the publisher nor the author(s)/editor(s) assume any liability for any injury and/or damage to persons or property arising from or related to use of material in this book.

This book is sold on the understanding that the publisher is not engaged in providing professional medical services. If such advice or services are required, the services of a competent medical professional should be sought.

Every effort has been made where necessary to contact holders of copyright to obtain permission to reproduce copyright material. If any have been inadvertently overlooked, the publisher will be pleased to make the necessary arrangements at the first opportunity. The **CD/DVD-ROM** (if any) provided in the sealed envelope with this book is complimentary and free of cost. **Not meant for sale**.

Inquiries for bulk sales may be solicited at: jaypee@jaypeebrothers.com

MCQs in Medical Surgical Nursing (With Explanatory Answers)

First Edition: 2007

Second Edition: 2019, Reprint: **2026**

ISBN: 978-93-5270-539-9

Printed in India

Preface to the Second Edition

The second edition of my book incorporates the most current pharmacological treatment modalities used in the Indian scenario, amongst the others discussed in the previous edition. The comprehensive and brainstorming Multiple Choice Questions (MCQs) in medical surgical nursing would help the students in general nursing and BSc nursing programs, preparing for competitive examinations.

I am highly indebted to my colleagues and friends for the invaluable support they have provided me. I also dedicate this book to all my students over the years.

Srinanda Ghosh

Preface to the First Edition

The constant element in life and nature is "change", and never more than now have I felt this truth, in the trends of changing examination papers for various admission tests. Multiple choice questions (MCQs) are the mainstay of any competitive examinations and students who have scored well in this examination have avenues opened to them.

In my 28 years of academic experience, I have witnessed that a comprehensive book of MCQs on nursing in India is lacking. Taking cue from this, I have decided to write this book of MCQs on Medical Surgical Nursing (which I have taught for many years). The book would pave the path for detailed reviewing of the conditions, symptoms and management of the diseases.

The book covers the 12 major areas, namely circulatory, hematological, urinary, respiratory, reproductive, endocrine, integumentary, musculoskeletal, gastrointestinal and nervous systems and immunology and oncology. They are mainly targeted to the BSc students and graduate nurses of both collegiate and diploma program, appearing for competitive examinations.

There are some areas which I have not been able to touch upon in this book, and which I intend to cover in my next edition of MCQs.

I am highly indebted to my family and friends for the invaluable support they have provided me, while I struggled on with the book for the last two years. I also dedicate this book to all my students over the years.

Srinanda Ghosh

Contents

1
CHAPTER

Nervous System Including Special Senses (Eye and Ear)

Q1. Which of the following statements is not true about neurotransmitters?

A. Chemicals that are manufactured in the nerve cell body
B. Chemicals that are manufactured by the myelin sheath of axon
C. Transfer information from one neuron to another across synapse
D. Exhibit both excitatory and inhibitory action

Q2. Which of the following neurotransmitters exhibits excitatory action, transmits pleasurable sensation and inhibits pain transmission?

A. Gamma-aminobutyric acid (GABA)
B. Dopamine
C. Serotonin
D. Endorphin

Q3. The lobe of the brain that contains the primary sensory cortex, which analyzes sensory information is the:

A. Frontal lobe
B. Parietal lobe
C. Temporal lobe
D. Occipital lobe

Q4. The part of the brain, which is responsible for coordination of movement is:

A. Brainstem
B. Cerebellum
C. Thalamus
D. Hypothalamus

Q5. After a head injury a patient has lost his recent memory. Which lobe of the brain is affected?

A. Frontal
B. Occipital
C. Parietal
D. Temporal

Q6. The heat regulatory center is located in the:

A. Thalamus
B. Hypothalamus
C. Limbic system
D. Medulla

Q7. What is the function of the cranial nerve IV?

A. Hearing
B. Vision
C. Eye movement
D. Chewing

Q8. The cranial nerve that is responsible for hearing and maintaining balance is the:

A. Trochlear
B. Vestibulocochlear
C. Trigeminal
D. Vagus

Q9. Drooping eyelid (Ptosis) is a disorder of which cranial nerve?

A. CN III
B. CN V
C. CN VI
D. CN VIII

Q10. Bell's palsy is a disorder of which cranial nerve?

A. CN IV
B. CN VII
C. CN IX
D. CN XII

Q11. What is the first thing a nurse should assess to determine the presence of neurological changes?

A. Vital signs
B. Level of consciousness
C. Mental status
D. Reflexes

Q12. Objective measurement of patient's level of consciousness is best determined by using Glasgow:

A. Consciousness scale
B. Communication scale
C. Coma scale
D. Stimuli scale

Q13. During neurological assessment the nurse asks the patient to close his eyes and then to smell and identify different odors. Ability to correctly perceive any one smell signifies proper functioning of which of the following cranial nerves?

A. Cranial nerve I
B. Cranial nerve II
C. Cranial nerve V
D. Cranial nerve VII

Q14. The nurse is assessing a patient to detect the status of cranial nerves. Which of the following findings is an abnormality noted with cranial nerve VII dysfunction?

A. Face movements symmetrical with smiling
B. Increased tearing
C. Inability to differentiate different taste
D. Presence of nasolabial fold

Q15. Which of the following assessment findings indicates dysfunction of cranial nerve XI?

A. Inability to swallow
B. Hoarse voice
C. Inability to move the tongue from side to side
D. Inability to shrug shoulders

Q16. The nurse is performing a routine neurological assessment of a patient. To assess the function of the cranial nerve XII (hypoglossal) the nurse should ask the patient to:

A. Make chewing movements
B. Drink a small amount of water
C. Taste different food items
D. Stick out the tongue and move it from side to side and in and out

Q17. Nurse understands that assessment of mental status is an essential component of neurological assessment. Which part of the brain is evaluated by mental status examination?

A. Cerebrum
B. Cerebellum
C. Midbrain
D. Thalamus

Q18. One of the important components of neurological assessment is examination of motor system. Motor system examination includes:

A. Assessment of bulk, tone, and power of the major muscle groups of the body
B. Assessment of mechanical sensation
C. Assessment of balance and coordination
D. All except B

Q19. The heel-to-shin test assesses:

A. Muscle strength of lower extremities
B. Muscle coordination of lower extremities

C. Involuntary movements of lower extremities
D. All of the above

Q20. Which of the following assessment findings indicates cerebeller disease?

A. Pronator drift
B. Spasticity
C. Ataxic gait
D. Chorea

Q21. Which of the following terms describes discrete, jerky, purposeless movements in distal extremities and face?

A. Chorea
B. Myoclonus
C. Tic
D. Tremors

Q22. Which of the following terms refers to inability to carry out a learned movement on command in the absence of weakness or paralysis?

A. Akinesia
B. Athetosis
C. Apraxia
D. Agnosia

Q23. The nurse is assessing best motor response in an unconscious patient. With painful stimuli the patient flexes, adducts and internally rotates the wrists and arms to the chest and rigidly extends the legs. She records her findings as:

A. Normal posturing
B. Spastic posturing
C. Decorticate posturing
D. Decerebrate posturing

Q24. All of the following reflexes are examples of superficial reflexes *except:*

A. Planter
B. Corneal
C. Patellar
D. Pharyngeal or Gag

Q25. Which of the following reflexes if found in a patient during neurological examination is considered abnormal?

A. Corneal
B. Pupillary
C. Achilles or ankle jerk
D. Chewing

Q26. A patient with a space-occupying lesion is scheduled for a CT scan of head. The nurse prepares the patient for the test by:

A. Keeping the patient NPO 4–6 hours before the test
B. Ensuring that the patient is not allergic to iodine, contrast medium or shellfish
C. Obtaining an informed consent
D. Both B and C

Q27. A patient with suspected brain tumor is scheduled for a CT scan. To prepare the patient for this test the nurse should:

A. Describe the equipment involved in this procedure
B. Shampoo patient's hair
C. Explain that no radiation will be involved in this test
D. Withhold routine medication before the test

Q28. Which of the following tests enables visualization of physiologic functions in body areas?

A. Computed tomography (CT)
B. Magnetic resonance imaging (MRI)
C. Positron emission tomography (PET)
D. Doppler scanning

Q29. X-ray examination of the spinal cord and vertebral canal following introduction of a contrast material into the spinal subarachnoid space is known as:

A. Angiography
B. Myelography
C. Spinal tap
D. Electromyography

Q30. All of the following statements regarding lumbar puncture is true *except:*

A. The needle is inserted into the lumbar subarachnoid space of the spinal canal
B. Purposes may be diagnostic or therapeutic
C. Strict aseptic technique must be observed
D. Should immediately precede encephalography or myelography

Q31. Which of the following nursing interventions after a lumbar puncture will prevent spinal headache in patient?

A. Instruct the patient to lie in bed for 3–4 hours
B. Encourage drinking extra fluids
C. Withheld food and fluids for 3–4 hours
D. Both A and B

Q32. A patient who had an episode of seizure for the first time has been ordered an electroencephalogram (EEG). The nurse is instructing the patient regarding preprocedure care. Which of the following instructions is not appropriate?

A. "You can have normal food and fluids before the test"
B. "Avoid taking stimulants, e.g. tea, coffee, alcohol, cola and cigarettes for 24–48 hours"
C. "Avoid shampooing your hair for 3 days before the test"
D. "Withheld anticonvulsant 48 hours before the test"

Q33. A patient has to undergo a lumbar puncture. The nursing responsibilities will include all of the following *except:*

A. Obtaining an informed consent
B. Encouraging the patient to evacuate bladder and rectum
C. Placing the patient laterally with the knees drawn-up to the abdomen and the chin drawn to the chest
D. Asking the patient to cough when the needle has been inserted

Q34. A patient who demonstrates a stuporous level of consciousness:

A. Is oriented but sleeps often, has slowed speech
B. Sleeps almost constantly, can be aroused, follows simple command
C. Awakens only with vigorous stimulation
D. Does not respond to environmental stimuli

Q35. A patient has been admitted in medical surgical unit in a comatose state. Coma in an individual may be caused by:

A. Structural lesions in the brain affecting reticular activating system (RAS)
B. Functional lesions in the brain
C. Metabolic disorders
D. Both A and C

Q36. The following types of seizures are all examples of generalized seizures *except:*

A. Myoclonic
B. Tonic
C. Clonic
D. Myoclonic-tonic

Q37. Which of the following types of seizure is most common?

A. Partial seizures
B. Tonic-clonic
C. Atonic
D. Absence

Q38. In which of the following types of seizures there is sudden uncontrollable jerking movements of single or multiple muscle groups, sometimes causing the patient to fall?

A. Tonic-clonic
B. Tonic
C. Myoclonic
D. Clonic

Q39. A patient who had an attack of seizures reports seeing a flashes of light before his seizures. Which of the following terms describes this condition?

A. Autonomic manifestation
B. Precipitating factor
C. Aura
D. Postictal experience

Q40. While assessing vital signs of a patient having recurrent attacks of seizures the nurse should:

A. Take an axillary temperature every 4 hourly
B. Observe for bradycardia
C. Observe for bradypnea
D. All of the above

Q41. A patient admitted with epilepsy for investigation suddenly started having a tonic-clonic seizure. The nurse should:

A. Lay the patient to the bed, remove pillows, raise side rails and insert an oral airway
B. Lay the patient to the bed, remove pillows, raise side rails and restrain his arms
C. Lay the patient on bed, place the patient on one side, remove pillows, raise side rails, and ensure patent airways
D. Lay the patient on bed, place the patient on his back, remove pillows, raise the side rails, and insert an oral airway

Q42. The nurse teaching the family members of a patient who has recently been diagnosed as a case of idiopathic epilepsy, regarding precaution to be taken during a seizure. Which of the following the nurse should include in the teaching?

A. Lay the patient on a flat surface, insert a padded spoon between the teeth
B. Lay the patient on a flat surface, turn him on his side and protect his head
C. Lay the patient on a flat surface, remove all furniture out of his way
D. Lay the patient and hold his arms and legs still

Q43. A patient with new onset tonic clonic seizures has been prescribed phenytoin 100 mg BD. The nurse should teach which of the following regarding treatment with phenytoin?

A. Discontinue to the drug if you experience palpitation
B. If you continue to feel sleepy reduce the dose by half of the daily dose
C. Attend regular follow-up visits and periodical assessment of plasma concentration of the drug
D. Stop taking the drug once you are symptom free for 3 months

Q44. A patient with seizure disorder is being taught about self-care. Which of the following statements by the patient indicates further teaching?

A. "I should not go for swimming alone"
B. "I need to avoid alcohol, coffee and tea"
C. "Meditation and relaxation therapy will be good for me"
D. "I can continue driving my two wheeler as much as I like"

Q45. The patients with seizures are usually advised to refrain from alcoholic beverages. Which of the following statements supports the rationale behind this advice?

A. Alcohol lowers seizure threshold
B. Alcohol is detoxified by the liver, interrupting metabolism of anticonvulsant drugs
C. Alcohol necessitates increase dosing of antiepileptic drugs
D. Both A and B

Q46. Which of the following side effects may occur during phenytoin therapy?

A. Thickened gum
B. Dry mouth
C. Drowsiness
D. Tachycardia

Q47. The nurse is reviewing the laboratory finding of plasma level of phenytoin and finds it as 30 mg/dL. What adverse effect may occur?

A. Water retention and hyponatremia
B. Ataxia and visual disturbance
C. Facial tics
D. Hypertension and tachycardia

Q48. A patient has been admitted in the hospital emergency department with status epilepticus. The nurse has administered diazepam10 mg IV stat as prescribed. At what time she may administer the second dose of diazepam if needed and prescribed?

A. After 5 minutes
B. After 15 minutes
C. After 30 minutes
D. After 1 hour

Q49. For a patient admitted in the hospital with status epilepticus, physician has prescribed injection diazepam10 mg IV stat and injection phenytoin 100 mg slow IV push. What precaution the nurse must take during the administration of these drugs?

A. Diazepam may be mixed with phenytoin and administered together
B. Diazepam may be administered at a rate of 5 mg/minute and phenytoin at a rate of 50 mg/minute
C. Keep ready resuscitative measures before injecting these drugs
D. Both B and C

Q50. What surgical procedure involves resection of dispensable areas of the cerebral cortex designed to cure complex partial seizures?

A. Corpus callosotomy
B. Temporal lobectomy
C. Hemispherectomy
D. None of the above

Q51. A patient with a space occupying lesion in brain is to undergo a magnetic resonance imaging (MRI) study. Which of the following nursing actions is indicated in preparing the patient for this test?

A. Keeping patient on NPO status for 6 hours before the test
B. Take history of allergy to shellfish
C. Shave the groin for insertion of a femoral catheter
D. Remove all metal containing objects from the patient

Q52. Which of the following is not a classic manifestation of brain tumor?

A. Headache
B. Vertigo
C. Nausea
D. Vomiting

Q53. Which of the following is not a major goal of treatment of malignant brain tumor?

A. Identifying the tumor type and location
B. Removing or decreasing tumor mass
C. Preventing or managing increased intracranial pressure
D. Identifying and locating metastatic lesions in other parts of the body

Q54. A patient with a space occupying lesion in brain is to undergo a magnetic resonance imaging (MRI) study. Which of the following nursing actions is indicated in preparing the patient for this test?

A. Keeping patient on NPO status for 6 hours before the test
B. Take history of allergy to shell fish
C. Shave the groins for insertion of a femoral catheter
D. Remove all metal containing objects from the patient

Q55. After a supratentorial craniotomy the patient should be placed in which of the following positions?

A. Side-lying
B. Prone
C. Supine
D. Semi-Fowler

Q56. A patient has had a craniotomy to remove a brain tumor. Hospital's protocol for positioning the patient includes, maintaining the head of bed at 45° and turning from side to side. Which of the following actions during positioning is contraindicated?

A. Placing patient on a side with neck in neutral position and hips flexed
B. Placing patient on a side, neck in neutral position, and a pillow between the patient's knees
C. Placing the patient on the back with both arms slightly elevated on pillows
D. Placing the patient on the back, neck in neutral position and arms slightly elevated

Q57. The primary goal of nursing care after a craniotomy is:

A. Preventing infection
B. Preventing increased intracranial pressure
C. Teaching patient and family members ambulatory care
D. Promoting improved body image

Q58. The nurse is assessing a patient who had undergone a transsphenoidal hypophysectomy in the immediate postoperative period. Which of the following signs indicates that the patient is bleeding from the operative site?

A. Bloody drainage from the ears
B. Frequent swallowing
C. Hematuria
D. Guaiac-positive stools

Q59. The nurse is assessing a patient admitted with bacterial meningitis. She is expected to find all of the following signs *except:*

A. Trismus
B. Nuchal rigidity
C. Kernig's sign
D. Brudzinski's sign

Q60. Physician has performed a lumbar puncture for cerebrospinal fluid (CSF) analysis for a patient with suspected meningitis. Which of the following findings of CSF analysis is expected in a patient with bacterial meningitis?

A. CSF turbid
B. Elevated protein level
C. Decreased glucose level
D. All are correct

Q61. Of the following patients, the one with the highest risk for a stroke is:

A. A 45-year-old obese man who takes moderate amount of alcohol
B. A 35-year-old physically inactive woman on oral contraceptive
C. A 60-year-old man with hypertension
D. A 70-year-old man with a history of transient ischemic attack

Q62. The nurse is taking history from the wife of a patient admitted with stroke. Which of the following informations provided by the wife would help differentiate a thrombotic stroke from an embolic stroke?

A. History of hypotension
B. Symptoms appeared during sleep
C. History of unconsciousness
D. None of the above provides any clue

Q63. Which of the following conditions places a patient at risk for embolic stroke?

A. Atrial fibrillation
B. Deep vein thrombosis
C. Dehydration
D. Atherosclerosis

Q64. The primary causative factor for thrombus formation in people suffering from thrombotic stroke is:

A. Atherosclerosis
B. Arteritis
C. Hypertension
D. All of the above

Q65. Which of the followings is the common manifestation of hemorrhagic stroke?

A. Tends to occur during sleep
B. Severe occipital or nuchal headaches
C. Presence of motor weakness
D. All of the above

Q66. Which of the following conditions is the most important risk factor for intra-cerebral hemorrhage?

A. Coronary artery disease
B. Hypertension
C. Thrombolytic drugs
D. Shock

Q67. The nurse is assesing a patient who recently experienced CVA and finds that the patient is unable to form words that are understandable neither he can comprehend the spoken words. Which of the following conditions best describes the assessment findings?

A. Wernicke's (sensory/receptive) aphasia
B. Broca's (expressive or motor) aphasia
C. Global aphasia
D. Anomia

Q68. While communicating with the patient who has expressive aphasia the nurse should:

A. Speak loudly and clearly to the unaffected side
B. Allow the patient time to respond
C. Use simple sentences with appropriate gestures
D. Ask the patient to write what he wants

Q69. The nurse notices that a patient who had an attack of CVA has taken only a half of the food laid down on the right side of the table. The food laid down on the left side was ignored. The nurse understands that the patient is exhibiting:

A. Unilateral neglect
B. Homonymous hemianopia
C. Visual agnosia
D. Double vision

Q70. The nurse is taking care of a patient recovering from a stroke. In order to promote mobility of the patient the nurse should:

A. Encourage the patient to exercise while they are at bed rest
B. Teach the patient to sit up
C. Teach and demonstrate the patient and family member how to use a wheel chair
D. All of the above

Q71. A patient with left-sided hemiplegia has developed complete flaccidity of the left arm. Anticipating high-risk for shoulder subluxation the nurse should do which of the following?

A. Avoid lifting patient by the flaccid shoulder
B. Position flaccid arm on a pillow while the patient is seated
C. Provide a sling when the patient is ambulatory to prevent dangling of arm
D. All of the above

Q72. A patient with valvular prosthesis has suffered a transient ischemic attack (TIA). Which of the following medications may be prescribed to him to prevent a stroke?

A. Aspirin **B.** Ticlopidine
C. Streptokinase **D.** Warfarin

Q73. Which of the following statements shows the major difference between pathophysiology of a TIA (transient ischemic attack) and that of a stroke?

A. TIAs mostly occur due to hemorrhage in brain
B. In TIA there is rapid onset of unconsciousness with weakness in an arm or leg
C. TIA tend to occur repeatedly and give rise to permanent motor deficit
D. In TIA there is short duration of ischemia and complete recovery of neurological deficit

Q74. A patient is admitted in the hospital and is diagnosed as a case of thrombotic cerebrovascular accident. The physician is considering thrombolytic therapy. Thrombolytic therapy should be started within how many hours of the onset of clinical signs of stroke?

A. Within 3 hours
B. Within 6 hours
C. Within 12 hours
D. Within 24 hours

Q75. The drug of choice for thrombolytic therapy in ischemic stroke is:

A. Streptokinase
B. Heparin
C. Recombinant tissue plasminogen activator (rt-PA)
D. Any of the above

Q76. When caring for a patient with the nursing diagnosis of risk of aspiration related to decreased level of consciousness the nurse should:

A. Place the patient in supine position
B. Restrict dietary fluids
C. Ensure gag reflex returns before offering food and fluids
D. All of the above

Q77. The nurse is taking care of a patient recovering from stroke with residual dysphagia. Nursing intervention to promote adequate nutrition will include all of the following *except:*

A. Position the patient in an upright position
B. Allow the patient to have meal with other patient to encourage feeding
C. Offer thickened liquids or pureed foods
D. Provide pleasant and unhurried mealtime

Q78. The nurse is assessing a patient with brain tumor for increased intracranial pressure. Which of the symptoms if detected in the patient would indicate early sign of increased intracranial pressure?

A. Anorexia
B. Restlessness and irritability
C. Bradycardia
D. Hypotension

Q79. The nurse is assessing vital signs of a patient with head injury. Which of the following findings indicates increased intracranial pressure?

A. Tachycardia
B. Bradypnea
C. Widened pulse pressure
D. Decreased body temperature

Q80. A patient with head injury has increased intracranial pressure. The physician increased the ventilator setting to cause hyperventilation. Which of the following blood gas level should be maintained to reduce increased intracranial pressure?

A. $PaCO_2$ at 30–35 mm Hg, PaO_2 90-100 mm Hg
B. $PaCO_2$ at 35–40 mm Hg, PaO_2 80-90 mm Hg
C. $PaCO_2$ at 40–45 mm Hg, PaO_2 70-80 mm Hg
D. $PaCO_2$ at 45–50 mm Hg, PaO_2 60–70 mm Hg

Q81. The physician has ordered Inj. Mannitol 20% 1 g/kg of body weight to a patient with increased intracranial pressure. The nurse understands that this drug is given to:

A. Raise blood pressure and thus raise cerebral perfusion pressure
B. Reduce cerebral metabolism
C. Reduce intracranial pressure by reducing cerebral edema
D. Meet increased need of glucose by the brain cells

Q82. Which of the following methods of intracranial pressure monitoring provides most accurate results?

A. Epidural catheter
B. Intraventricular catheters
C. Subarachnoid catheter
D. Intravertebral catheter

Q83. Which of the following is a major complication of continuous intracranial pressure (ICP) monitoring?

A. Intracranial hypertension
B. Infection
C. Leakage of CSF (cerebrospinal fluid)
D. Seizures

Q84. A patient with hemorrhagic stroke has undergone evacuation of the hematoma and is recovering in the ICU. Which of the following nursing interventions is not approppriate and may increase intracranial pressure?

A. Placing patient in supine position with head elevated to 30°
B. Maintaining a patent airway by suctioning every hour
C. Maintaining PaO_2 at 100 mm Hg.
D. Administering prophylactic anticonvulsant as prescribed

Q85. A 15-year-old girl with a concussion is being discharged from the hospital. During discharge the nurse is teaching the mother of the girl to report to emergency department immediately if the girl:

A. Complains of headache
B. Is anorexic
C. Complains of pain in leg
D. Is confused

Q86. During assessment of a patient with head injury the nurse notices blood tinged fluid is draining from the nose of the patient. Which of the following the nurse should do?

A. Test the fluid for Halo sign
B. Test the fluid for glucose with a dextrostix strip
C. Raise the headend of the bed at 60°
D. Pack the anterior nares with sterile gauze

Q87. Which of the following statements about myasthenia gravis is not true?

A. The disease is caused by viral infection of neuromuscular junction
B. Antibodies against acetylcholine receptors are detected amongst majority of patients
C. The disease is more common in women
D. Destruction of acetylcholine receptors causes muscle weakness

Q88. The most common early manifestation of myasthenia gravis is:

A. Paresthesia of lower extremities
B. Absent pupillary reflex
C. Ptosis
D. Dysphagia

Q89. The diagnosis of myasthenia gravis is established by:

A. Typical symptoms of the patient
B. Presence of Halo sign
C. Presence of Brudzinski's sign
D. Observing response of the patient to edrophonium test

Q90. A patient with suspected myasthenia gravis is undergoing tensilon (Edrophonium chloride) test. The nurse understands that the response of the patient that will decide the diagnosis is:

A. Increase of symptoms for a short period
B. Immediate improvement in muscle strength for a short period
C. Quite a lot of improvement in muscle strength lasting for 2-3 hours
D. Change in heart rate and rhythm

Q91. A patient has just been diagnosed with myasthenia gravis. The nurse anticipates that the patient will be treated with:

A. Atropine sulfate
B. Neostigmine (prostigmine)
C. Edrophonium chloride (tensilon)
D. All of the above

Q92. The physician orders neostigmin for a patient with MG. Which of the following teachings by the nurse is appropriate?

A. Keep the drug in the refrigerator

B. Strictly maintain the timings of the drug ordered
C. Take the drug in between meals for better absorption
D. Peak action of the drug occurs after 2–3 hours of taking the drug

Q93. A 35-year-old patient with myasthenia gravis is scheduled to undergo plasmapheresis. The mechanism by which the procedure yield short-term relief to the patient is:

A. Removing anticholinesterase drugs bound to plasma caused by overdose of medication
B. Remove T lymphocytes that attack acetylcholine receptors from blood
C. Remove viral antigen causing the disease
D. Remove acetylcholine receptor antibodies from blood

Q94. The nurse is teaching a patient with myasthenia gravis attending hospital outpatient department with the complaint of difficulty in chewing and swallowing. Which of the following instructions is not appropriate?

A. Take semisolid and pureed foods
B. Take the medication prescribed 45 minutes before meal
C. Hyperextend the neck during swallowing
D. Suction when needed

Q95. A patient with MG is brought to the emergency department in crisis. To distinguish between myasthenia crisis and cholinergic crisis the physician would order which of the following drugs?

A. Atropine sulfate
B. Protamine sulfate
C. Edrophonium chloride
D. Lignocaine hydrochloride

Q96. Which nursing diagnosis takes highest priority for a patient with myasthenic crisis?

A. Disturbed sensory perception
B. Ineffective breathing pattern
C. Imbalanced nutrition: less than body requirement
D. Activity intolerance

Q97. Parkinson's disease is caused by:

A. Ischemia in the brainstem producing motor disorder
B. A post-viral illness causing ascending paresthesias
C. Degeneration of substantia nigra depleting dopamine production
D. An autoimmune disorder that destroy acetylcholine receptors

Q98. Parkinson's disease is:

A. A progressive disorder of motor, cognitive, psychiatric disturbances
B. A progressive disorder characterized by resting tremor, akinesia, rigidity and impaired postural reflexes.
C. Early onset of progressive impairment of memory, judgment and language
D. A disease starting with ascending paresthesias to generalized paralysis

Q99. The early sign of Parkinson's disease is:

A. Masked facies
B. Pill rolling movements of the hands
C. Difficulty in initiating movement
D. Shuffling gait

Q100. The three cardinal features the nurse would expect to find in a patient with Parkinson's disease are:

A. Amnesia, echolalia, apraxia
B. Paresthesias, drowsiness, incontinence
C. Tremor, rigidity, bradykinesia
D. Diplopia, dysphagia, dysarthria

Q101. Which of the following medications may be prescribed to a patient with Parkinson's disease to give him relief from distressing symptoms?

A. Levamisole
B. Levodopa
C. Levothyroxine
D. Levofloxacin

Q102. Which of the patients are at risk for developing drug induced Parkinsonism?

A. A patient with manic depressive psychosis on lithium carbonate
B. A 45-year-old lady with diabetes on sulfonylurea
C. A 60-year-old patient on aminophylline for bronchial asthma
D. A 50-year-old patient with angina on ecosprin

Q103. An appropriate nursing intervention for a patient with Parkinson's disease is:

A. To provide a weight reducing diet
B. To promote physical exercise
C. Teaching patient to avoid high fiber foods
D. Teaching patient to take the antiparkinsonian drug prescribed, e.g. levodopa in empty stomach

Q104. The incidence of Parkinson's disease is more in:

A. Male person of 50 years and above
B. Female person of 50 years and above
C. Male person of 60 years and above
D. Female person of 60 years and above

Q105. Which of the following diseases results from degenerative changes in the basal ganglia leading to a depletion of acetylcholine and gamma-aminobutyric acid and a relative increase of dopamine?

A. Parkinson's disease
B. Huntington's disease
C. Restless leg syndrome
D. None of the above

Q106. Which of the following persons is at highest risk of developing multiple sclerosis?

A. 18-year-old African boy
B. 30-year-old European lady
C. 55-year-old Indian man
D. 65-year-old North American woman

Q107. The nurse is assessing a 35-year-old female patient recently diagnosed with multiple sclerosis. Which of the following symptoms she is expected to find?

A. Diplopia
B. Dementia
C. Flaccid paralysis
D. Absent deep tendon reflexes

Q108. Which of the following disease is a chronic progressive genetically transmitted degenerative neurologic disease resulting into abnormal movements (chorea), dementia and emotional disturbances?

A. Alzheimer's disease
B. Parkinson's disease
C. Huntington's disease
D. Creutzfeldt-Jakob disease (CJD)

Q109. Which of the following organisms is most often implicated for causing Guillain-Barré (GB) syndrome?

A. *Helicobacter pylori*
B. *Campylobacter jejuni*
C. *Pneumocystic carinii*
D. None of the above

Q110. Respiratory paralysis in GB syndrome is believed to be caused by:

A. The effects of a potent neurotoxin released by the *Campylobacter jejuni* on the respiratory center.
B. Complication arising from immobility resulting from acute paralysis
C. Paralysis ascending to the nerves that stimulates the thoracic area
D. Degenerative changes in the spinal cord and brainstem

Q111. The nurse is assessing a patient admitted with GB syndrome. She is expected to find all of the following sign and symptoms *except:*

A. Hypertonia
B. Areflexia
C. Paresthesia
D. Urinary retention

Q112. The nurse is preparing a nursing care plan for a patient with GB syndrome. Which of the following plan of action is *not* appropriate?

A. Check vital signs every 2 to 4 hours
B. Give clear liquid diet
C. Perform passive range of motion exercises
D. Measure bilateral calf circumference

Q113. The most common risk factor for Alzheimer's disease is:

A. Increasing age
B. Head trauma
C. Myocardial infarction
D. Environment

Q114. Which of the following elements of the nervous system is affected in Alzheimer's disease?

A. Neurotransmitters
B. Neuronal dendrites
C. Peripheral nerves
D. Monoamine oxidase

Q115. The most common visual problem in India is:

A. Cataract
B. Refractive error
C. Nutritional deficiency
D. Eye injury

Q116. The visual defect that occurs from a decrease in the accommodative ability of the eye due to aging is termed as:

A. Myopia
B. Hyperopia
C. Presbyopia
D. Amblyopia

Q117. The cause of presbyopia is:

A. Degeneration of retina in the elderly
B. Decreased refractive ability of the cornea
C. Reduced elasticity of the lens with aging
D. Onset of early opacity in crystalline lens

Q118. Presbyopia is treated by:

A. Convex lens
B. Concave lens
C. Both convex and concave
D. Refractive surgery

Q119. A sty is:

A. An infection of a sebaceous gland in the eyelid margin
B. An inflammation of a sebaceous gland in the lid
C. A bilateral inflammation of the lid margin
D. Both A and B

Q120. A chalazion is treated by:

A. Application of antibiotic ointment
B. Injection of corticosteroids in the lesion
C. Incision and curettage
D. Either B or C

Q121. In corneal transplantation the corneal graft used is:

A. A synthetic polymer
B. Taken from a human cadaver eyes
C. Taken from pig's eyes
D. Taken from monkey's eyes

Q122. Which of the following symptoms a patient with cataract may report?

A. Loss of peripheral vision
B. Glare which is worse at night
C. Floaters in eyes
D. Halos around lights

Q123. A patient has undergone cataract extraction by phacoemulsification followed by an intraocular lens implantation. Postoperatively after how many weeks the corrective lens will be prescribed?

A. 2 weeks
B. 4 weeks
C. 8 week
D. 12 weeks

Q124. A patient who has had an extracapsular cataract extraction followed by an intraocular lens implantation in the left eye complains of increasing pain and nausea 4 hours after operation. Which of the following actions the nurse should take first?

A. Elevate the headend of the bed
B. Remove dressing and assess for intraocular hemorrhage
C. Administer aspirin as advised
D. Notify physician

Q125. The nurse is teaching an elderly patient after cataract surgery regarding home care. Which of the following instructions is most appropriate?

A. Elevate the head of your bed when sleeping
B. Keep the room environment cool and dry
C. Avoid climbing stairs
D. Take a stool softener daily at night

Q126. Three days after cataract surgery a patient makes all of the following statements to a public health nurse visiting her. Which statement would indicate that the patient needs further teaching regarding self-care after cataract surgery?

A. "I wear sunglasses most of the time as advised."
B. "I take assistance while climbing stairs".
C. "I use a portable lavatory seat on my Indian style latrine"
D. "Today I went to market to buy vegetables and fruits for the family"

Q127. Which of the following advice is not appropriate for a patient after cataract surgery?

A. Avoid bending and straining
B. Avoid high salt diet
C. Do not sleep on the affected side
D. Do not use eye make up

Q128. Aqueous humor is formed by:

A. Iris
B. Lacrimal apparatus
C. Ciliary processes
D. Choroid

Q129. The nurse instills atropine drops into both eyes for a patient undergoing eye examination. Which of the following instructions is appropriate?

A. Avoid injury to your eyes as blink reflex is paralyzed
B. Wear dark glasses in bright light as the pupils are dilated
C. Use bright light while studying
D. You may continue to drive as before

Q130. The most common symptom experienced by a patient with untreated chronic open angle glaucoma is:

A. Constant blurred vision
B. Pain around the eye
C. Tunnel vision
D. Both B and C

Q131. Which of the following additional symptoms would help the nurse to suspect acute angle closure glaucoma?

A. Hazy vision
B. Watering of eyes
C. Floaters in the field of vision
D. Halos around lights

Q132. All of the following drugs may be used in the treatment of glaucoma *except:*

A. Betaxolol
B. Pilocarpine
C. Acetazolamide
D. Atropine sulfate

Q133. The nurse is teaching a patient with glaucoma regarding self-care. Which of the following teachings is appropriate?

A. Avoid watching television more than 1 hour
B. Avoid lifting heavy weights
C. Avoid caffeinated and carbonated beverages
D. To come to the ophthalmologist when symptoms increase

Q134. The nurse is teaching a patient with glaucoma regarding the need of taking his prescribed medication regularly. Which of the following conditions may occur due to non-compliance of treatment?

A. Permanent loss of vision
B. Progressive loss of peripheral vision
C. Loss of color vision
D. Nystagmus

Q135. Which of the following measures is the treatment of choice in elderly persons with aphakia?

A. Eye glasses (spectacles)
B. Contact lenses
C. Intraocular lenses
D. Corneal grafts

Q136. Which of the following persons is at risk of developing retinal detachment?

A. Adolescent boys
B. Persons with hyperopia
C. Persons with severe myopia
D. Persons with vitamin A deficiency

Q137. The sign and symptoms of retinal detachment include all of the following *except:*

A. Sudden severe pain in the eye
B. A curtain falling across the field of vision
C. Light flashes in the visual field
D. Floaters in the field of vision

Q138. The length of the external auditory canal in adult is approximately:

A. 1.5 cm **B.** 2.5 cm
C. 3.5 cm **D.** 1 cm

Q139. Which part of the external auditory canal contains hair follicle?

A. Outer half of the canal
B. Inner half of the canal
C. Middle one-third of the canal
D. Throughout the ear canal

Q140. While performing a tuning fork test in a patient the nurse is aware that bone conduction is lengthened in:

A. Conductive deafness
B. Sensorineural deafness
C. Normal hearing
D. None of the above

Q141. Which of the following statements about pure tone audiometry is not correct?

A. It is simple, reliable and commonly performed test to measure hearing
B. Can diagnose both conductive and sensorineural hearing loss
C. It tests sound frequencies from 250–8,000 Hz
D. It gives conclusive evidence of deafness in children below 1 year

Q142. Caloric test is done to assess:

A. Auditory function
B. Vestibular function
C. Brainstem function
D. Cochlear function

Q143. The nurse is planning to irrigate a child's ear to remove foreign body. To irrigate the ear she should use water at which of the following temperature?

A. 25° centigrade
B. 30° centigrade
C. 37° centigrade
D. 45° centigrade

Q144. In which of the following conditions ear irrigation is contraindicated?

A. Pain in ear
B. Loss of hearing
C. Otitis externa
D. Perforated tympanic membrane

Q145. The most common cause of conductive hearing loss is:

A. Foreign body in external ear
B. Otitis media with effusion
C. Noise pollution
D. Ototoxic drugs

Q146. Otalgia is one of the first signs of external otitis. Otalgia means:

A. Itching in the ear
B. Foul smell in the ear
C. Pain in ear
D. Bleeding from ear

Q147. Myringoplasty involves:

A. Incision into the tympanic membrane for removal of fluid
B. Closure of a simple perforation of tympanic membrane
C. Surgical correction of the tympanic membrane with ossicular chain
D. Surgical reconstruction of the ossicular chain

Q148. The nurse is teaching a patient who has undergone tympanoplasty during immediate postoperative period. Which of the following instructions is not appropriate?

A. "Lie down with operated ear up for several hours"
B. "If necessary blow nose gently one at a time"
C. "If at all necessary sneeze or cough with the mouth open"
D. "Inform if you experience noises in the ear such as cracking or popping"

Q149. During assessment of a patient with otosclerosis, the nurse is expected to find all of the following symptoms *except:*

A. Progressive deafness
B. Tinnitus
C. Vomiting
D. Schwartz's sign

Q150. Otosclerosis is fixation of the footplate of the stapes in the oval window by:

A. Abnormal bony growth
B. Fibrous tissue formation secondary to bacterial invasion
C. Abnormal deposition of collagen and calcium secondary to trauma
D. None of the above

Q151. The clinical features of acute otitis media in adults include:

A. Otalgia, fever, hearing loss and bulging tympanic membrane
B. Bilateral otalgia, hearing loss, tinnitus and fever
C. Hearing loss, vomiting, discharge from ear and vertigo
D. Pain and tenderness on movement of auricle, fever, and hearing loss

Q152. The term presbycusis refers to:

A. Sudden hearing loss
B. Progressive hearing loss with aging
C. Congenital hearing loss
D. Noise induced hearing loss

Q153. A person with sensorineural hearing loss:

A. Has difficulty understanding speech
B. Speaks softly as he hears his voice loud
C. Is benefited by use of hearing aid
D. Has all of the above symptoms

Q154. The nurse taking care of a patient with chronic suppurative otitis media assesses the patient for development of possible complications. Which of the following she should assess in this patient?

A. Anosmia
B. Balance disorder
C. Facial paralysis
D. Dysphagia

Q155. The nurse is caring for an elderly patient with hearing impairment. Which nursing intervention will be most useful in establishing communication with the patient?

A. Use visual cues and written instructions
B. Provide a hearing aid
C. Speak slowly and articulate clearly
D. Allow time for understanding and a response

Q156. Which of the following methods to be adopted by the nurse to instill eardrops in a 30-year-old patient?

A. Pull the pinna up and back
B. Pull the pinna down and back
C. Pull the pinna down
D. Pull the pinna up

Q157. The clinical features of Méniére's disease is:

A. Otalgia, fever and aural fullness
B. Episodic vertigo, tinnitus, hearing loss and aural fullness
C. Vertigo accompanied by nystagmus, vomiting
D. Otalgia, loss of balance and unilateral hearing loss

Q158. The nurse is assessing a patient diagnosed with Méniére's disease. Which of the following assessment findings she is expected to find?

A. Pain and tenderness on application of pressure over tragus (directly in front of the ear)
B. Schwartz's sign
C. Sensorineural hearing loss
D. Conductive hearing loss

Q159. The nurse is teaching a patient with Méniére's disease regarding diet. Which of the following he should avoid?

A. High salt diet
B. High protein and fat diet
C. Alcohol, caffeine and nicotine
D. A and C

Q160. The priority nursing diagnosis for a patient with newly diagnosed Meniere's disease is:

A. Risk for infection
B. Risk for injury
C. Impaired social interaction
D. Altered nutrition: Less than body requirement

ANSWERS AND RATIONALES OF NERVOUS SYSTEM INCLUDING SPECIAL SENSES (EYE AND EAR)

1. **B.** Neurotransmitters are chemical substances that are manufactured by the cell body of neuron and not axon. These substances are discharged into the space between two neurons and propel the message on to the next neuron. The neurotransmitters excite, inhibit or modify signals to the second neuron (post-synaptic neuron) by interacting with the receptors on its membrane.

2. **D.** Endorphin exhibits excitatory action, transmits pleasurable sensation and inhibits pain transmission. The sources of endorphin are nerve terminals in the spine, brainstem, thalamus and hypothalamus. Another neurotransmitter having similar action is enkephalin. Gamma-aminobutyric acid (GABA) is inhibitory, conveys muscle and nerve transmission. Dopamine also is inhibitory, affects behavior and fine movement. Serotonin is inhibitory, helps control mood and sleep, and inhibits pain pathways.

3. **B.** Parietal lobe is predominantly sensory lobe. Contains the primary sensory cortex. Analyzes sensory information and relays to the thalamus and other cortical areas. It is also responsible for proprioception. Frontal lobe is the largest and controls abstract thought, concentration, information storage or memory and motor function. Temporal lobe contains the auditory receptive area and is the interpretive area. Occipital lobe is responsible for visual interpretation.

4. **B.** Cerebellum is largely responsible for coordination of movement. It also controls fine movement, balance, position sense and integration of sensory input. Brainstem consists of midbrain, pons and medulla and contains cardiac, vasomotor and respiratory centers. Thalamus is a relay station for all sensation except smell. Hypothalamus is the center for temperature control, water metabolism, control of hormonal secretion, heart rate, peristalsis, and appetite control, thirst and sleep-wake cycle.

5. **D.** The part of brain, which plays an essential role in the process of memory is hippocampus and is situated in the medial section of the temporal lobe. Frontal lobe primarily functions in thinking, planning, judgment and past memory. Occipital lobe is the center of vision. Parietal lobe is mainly responsible for sensory functions.

6. **B.** The heat regulatory center is located in hypothalamus. Thalamus channels all sensory information except smell. Limbic system is the center for emotional expression and feelings. Medulla is the motor and sensory pathway between brain and spinal cord.

7. **C.** Cranial nerve IV or trochlear nerve is responsible for extraocular eye movement. Cranial nerve VIII, vestibulocochlear, is responsible for hearing, cranial nerve II, optic, is responsible for vision and cranial nerve V or trigeminal nerve is responsible for chewing.

8. **B.** Vestibulocochlear nerve is responsible for hearing and

maintaining equilibrium or balance. Trochlear nerve functions in eye movement. Trigeminal nerve is for somatic sensation of face and chewing and vagus nerve is responsible for pharynx, respiratory, cardiac and circulatory reflexes.

9. A. Cranial nerve III, oculomotor, if damaged gives rise to ptosis or drooping eyelids. Disorder of cranial nerve V or trigeminal nerve is trigeminal neuralgia causes face pain. Disorder of the cranial nerve VI, abducens will cause inability of the eye to move laterally outward. Disorder of the cranial nerve VIII, vestibulocochlear is seen in Méniére's syndrome.

10. B. Bell's palsy is paralysis of the facial muscles due to damage of cranial nerve VII or facial nerve. Damage of cranial nerve IV or trochlear will give rise to inability to look down or walk down steps. Disorder of cranial nerve IX, glossopharyngeal gives rise to loss of taste and sensations and disorder of cranial nerve XII, hypoglossal nerve will give rise to inability of the tongue to move.

11. B. Patient's level of consciousness is the best early indicator of changes in neurologic status. Neurological disorders can cause life-threatening changes in vital signs, which are assessed next. Variations in patient's age, physical condition and level of consciousness determine the nature and extensiveness of further examinations.

12. C. Glasgow Coma Scale is the most commonly used neurologic assessment tool. This scale provides objective measurement of 3 essential components of the neurologic examination, e.g. spontaneity of eye opening, best verbal response and best motor response.

13. A. Ability to correctly perceive any one smell signifies proper functioning of the cranial nerve I, i.e. olfactory nerve. Other cranial nerves listed do not have any function with olfaction.

14. C. Cranial nerve VII has both motor and sensory functions. Sensory functions include differentiation of different taste, e.g. sweet, sour and bitter, etc. by anterior two-third of the tongue. So dysfunction of the nerve will result in inability to differentiate various taste. Symmetrical facial movement, presence of nasolabial fold, tearing are findings of a functioning nerve.

15. D. Cranial nerve XI, spinal accessory nerve is a motor nerve, innervates sternocleidomastoid muscle. Dysfunction of the nerve will result in inability to elevate the shoulders. Inability to swallow is the result of dysfunction of cranial nerves VII and IX. Hoarse and weak voice results from dysfunction of cranial nerve X and inability to move the tongue from side to side results from dysfunction of cranial nerve XII.

16. D. Cranial nerve XII, hypoglossal, innervates the tongue. So to test the functioning of the nerve the patient is asked to do various movement of the tongue. Muscles of mastication are innervated by cranial nerve V, trigeminal. So to test the functioning of cranial nerve V the patient is asked to do chewing movements. Gag reflex and swallowing ability is the function of both cranial nerves VII, facial and IX, glossopharyngeal. Differentiation of taste is the function of cranial nerves VII and IX.

17. A. Mental status includes level of consciousness, orientation, memory, mood, intellectual functioning, judgment and insight, language and communication. So by performing a thorough examination of the mental status different areas of the cerebral cortex are evaluated. Other areas of the brain are not related with mental status of an individual.

18. D. Motor system examination includes assessment of bulk, tone and power of major muscle groups of the body as well as balance and coordination. Assessment of mechanical sensation is a part of sensory function examination.

19. B. The heel-to-shin test involves having the patient place one heel on the opposite shin below the knee and moving the heel down the shin to the ankle. This is repeated for the other leg. An individual with coordination will perform these movements smoothly without jerking or hesitation.

20. C. Standing and walking require good muscle power and balance. Assessment for cerebeller disease involves observation of the patient's stature and gait. Ataxic gait may be noted in a patient with cerebeller disorder. Pronator drift is noticed in mild weakness of the arm. Spasticity is due to abnormal or hypertonicity of muscles. Chorea is a finding of abnormal muscle movement, associated with extrapyramidal disease.

21. A. Chorea is discrete, jerky, purposeless movements in distal extremities and face. Myoclonus describes sudden muscle contraction of varying intensity involving a part or the entire body. Tic is involuntary movement of groups of muscles in stereotypic patterns and a tremor is involuntary trembling or quivering of muscles.

22. C. Inability to carry out the learned movement on command in the absence of weakness or paralysis is apraxia. Akinesia is reduced body movements in the absence of weakness or paralysis. Athetosis is gross, writhing, worm like movements of the body, face or extremities. Agnosia refers to failure to recognize familiar objects perceived by the senses.

23. C. Decorticate posturing is a posture of abnormal flexion. In this the patient flexes, adducts and internally rotates the arms and wrists to the chest and rigidly extends legs. When muscles are rigid and resist to move is called spastic. Decerebrate posturing is a posture of abnormal extension. In this posturing patient extends and pronates the arms while rigidly extending the legs. This may occur spontaneously, intermittently, or in response to a stimulus.

24. C. Patellar reflex or a knee-jerk or a quadriceps jerk is produced by tapping the quadriceps femoris tendon just below the patella and is an example of deep tendon or muscle-stretch reflexes.

25. D. In chewing reflex a tongue blade placed between the teeth results in the tight closing of the jaw. Positive chewing reflex is pathological.

26. D. CT scan may require use of a contrast dye. Some contrast agents are iodine based and produces allergic reactions to susceptible individual. If a contrast material is used an informed consent is necessary. Fasting is usually not required unless the patient is nauseated.

27. A. Knowing what to expect during the test beforehand reduces anxiety. A small amount of radiation is emitted during the scan but patient should be reassured that the procedure is safe. Patient need not shampoo his hair. Routine medication may not be withheld unless ordered by the physician.

28. C. PET scanning enables visualization of physiologic functions in body areas, e.g. amount of blood flow to specific body tissues; utilization of blood and other nutrients, e.g. glucose and oxygen by tissues and mapping specific receptors, e.g. medications and neurotransmitters. CT scanning provides visualization of anatomical structures and MRI provides more anatomically detailed pictures than are available with CT. In Doppler scanning visual representation of moving blood is obtained.

29. B. Myelography is a X-ray examination of the spinal cord and vertebral canal after introduction of a contrast material in to the spinal subarachnoid space. Angiography is X-ray visualization of vertebral structures after injection of contrast material into an artery. In spinal tap or lumbar puncture a needle is inserted in to the sub-arachnoid space below the level of the spinal cord in the lumbar region. Spinal tap precedes myelography. Electromyography measures and documents electrical currents (action potential) produced by skeletal muscles.

30. D. Encephalography or electroencephalography is the study of electrical activity of the superficial layers of the cerebral cortex by placing electrodes on specific areas of skull. It is a noninvasive study and does not require a lumbar puncture. All other statements about lumbar puncture are true.

31. D. Post-lumbar puncture headache or spinal headache is due to leakage of CSF (cerebrospinal fluid) from the puncture site in dura resulting in depletion of CSF volume and pressure. Keeping the patient lying in bed for several hours, average being 3 hours and encouraging additional fluid intake to restore CSF volume may reduce risk of headache. Patient need not withheld food and fluid after the test.

32. C. Before EEG is performed hair must be shampooed because the electrodes must be applied on a clean scalp. Patient should have normal meals before the test to avoid hypoglycemia, which may alter test result. Stimulants and drugs like anticonvulsant, antidepressants, etc. must be withheld for 24–48 hours as they may interfere with the accuracy of test result.

33. D. Before the procedure the patient must be instructed about the purpose of the lumbar puncture, what the patient will feel and his role during the procedure. Patient must lie still during the test. Coughing when the needle has been inserted will cause injury and dislodgment of the needle from its proper place, i.e. subarachnoid space.

34. C. A stuporous patient awakens only to vigorous stimulation, e.g. shaking. Lethargic patient is oriented to time, place and person, but sleeps often, has a slowed speech and thought processes. A patient in obtunded level of consciousness sleeps almost constantly, can be aroused and follow simple commands. Patient who does not respond to environmental stimuli is comatose.

35. D. Two kinds of disorders produce sustained unconsciousnes or coma. (1) Structural lesions in the brain, e.g. brainstem, posterior cranial fossa including the cerebellum, midbrain, pons and medulla. These lesions affect reticular activating system. A functioning reticular activating system is essential for consciousness. (2) Metabolic disorders reducing supply of oxygen and glucose or accumulating waste products in the brain. Structural lesions can affect the functioning of brain, but functional lesions do not exist.

36. D. According to the international classification of epileptic seizures, generalized seizures are classified as (1) absence, (2) myoclonic, (3) clonic, (4) tonic, (5) tonic-clonic, and (6) atonic. There is no myoclonic-tonic seizure.

37. A. Partial seizures are most common. Tonic-clonic, absence and atonic, are included in generalized seizures. Generalized seizures are about one-third of all seizures.

38. C. In myoclonic seizures there is sudden uncontrollable jerking movements of single or multiple muscle groups causing the patient to fall. Patient looses consciousness for a moment and remains confused postictally. Tonic-clonic seizures are most closely associated with grand mal epilepsy and proceeds as aura, loss of consciousness, tonic phase, clonic phase and postictal phase. In tonic seizures, there is an abrupt increase in muscle tone and muscular contraction and in clonic seizures there is rhythmic contraction and relaxation lasting several minutes.

39. C. An aura occurs in some patients before the onset of seizures. The person may experience a certain smell or sensation or seeing a flash of light and these symptoms may serve as a warning symptom of seizures. Certain partial seizures are accompanied by autonomic manifestations, e.g. epigastric sensation, pallor, sweating, flushing, etc. Seeing flashes of light is not a precipitating factor, but observing flushing lights for some time may precipitate absence seizures. Post-ictal experience happens after the seizures not before seizures.

40. A. During assessment of vital signs the nurse should take axillary temperature instead of oral temperaure to prevent injury if a seizure occurs. Heart rate and respiratory rate is usually not altered after the patient has recovered from seizure episode.

41. C. When the patient has already started with a tonic-clonic seizure, the nurse should lay the patient in bed on his side, raise the side rails of the bed, remove pillows and ensure a patent airway. Nothing should be placed inside his mouth if he has already started with the seizures and hands and legs should not be restrained.

42. B. In the home or community the victim should be eased on a flat surface and turned on his side that would result in a patent airway and a folded towel or a sheet is placed under the head for protection. Care should be taken not to flex the head sharply or close the airway. Furniture should be moved from his way but placing the patient on his side over a flat surface is the priority. Trying to insert a padded spoon between the teeth during seizure can cause injury and block the airway by pushing the tongue back. Arms and legs should never be restrained during seizures as it may cause fractures.

43. C. The patient should take medicine daily as prescribed to maintain blood levels of the drug. He should attend follow-up visits and have the blood tested for plasma levels as directed to regulate the dose of the drug. The patient should never discontinue the drug or reduce the dose on his own because of annoying side effects, but should report to physician.

Palpitation is not an adverse effect of this drug. Some sedation occurs with phenytoin therapy, but this does not increase further with dose.

44. D. Patients with epilepsy have to live a life with moderation. Activities that require alertness, e.g. driving or operating machinery must be avoided. Patients should not go for swimming alone nor they should have tub bath at home. Alcohol, coffee and tea, etc. are considered to be seizure trigger and need to be avoided. Patient should take regular meal, avoid hypoglycemia, must develop a regular sleep pattern to prevent insomnia. Meditation and relaxation therapy helps reduce stress and the potential to seizures.

45. D. Alcoholic beverages are contraindicated in patients with epilepsy because (1) alcohol lowers seizure threshold. (2) alcohol is detoxified by liver, most of the antiepileptic drugs also metabolized by liver. Consuming alcohol while on anticonvulsant places an increased strain on the liver and on its metabolic function.

46. A. The most common side effect of phenytoin is gum hypertrophy, which can be minimized by good oral care. Phenytoin may cause nervous stimulation leading to insomnia, nervousness and twitching. Dry mouth and tachycardia are not related to phenytoin therapy.

47. B. The dose related adverse effects of phenytoin include, ataxia, vertigo, diplopia, nystagmus, drowsiness, confusion, behavioral alterations, etc. Hypotension not hypertension and bradycardia not tachycardia may occur with IV injection of phenytoin. Water retention and hyponatremia in elderly can occur with carbamazepine therapy. Phenytoin does not cause facial tics.

48. B. Status epilepticus is treated with diazepam 5–10 mg IV at every 10–20 minutes for a total dose of up to 30 mg in an 8 hours period. Repeating the dose after 5 minutes is too early and after 30 minutes and 1 hour are too late because of increasing risk of complications from uncontrolled status epilepticus.

49. D. Injection diazepam and injection phenytoin should be given by slow IV push. Diazepam should be administered no faster than 5 mg/minute and phenytoin 50 mg/minute. Marked fall in blood pressure and respiration may occur during the IV administration of these drugs. So resuscitative measures should be ready at hand before administration of these drugs. Diazepam should never be mixed with any other drugs, as it is incompatible with all other medications in solution.

50. B. The safest and most effective (curative) surgical treatment for complex partial seizure is cortical resection of the anterior temporal lobe or temporal lobectomy. The area in which seizures begin is removed without causing neurologic or cognitive deficits. This is done when the focus of abnormal discharge is located in the dispensable areas (areas for which there are duplicate areas in the cortex) and are easily accessible. Corpus callosotomy and hemispherectomy are palliative surgeries to control intractable seizures.

51. D. In MRI powerful magnetic fields and radiofrequency pulses are used to produce the image. All metal containing objects such as watches, ornaments are removed and it is ensured that the patient does not have any metallic internal devices such as pacemaker, orthopedic appliances. NPO status is not required for MRI of brain. It is required for MRI of abdomen.

52. B. The classic clinical manifestations of brain tumor result from edema and increased intracranial pressure and include headache, nausea and vomiting. These symptoms are considered as the classic triad. Other general clinical manifestations are mental status changes, seizure, and papilledema. Vertigo as a localized manifestation is seen in tumors located in the brainstem or cerebellum and is not considered as a classic manifestation.

53. D. Identifying and locating metastatic lesions in other parts of the body is not a treatment goal because malignant tumors of brain rarely metastasize outside the central nervous system because they are contained by structural (meninges) and physiologic (blood-brain) barriers. All other goals of treatment are appropriate.

54. D. In MRI powerful magnetic fields and radiofrequency pulses are used to produce the image. All metal containing objects such as watches, ornaments are removed and it is ensured that the patient does not have any metallic internal devices such as pacemaker, orthopedic appliances. NPO status is not required for MRI of brain. It is required for MRI of abdomen.

55. D. After a craniotomy the head of the patient's bed is elevated to 30 degrees to promote venous return. Other positions are incorrect after this surgery.

56. A. Proper positioning after craniotomy involves raising the head of the bed elevated at 30–45° angle, the head and neck in neutral position. Hip flexion should be avoided as it may cause increase in intracranial pressure. During turning the patient should be turned as a unit, placing a pillow in between the knees and avoiding sharp flexion of the upper thigh. All other actions during positioning are appropriate after craniotomy.

57. B. Preventing increased intracranial pressure after cranial surgery is the primary goal of nursing care as increased intracranial pressure is life-threatening. Preventing infection is a major goal of care after any surgery. After cerebral edema and increased intracranial pressure subsides, rehabilitative potential of the patient is determined and measures for ambulation started. Objective of enhancing body image also may be met during recovery phase.

58. B. Frequent swallowing after brain surgery indicates fluid or blood leaking from the sinuses into the oropharynx. Bloody drainage from the ears occurs in basilar skull fracture. Hematuria in absence of other signs of bleeding indicates urological problems. Guaiac-positive stools indicate gastrointestinal bleeding.

59. A. Trismus or locked jaw is a sign of tetanus and not of bacterial meningitis. Nuchal rigidity or Stiff neck, Kernig's sign and Brudzinski's sign are seen in meningitis.

60. D. Meningitis is often confirmed by examination of CSF. In bacterial meningitis CSF is purulent and turbid. Protein levels in the CSF are usually elevated (normal is 15–45 mg/dL) and are higher than in viral meningitis. Decreased CSF glucose concentration is common in bacterial meningitis and may be normal in viral meningitis. The CSF is turbid and purulent in bacterial meningitis but it is same or clear in viral meningitis.

61. D. The most important nonmodifiable risk factor for stroke is age. Two-thirds of all stroke occur in individual over age 65 years. A history of transient ischemic attack also increases the risk of stroke. Heavy alcohol consumption increases the risk of stroke but moderate alcohol consumption is protective. Oral contraceptives are associated with increased stroke risk, but absolute risk is low in this group of individual being younger in age. Hypertension is the single most important modifiable risk factor. A 60-year-old man with hypertension has increased risk of stroke but the risk decreases with appropriate treatment of hypertension.

62. B. Thrombotic stroke tends to appear during sleep or within 1 hour of arising. Patient is hypertensive or diabetic, may have a history of transient ischemic attack (TIA). Patient with thrombotic stroke does not have a decreased level of consciousness in the first 24 hours unless it is due to a brainstem stroke. Embolic stroke can occur at any time and may not be related to activity. Manifestations appear rapidly with severe clinical symptoms. Patient is relatively conscious, may have a headache. Patient is usually normotensive.

63. A. Atrial fibrillation occurs with the irregular and rapid discharge from multiple ectopic atrial foci that causes quivering of the atria without contraction resulting into stagnation, which predisposes to mural thrombi, leading to a CVA (cerebrovascular accident or stroke). Deep vein thrombosis will cause pulmonary embolism. Dehydration is not related to stroke. Atherosclerosis is the cause of thrombotic stroke.

64. A. The primary cause for thrombous formation is atherosclerosis. Atherosclerosis causes fatty material to deposit and form plaques on vessel walls. These plaques continue to enlarge and cause stenosis of the vessel lumen. When blood flows through the irregular surfaces of the plaques, platelets adhere to the plaques eventually obstructing the vessel. Inflammation of the arteries called arteritis is a rare cause of thrombus formation. Two-thirds of thrombotic strokes are associated with hypertension or diabetes mellitus, both of which accelerate atherosclerosis. Hypertension is the most important cause of hemorrhagic stroke.

65. B. Onset of hemorrhagic stroke occurs rapidly. Common manifestations include severe occipital or nuchal headaches, vertigo or syncope, paresthesias, transient paralysis, etc. It commonly occurs during periods of activity and not during sleep. Rapid onset of complete hemiplegia occurs within minutes to 1 hour, not only weakness.

66. B. Intracerebral hemorrhage is the bleeding within the brain caused by a rupture of a vessel. Hypertension is the most important cause of intracerebral hemorrhage. Other causes include, vascular malformation, trauma, brain tumors, ruptured aneurysms, coagulation disorders, anticoagulant and thrombolytic drugs. Coronary artery disease may be associated with thrombotic stroke. Shock is not a cause of intracerebral hemorrhage.

67. C. In global aphasia the patient cannot form words that are understandable nor comprehend the spoken words. In Wernicke's aphasia, the patient neither understands the sound of speech nor its meaning. In Broca's aphasia, the patient has difficulty in speaking and writing and in anomia patient has difficulty in selecting appropriate words, particularly nouns.

68. D. In expressive aphasia patient has difficulty in producing spoken words. So nurse should encourage non-verbal communication and ask the patient to write out what he or she wants. Nurse should speak in normal volume and tone and not speak loudly. Allowing patient time to respond and speaking simple sentences with gestures will promote comprehension and help a patient with receptive aphasia.

69. B. The patient has left out food laid down on his left side of the table as he could not see objects in the left half of his visual field with both eyes. This condition is called homonymous hemianopia. Homonymous hemianopia can be either side. Unilateral neglect is the inability of the person to respond to stimulus on the contralateral side of a cerebral infarction. In visual agnosia, the patient sees objects but is unable to recognize or attach meaning to them. In this situation patient is not having visual agnosia since he has taken what he could see. This is not due to double vision also.

70. D. A patient with hemiplegia may achieve maximal physical mobility within the limitations imposed by stroke by gaining muscle strength and by using adaptive devices. The nurse plays a crucial role in encouraging the patient to exercise to gain muscle strength, teaching and helping the patient to first sit up on bed, then on the edge of bed while maintaining balance and then to move into a wheel chair gradually.

71. D. Subluxation or incomplete dislocation at the shoulder can occur from overstretching the joint capsule and musculature by the force of gravity when the patient sits or stands in the early stages after a stroke. This problem can be prevented by proper patient movement and positioning as mentioned.

72. D. The cause of TIA in a patient with valvular prosthesis is due to a dislodged thrombus formed around the valvular prosthesis due to inadequate anticoagulation. So anticoagulant drugs like warfarin is the treatment of choice to prevent further embolization and embolic stroke. Antiplatelet agents like aspirin and ticlopidin is prescribed to prevent stroke related to atherosclerosis. Streptokinase is a thrombolytic drug used to lyse a clot already formed.

73. D. Symptom of TIA usually result from a transient lack of oxygen to the brain. The focal loss of neurologic function resulting from ischemia lasts less than 24 hours and recovery is complete. A microthromboemboli is the most common cause of TIA and not hemorrhage. TIA does not cause unconsciousness. TIA may occur repeatedly but there is no permanent loss of neurological function.

74. A. Thrombolytic therapy in ischemic stroke must be given within 3 hours of the onset of clinical signs and symptoms of stroke to reduce the disability without increasing mortality. Beyond this time thrombolytic therapy will be ineffective to bring about desired outcomes.

75. C. The drug of choice in the treatment of ischemic stroke is recombinant tissue plasminogn activator. Since- this is a clot specific drug, it is less likely to cause hemorrhage and is used in the management of stroke. Heparin is given after 24 hours of thrombolysis to prevent further clot formation. Streptokinase is not used in cerebrovascular accident because of the risk of hemorrhage.

76. C. The patient whose level of consciousness is decreased is a high risk of aspiration. The nurse must ensure that the patient's gag reflex returns before offering food and fluids. The patient with decreased level of consciousness must not be placed in supine position, but should be placed in Fowler's or semi-prone position. Restriction of fluids does not minimize the problem and is not indicated.

77. B. The dysphagic patient must concentrate on swallowing. So a quiet environment free from distractions should be provided. Presence of other patients can cause distractions. A dysphagic patient should sit upright as close to 90 degrees as possible to aid in swallowing. Hyperextension may cause aspiration and should be avoided. Foods should be such that they require no chewing and easy to swallow. Thickened liquid, semisolid foods are easy to swallow.

78. B. The most important early clinical manifestations of increased intracranial pressure (ICP) that is exhibited by the patient is change in level of consciousness, e.g. restlessness, irritability, confusion or decreased responsiveness. Bradycardia and increased systolic blood pressure not hypotension occur as a late response in severe increased intracranial pressure. Patients with increased ICP may report nausea and vomiting, not anorexia.

79. C. Signs and symptoms of severe increased intracranial pressure include increased systolic blood pressure with widened pulse pressure, bradycardia, rapid respiration and hyperthermia. Tachycardia, bradypnea and decreased body temperature are not associated with increased intracranial pressure.

80. A. Carbon dioxide causes cerebral vasodilation. By increasing the ventilator settings to cause hyperventilation, a hypocarbic (low CO_2) blood level is created. A partial pressure of CO_2 ($PaCO_2$) level between 30–35 mm Hg (normal PaCO2 35–45 mm Hg) causes cerebral vasoconstriction and thus lowers increased intra-cranial pressure (ICP). It is also important to maintain optimum oxygenation as the injured brain has an increased need for oxygen and glucose.

81. C. Mannitol acts by increasing intravascular pressure by drawing fluid from the interstitial spaces and from the brain cells. Therefore, intracranial pressure is reduced by a decrease in the total brain fluid content. To maintain optimal cerebral perfusion pressure blood pressure may have to be raised or lowered by vasoactive substances and not by mannitol. Medications, e.g. barbiturates are given to reduce cerebral metabolism. Mannitol does not provide glucose, as the body does not metabolize it.

82. B. Several methods of intracranial pressure monitoring are available. Among them the most accurate results are obtained from intraventricular catheters. Others are brain parenchyma or subarachnoid catheters and epidural catheters.

83. B. The major complication of continuous intracranial pressure (ICP) monitoring includes infection. Intracranial hypertension is increased intracranial pressure to 20–25 mm Hg, is not a complication but an indication of continuous ICP monitoring. Sometimes there may be leaks in the system giving inaccurate results. Seizures increase ICP but it is not a complication of ICP monitoring.

84. B. These patients must have a patent airway. So suctioning should be done whenever needed instead of a 1 hourly schedule, as these patients poorly tolerate suction. Patient should be adequately oxygenated before suction, in between suction and after suction. Suctioning should be limited to 3 passes and each pass to 10 seconds. Supine position with the head elevated to 30 degrees facilitates venous drainage from brain and reduces intracranial pressure. Adequate oxygenation should be maintained to meet the increased need for oxygen. Prophylactic anticonvulsant should be administered to prevent seizures as seizures increase metabolic requirements and cerebral blood flow and volume and thus increase intracranial pressure.

85. D. Patient with concussion without loss of consciousness is usually discharged with advice to come back if symptoms persist or behavioral changes are noticed. Increasing drowsiness, e.g. difficulty arousing, confusion signifies beginning of a more serious problem, e.g. increased intracranial pressure. Headache is a normal complain after concussion. Anorexia is not related to concussion. Weakness in arms and legs is an alarming sign not pain in legs.

86. A. If blood stained fluid comes from ear or nose the nurse should look for halo or ring sign. When clear fluid comes out, the nurse should check for glucose as CSF (cerebrospinal fluid) contains glucose. Head of the bed should be raised to 30 degrees to allow drainage of CSF, and not 60 degrees, which increases ICP (intracranial pressure). The nose or ear should never be packed.

87. A. Myasthenia gravis is an autoimmune disease of the neuromuscular junction and not a viral infection. Antibodies attack acetylcholine receptors, destroying and reducing acetylcholine receptor sites at the neuromuscular junction. Anti-acetylcholine receptor antibodies are detectable in the serum of 85 to 90% patients with generalized myasthenia gravis.

88. C. In 90% of patients eyelid muscles or extraocular muscles are involved giving rise to ptosis. Dysphagia, respiratory difficulty occur later. Muscles of the distal part of the body are less affected so paresthesia of lower extremity is less common. Pupillary reflexes and other reflexes are normal.

89. D. The diagnosis of myasthenia gravis is confirmed by observing objective signs of improvement in muscle strength after an intravenous injection of edrophonium (tensilon), a short-acting anticholinesterase drug. Typical symptoms of the patient help to suspect the presence of the disease, but cannot establish the diagnosis. Halo sign is present in head injury with skull fracture. Brudzinski's sign is present in meningitis

90. B. Intravenous injection of edrophonium chloride, a short acting anticholinergic drug (Tensilon test) in a dose of 10 mg results in immediate improvement of muscle strength for a short period lasting about 3-5 minutes. Tensilon does not increase symptoms. The drug, which increases muscle strength for a duration of 1-2 hours is neostigmine methylsulfate. Change in heart rate and rhythm is an adverse reaction of tensilon.

91. B. Drug therapy for myasthenia gravis includes anticholinesterase drugs, e.g. neostigmine and pyridostigmine (mestinon). Other drugs used in this disease are corticosteroids and immunosuppressants. Atropine sulfate and anticholinergic drug is used to antagonize overdose of anticholinesterase medications. Edrophonium chloride has a short duration of action (10-30 minutes) and is not used in the treatment. It is used for diagnostic purpose.

92. B. Patient should take the drug at exact time ordered by the physician, usually it should be taken 30-60 minutes before meals to facilitate swallowing and prevent aspiration. The drug may be kept at room temperature. It is usually taken with milk to reduce gastric irritation.

93. D. The purpose of plasmapheresis in myasthenia gravis is to remove plasma proteins containing antibodies that are believed to cause the disease. The disease is not due to virus, so the question of removing viral antigen does not arise. To counteract overdose of medication plasmapheresis is not done. The procedure does not remove T lymphocytes.

94. C. The patient with myasthenia gravis should be instructed to swallow only when the chin is tipped downward toward the chest. Hyper-extension of neck will facilitate aspiration and is contraindicated. Eating will be easier if the patient schedule his medication before meal, so that peak action is reached at mealtime. Soft or pureed foods are easier to swallow than solid foods. In extreme cases suction may be necessary and patient should learn to suction if aspiration occurs.

95. C Myasthenic crisis is an acute exacerbation of the disease process giving rise to generalized muscle weakness affecting breathing and swallowing. Cholinergic crisis is due to overmedication of anticholinergic drug and gives rise to symptoms like myasthenic crisis. Differentiation between these two conditions may be done by administration of edrophonium chloride (tensilon test). The patient with myasthenic crisis improves immediately after administration of edrophonium but the patient with cholinergic crisis does not improve or deteriorates. Atropine sulfate is the treatment of cholinergic crisis. Protamine sulfate is the antidote for heparin. Lignocaine hydrochloride is anti-arrhythmic drug.

96. B. Myasthenic crisis is an acute exacerbation of muscle weakness in areas that affect swallowing and breathing resulting in aspiration, respiratory insufficiency and respiratory infection. Because of these the nursing diagnosis of 'ineffective breathing pattern' should receive highest priority. Other diagnoses are also appropriate but they are not life-threatening and immediate.

97. C. Parkinson's disease is caused by degeneration of the substantia nigra in the basal ganglia of the brain, where dopamine is produced and stored. Ischemia in brainstem is ischemic stroke. A post-viral illness causing ascending paresthesias is Guillain-Barré syndrome. An autoimmune disorder that destroys acetylcholine receptors is the cause of myasthenia gravis.

98. B. Parkinson's disease is a progressive disorder characterized by disability from resting tremor, akinesia and rigidity. A progressive disorder of motor, cognitive and psychiatric disturbances is Huntington's disease. In early onset familial Alzheimer's disease there is progressive impairment of memory, judgment and language. Guillain-Barré syndrome begins with ascending paresthesias to generalized paralysis.

99. B. The early sign of Parkinson's disease is resting tremor in one of the upper limbs, and involves a coarse pill rolling movement of the thumb against the fingers. Other symptoms being bradykinesia, a general feeling of stiffness along with mild diffuse muscular pain. Masked facies, difficulty in initiating movement and shuffling gait appears late in the course of the disease.

100. C. The three cardinal features of Parkinson's disease are tremor, rigidity and bradykinesia, also known as classic triad. Other neurological symptoms are not associated with Parkinson's disease.

101. B. Levodopa and various other drugs are used in the treatment of Parkinson's disease. Levodopa augments body's dopamine level, which is depleted in Parkinson's disease. Dopamine is essential in neurotransmission. Levamisole is an antihelmintics, levothyroxine is thyroid hormone replacement, levofloxacin is an antibiotic and none has effect on neurotransmission.

102. A. Drug-induced Parkinsonism can follow lithium carbonate therapy. Other drugs believed to cause Parkinsonism include reserpine (serpasil), methyldopa (aldomet), haloperidol, and phenothiazine. Sulfonyluria (oral antidiabetic), aminophyllin (bronchodilator), and ecospirin (antiplatelet drug) are not known to cause Parkinsonism.

103. B. Promotion of physical exercise is one of the major concerns for nursing care. Individual exercise plan should be designed to achieve overall muscle tone and strengthening and stretching specific muscles involved. Another major concern for nursing care is providing adequate nutrition, maintaining ideal body weight and preventing constipation. Since these patients have dysphagia and bradykinesia promoting adequate nutrition is a challenge. So providing weight-reducing diet is not appropriate for these patients. Adequate food along with fibers must be provided to prevent malnutrition and constipation. Levodopa should be taken with meals and not in empty stomach to prevent the side effect of the drug.

104. C. The incidence of Parkinson's disease increases with age, with the peak onset in the sixth decade. The disease is more common in men by a ratio of 3:2.

105. B. Huntington's disease involves degeneration of basal ganglia leading to a depletion of several neurotransmitter, e.g. gamma aminobutyric acid and acetylcholine. This depletion results in relatively higher concentration of other neuro-transmitters like dopamine and norepinephrine. This relative increase of dopamin is responsible for excessive movement in Huntington's disease, whereas in Parkinson's disease there is a lack of dopamine giving rise to lack of movement. The exact pathological mechanism in restless leg syndrome is not yet understood.

106. B. Multiple sclerosis usually occurs between ages 20 and 40 and it affects women twice as often as men. Whites are affected more often than

Hispanics, blacks or Asians. The disease is more prevalent in colder climates of North America and Europe.

107. A. Vision changes, e.g. diplopia, blurred vision, or patchy blindness (scotomas) may be the early manifestations of multiple sclerosis. Dementia is not associated with multiple sclerosis. In multiple sclerosis affected muscles are spastic not flaccid. Deep tendon reflexes are exaggerated rather than absent.

108. C. Huntington's disease is a chronic progressive genetically transmitted degenerative disease of the nervous system. It is characterized by abnormal movements (chorea), intellectual decline, and emotional disturbances. Alzheimer's disease is a chronic progressive degenerative disease of the brain, clinically characterized by dementia and severe impairment of decision making that begins insidiously and can progress for a decade or so. Parkinson's disease is characterized by disability from tremor and rigidity. Creutzfeldt -Jakob disease (CJD) is a subacute CNS disorder that produces progressive dementia, myoclonus and distinctive EEG changes.

109. B. Guillain-Barré syndrome is often preceded by immune system stimulation by infection, trauma, surgery, immunizations or lymphoproliferative neoplasms. *Campilobacter jejuni* is the most frequently implicated organism. CJ gastroenteritis is thought to precede GB syndrome in about 30 percent cases. The disease is not related to infections by Helicobacter pylori and Pneumocystic carinii.

110. C. GB syndrome is an acute rapidly progressing polyneuritis. It affects the peripheral nervous system and results in loss of myelin, and edema and inflammation of the affected nerves, causing a loss of neurotransmission to the peripheri. The muscles innervated by the damaged peripheral nerves undergo denervation and atrophy. Respiratory paralysis is due to affection of nerves innervating the thoracic region. It is due to a cell-mediated immunologic reaction directed at the peripheral nerves and not due to neurotoxin affecting the respiratory center, immobility or degeneration of spinal cord and brainstem.

111. A. Sign and symptoms of GB syndrome include paresthesia followed by paralysis, hypotonia (reduced muscle tone) and areflexia (loss of deep tendon reflexes). The two most dangerous features of the disease are respiratory muscle weakness and autonomic neuropathy, involving both the sympathetic and parasympathetic systems. Urinary retention may be present if there is autonomic neuropathy. Other symptoms of autonomic neuropathy being orthostatic hypotension, hypertension, pupillary disturbances, sweating dysfunction, cardiac dysrhythmias, paralytic ileus and urinary retention.

112. B. Patient with GB syndrome has dysphagia. Patient with dysphagia is more likely to aspirate clear liquids than thick liquids or semisolid foods. Frequent monitoring of vital signs are required as the patient may develop bradycardia, hypotension or hypertension and respiratory depression. Passive range of exercise will prevent contracture. Regular measurement of calf circumference of both limbs will help detect deep vein thrombosis early.

113. A. Increasing age is the most common risk factor for Alzheimer's disease.

10% of people over the age 65 and 50% of those over the age 85 have Alzheimer's disease. Genetic factors also play a role in the causation of disease. Head trauma, myocardial infarction, environment have been linked with Alzheimer's disease but these links are weak.

114. B Alzheimer's disease is characterized by changes in the dendrites of the neurons. The decrease in the number and composition of the dendrites is responsible for symptoms of the disease. Others are not related to the pathology of the disease.

115. B. The most common cause of visual problem in India or worldwide is refractive error. Cataract is the most common cause of blindness in India. Visual impairment or blindness due to nutritional deficiency or eye injury is less common.

116. C. The visual defect, i.e. farsightedness resulting from the decrease in accommodative ability of the eye in aged is presbyopia. Myopia is nearsightedness, light focusses in front of retina, occurs due to excessive refractive power of cornea or lens or too long eyeball. Hyperopia is farsightedness, light focusses behind the retina, results from too short eyeball, or inadequate refractive power of the lens or cornea. Amblyopia is reduced vision in the affected eye, may occur in children if their refractive error is not corrected.

117. C. The cause of presbyopia in individuals above the age of 40 years is reduced elasticity of the lens. With aging the crystalline lens becomes larger, firmer and less elastic. These changes decrease the eye's accommodative ability and results in difficulty focussing near objects. Presbyopia is not due to retinal degeneration, decreased corneal refractive ability or opacity in crystalline lens.

118. A. Presbyopia or farsightedness occurring in individual above the age of 40 years is corrected by use of convex lens. Glasses for presbyopia are often called reading glasses as they are usually worn for close vision only. Concave lens is used for correction of myopic vision. Both convex and concave lenses maybe used when presbyopic correction is combined with correction of myopia. Refractive surgery is most commonly employed in the correction of myopia.

119. A. A sty or hordeolum is an infection of a sebaceous gland in the lid margin. The most common bacterial agent causing the infection is *Staphylococcus aureus*. An inflammation of a sebaceous gland in the eyelid is chalazion. It occurs due to blockage of gland orifices and stagnation of sebaceous secretions. Bilateral inflammation of the lid margin is blepharitis, may result from staphylococcal infection and seborrhea of the scalp and eyebrows.

120. D. Treatment of a chalazion is surgical removal of the chronic lesion by incision and curettage or injection of corticosteroids into the lesion by an ophthalmologist. Application of antibiotic ointment is ineffective. Warm moist compresses may cause spontaneous drainage in the early stage.

121. B. The graft taken for corneal transplantation is from human cadaver eyes. Synthetic polymer and graft taken from pig or monkey are not used.

122. B. A cataract is opacity in the crystalline lense. Patients with cataract usually complain of decreased vision, abnormal color perception and glare, which is worse at night. Loss of peripheral vision is found in glaucoma. Floaters in eye is a symptom of retinal detachment.

Seeing halos around light is also a symptom of glaucoma.

123. A. Phacoemulsification being a sutureless surgery recovery is early and refraction can be done after 1–2 weeks of surgery. In conventional surgery where sutures are used refraction for correction of residual refractive error is done when eye is fully recovered and 2 weeks after suture removal, i.e. usually 8 weeks. 4 weeks is too early and 12 weeks is too late for this purpose.

124. D. Pain after cataract surgery is mild to moderate and is usually relieved by pain medication, e.g. acetaminophen. But increasing pain signals complication. So the nurse should immediately inform the physician. Elevation of head will not relieve pain and is not indicated. The nurse should not remove dressing. Aspirin is contraindicated after cataract surgery. Patient should be examined first before administering pain medication.

125. D. The patient must be instructed to avoid straining at stool (Valsalva's maneuver). Straining at stool, increases intraocular pressure. Since, the elderlies often remain constipated, they should take laxative every night to prevent constipation. The other activities, which increase intraocular pressure, are bending and coughing. The patient should avoid sleeping on the operated side. Elevation of bed is not needed after cataract surgery. Keeping room environment cool and dry is also not required after cataract surgery. The patient should get assistance during climbing stairs, not avoid climbing stairs.

126. D. The patient should not carry weight more than 2–2.5 kg for approximately 1 week after cataract surgery. So patient should be taught further regarding limitation of carrying weight after cataract surgery. All other statements by the patient indicate adequate knowledge, e.g. wearing sunglasses for comfort, getting assistance during climbing stairs to prevent injury and using elevated toilet seat to avoid bending head below the waist.

127. B. After cataract surgery there is no need to avoid salt in diet if it is not otherwise contraindicated. Other advice is appropriate after cataract surgery.

128. C. Ciliary processes, which constitute the terminal portion of the ciliary body, lying behind the peripheral part of the iris, secrete aqueous humor. Iris is the structure containing a small hole in the center, called pupil. By the action of the iris sphincter muscle and iris dilator muscle pupil constricts and dilates respectively. Iris provides color of the eyes. Lacrimal apparatus produces tear, not aqueous humor. Choroid is a highly vascular structure that nourishes the ciliary body, the iris and the outer portion of the retina. It is not involved with aqueous humor production.

129. B. Atropine has mydriatic effects causing pupil dilation leading to photophobia. Dark glasses give relief from photophobia. Atropine does not paralyze blink reflex. Driving may be contraindicated in blurred vision.

130. C. A patient with chronic open angle glaucoma usually does not notice the gradual visual field loss until peripheral vision is severely compromised. If the patient remains untreated he is left with tunnel vision in which peripheral vision is totally lost and a small center field can be seen. Constant blurred vision is usually not associated with open angle glaucoma. It may be a symptom in angle closure glaucoma. Pain and pressure symptoms are not associated with open angle glaucoma. Sudden excruciating pain in or around the eye is associated with acute angle closure glaucoma.

131. D. The symptom of halos around lights along with the complain of sudden severe pain in and around eyes usually indicate acute angle closure glaucoma. Hazy vision is usually associated with cataract, watering of eyes is associated with conjunctivitis and floaters in the field of vision is associated with retinal detachment.

132. D. In glaucoma intraocular pressure rises due to impaired drainage of aqueous humor. Treatment aims at increasing the drainage of aqueous humor and decrease production of aqueous humor. Atropine sulfate causes pupillary dilation, which further obstructs aqueous humor drainage. So atropine sulfate is not given in the treatment of glaucoma. Betaxolol, a beta adrenergic blockers, decreases aqueous humor production; pilocarpine, a miotic causes pupillary constriction and opening of trabecular meshwork, facilitates aqueous humor outflow; and acetazolamide, a systemic carbonic anhydrase inhibitor decreases aqueous humor production and are used in the treatment of glaucoma.

133. B. In glaucoma intraocular pressure (IOP) increases. So the patient should avoid activities that increase intraocular pressure. Activities that increase IOP are bending head below waist, coughing, sneezing, Valsalva's maneuver and lifting heavy objects. Watching television, carbonated and caffeinated drinks are not associated with increase IOP. Since, it is a chronic disease patient should adhere to prescribed therapeutic regimen and follow-up schedule prescribed by the ophthalmologist and not only visit ophthalmologist when symptoms increase.

134. Without regular treatment patient with glaucoma may be permanently blind from damage of optic nerve. Progressive loss of peripheral vision is a typical symptom of glaucoma. Loss of color vision and nystagmus is not associated with glaucoma.

135. C. Absence of the lens is called aphakia. Aphakia may be corrected by the use of eyeglasses, contact lenses and intraocular lenses. Intraocular lens is the treatment of choice as it provides best visual correction with immediate return of binocular vision. Eyeglasses are cheap and safest but one has to wear very thick lenses. It also magnifies objects and causes difficulty in judging distances. Contact lenses are difficult to handle by the elderlies.

136. C. Persons with severe myopia is at risk of developing retinal detachment. The other risk factors of retinal detachment include increased age, cataract extraction, degeneration of the retina, trauma, previous retinal detachment in the other eye and a family history of retinal detachment.

137. A. Sudden severe pain in the eye is not the symptom of retinal detachment as no pain is associated with detached retina. All other symptoms are characteristic of retinal detachment.

138. B. The external auditory canal is a slightly S-shaped tube about 1 inch or 2.5 cm in length in the adult.

139. A. The outer half of the ear canal is covered with thick skin that contains hair follicles and ceruminous glands, but the skin of inner half of the canal lacks these structures.

140. A. In conductive deafness the patient hears the tuning fork louder and longer by bone conduction, i.e. negative Rinne test finding. In sensorineural hearing loss or in normal hearing the air conductions heard better and longer, i.e. positive Rinne test finding.

141. D. Pure tone audiometry is a subjective test and cannot be used in children who are unable to follow instructions. All other statements about pure tone audiometry are correct.

142. B. Caloric test is done to assess vestibular function. Auditory function is tested by audiometry. Brainstem function is assessed by auditory brainstem response (ABR). Cochlear function is assessed by electrocochleography.

143. C. The temperature of the irrigating solution should be at body temperature, i.e. 37° centigrade, which does not evoke caloric response in the patient. Temperature below or above body temperature stimulates endolymph of semicircular canal resulting in nystagmus, vomiting or vertigo.

144. D. Irrigation of ear canal is contraindicated in perforated tympanic membrane as solution may enter inner ear and cause infection, dizziness, nausea and vomiting. Other conditions are not contraindications to ear irrigation.

145. B. Conductive hearing loss occurs from interference of sound transmission through the external ear and middle ear. The most common cause of conductive hearing loss is otitis media with effusion. Foreign body in external ear may also cause conductive hearing loss but is not common. Noise pollution and ototoxic drugs cause sensorineural hearing loss.

146. C. Otalgia is the term for pain in ear. Otalgia is one of the first signs of external otitis and is caused by the swelling of the bony ear canal secondary to inflammatory process.

147. B. Myringoplasty involves repair or closure of a simple tympanic membrane perforation. In this operation surgical reconstruction is limited to repair of tympanic membrane perforation. Surgical correction or reconstruction of the tympanic membrane with ossicular chain is done in tympanoplasty. Surgical reconstruction of ossilar chain is done in ossiculoplasty. Myringotomy involves incision in the tympanic membrane for removal of fluid by suction.

148. D. Noises in the ear such as cracking or popping is a normal occurrence in the initial period after ear surgery, which should be explained to the patient. Patient need not report its occurrence, as this is a normal expectation after surgery. Other instructions are all appropriate and aim in preventing dislodgment of the graft from operated site.

149. C. The nurse is not expected to find vomiting in a patient with otosclerosis. The most important manifestation of otosclerosis involves progressive hearing loss. Patient may or may not complain of tinnitus. On examination Schwartz's sign (a reddish blush of the tympanum) is found.

150. A. In autosclerosis fixation of the stapes in the oval window results from repeated resorption and redeposition of abnormal spongy bone due to a genetic disorder. The condition does not occur from fibrous tissue formation secondary to bacterial invasion or abnormal deposition of collagen and calcium secondary to trauma.

151. A. The clinical features of acute otitis media in adults usually include otalgia, fever, hearing loss and drainage from the ear. On examination erythematous and bulging tympanic membrane is seen. In adults acute otitis media is usually unilateral, so bilateral otalgia is not a symptom of acute otitis media in adults. Tinnitus, vomiting, vertigo and pain and tenderness on movement of auricle are not found in acute otitis media.

152. B. The term presbycusis refers to progressive hearing loss associated with aging and is a form of sensorineural hearing loss. The term does not refer to sudden hearing loss, congenital hearing loss or noise induced hearing loss, which are other forms of sensorineural hearing loss.

153. A. A person with sensorineural hearing loss is able to hear sound but unable to understand speech. Ability to hear high-pitched sound diminishes. Consonants are high-pitched sounds that give intelligibility to speech. So words become difficult to distinguish and sound becomes muffled. Hearing aid reduces the strain of hearing but the sounds will be muffled. Patient with conductive type of hearing loss speaks softly as he hears his voice louder through bone conduction.

154. C. The nurse should assess development of facial paralysis in this patient. Chronic suppurative infection of middle ear may cause necrosis of the bone covering the facial nerve resulting in facial paralysis. Anosmia and dysphagia are not associated with chronic suppurative otitis media. Balance disorder is the symptom of inner ear involvement.

155. C. While communicating with a patient with sensorineural hearing impairment, the nurse should speak slowly and articulate clearly with normal tone of voice without shouting. She should also speak towards the patient's best ear, reduce background noises. Visual cues and written instructions are not necessary if the nurse speaks clearly and slowly. Providing hearing aid is not much helpful in understanding speech as patients with sensorineural hearing loss listens sound but have difficulty in understanding speech. The nurse should always allow patients, including the hearing impaired time to understand the spoken words before expecting a response.

156. A. To straighten the ear canal in an adult the pinna is pulled up and back. The other options are not appropriate to prepare ear for instillation of ear drops.

157. B. The characteristic symptoms of Ménière's disease are episodic vertigo, tinnitus, hearing loss and aural fullness. Episodic vertigo is commonly associated with nausea and vomiting and causes significant disability for the patient because of its sudden and severe nature. Otalgia and fever is associated with otitis media and vertigo accompanied by nystagmus and vomiting is associated with labyrinthitis. In Ménière's disease there is usually bilateral involvement. Otalgia and loss of balance is not associated with Ménière's disease.

158. C. Nurse will find evidence of sensorineural hearing loss in a patient with Ménière's disease. Pain and tenderness on application of pressure on tragus, Schwartz's sign and conductive hearing loss are not associated with Ménière's disease.

159. A. The patient with Ménière's disease should consume a low salt diet. He should also restrict fluid and avoid nicotine and caffeine.

160. B. Méniére's disease results in vertigo. So patient should be protected from falling. Social isolation due to hearing loss may occur with progress of disease but this is not a problem with this patient. Méniére's disease does not affect nutrition or cause infection.

2
CHAPTER

Circulatory System

Q1. A patient with the bicuspid valve disorder will have impaired blood flow between the:

A. Vena cava and right atrium
B. Right atrium and right ventricle
C. Right ventricle and pulmonary artery
D. Left atrium and left ventricle

Q2. The artery supplying the anterior wall of the heart is:

A. Right coronary artery
B. Circumflex artery
C. Left anterior descending artery
D. Left internal mammary artery

Q3. Blood flow through the coronary arteries primarily occurs during:

A. Inspiration
B. Expiration
C. Systole
D. Diastole

Q4. Which of the following areas of the heart will be affected by occlusion of right coronary artery?

A. Anterior wall
B. Posterior wall
C. Lateral wall
D. Inferior portion

Q5. Conduction disturbances arising out of ischemia developed in atrioventricular node and Purkinje fibers is the result of occlusion in which of the branch of coronary artery?

A. Left main coronary artery
B. Left anterior descending artery
C. Right coronary artery
D. Circumflex artery

Q6. The correct position to palpate the apical pulse is at the:

A. Left midclavicular line at the level of second intercostal space
B. Left midclavicular line at the level of the fifth intercostal space
C. Left axillary line at the level of fifth intercostal space
D. Left midclavicular line at the level of seventh intercostal space

Q7. One of the reasons for occurrence of murmur is turbulent blood flow across stenosed or incompetent valves. If a murmur is heard at the second intercostal space to the right of the sternum, which valve is stenosed or incompetent?

A. Aortic
B. Pulmonic
C. Mitral
D. Tricuspid

Q8. Which of the following blood tests for isoenzyme activity indicates cardiac damage?

A. CK-MM
B. CK-MB
C. CK-BB
D. LDH_3

Q9. A P wave on an ECG represents an impulse:

A. Originating at the SA node and depolarizing the atria
B. Originating at the SA node and repolarizing the atria
C. Originating at the AV node and depolarizing the atria
D. Originating at the AV node and spreading to the bundle of His

Q10. An important nursing responsibility for a patient after an invasive cardiovascular diagnostic study is:

A. Discourage fluid intake and place the patient in prone position
B. Apply heat to the puncture site and passively exercise the involved extremity
C. Limit motion of the affected extremity and assess the puncture site
D. Restrict fluid intake and encourage ambulation

Q11. A patient with history of chest pain has to undergo a thalium scan. The nurse understands that this test will be carried out to:

A. Determine the action of heart valves
B. Determine the direction and flow of blood through the heart
C. Determine intracardiac electrical activity
D. Determine myocardial muscle viability

Q12. In order to detect abnormal venous filling time and reveal valvular incompetence of the deep veins the nurse should perform which of the following tests?

A. Allen's test
B. Test for elevation pallor
C. Trendelenburg's test
D. Homan's test

Q13. The major determinant of diastolic blood pressure is:

A. Systemic vascular resistance
B. Blood volume
C. Renal function
D. Baroreceptors

Q14. Which of the following functions by the kidney helps to maintain the blood pressure at normal level?

A. Kidney's ability to retain sodium and excrete potassium
B. Kidney's ability to retain sodium and excrete excess water
C. Kidney's ability to excrete sodium and water
D. Kidney's ability to excrete sodium and retain water

Q15. The term used to describe elevated blood pressure without an identified cause that accounts for 90% of all cases of hypertension is:

A. Primary hypertension
B. Secondary hypertension
C. Malignant hypertension
D. Isolated systolic hypertension

Q16. Furosemide is often used to treat hypertension. The reason for furosemide administration is:

A. It blocks the sympathetic stimulation of the heart
B. It inhibits reabsorption of sodium and water in the kidney tubule and thus controls blood volume
C. It helps in reabsorption of sodium and excretion of potassium
D. It dilates peripheral blood vessels

Q17. Which of the following factors is found to be effective in lowering blood pressure and reducing cardiovascular risk factors?

A. Implementing lifestyle modification
B. Reducing environmental stressors
C. Increasing dietary fats
D. Maintaining routine lifestyle practices

Q18. Physician prescribes Lisinopril 10 mg daily to a patient. The drug is prescribed to treat:

A. Hypotension
B. Hypertension
C. Palpitation
D. Abdominal distension

Q19. A patient with hypertension has been prescribed an angiotensin-converting enzyme inhibitor and a loop diureti c. The expected outcome of this therapy is:

A. Excretion of calcium with diuretic effect
B. An increase in diastolic blood pressure
C. A decrease in blood pressure
D. Hypotension

Q20. A patient with hypertension on lisinopril complaints of dry nonproductive cough. The nurse tells the patient to:

A. Increase fluid intake
B. Take a cough medication
C. Avoid chills and drafts
D. Report to the doctor

Q21. A patient with hypertension is receiving diltiazem, a calcium channel blocker. The nurse understands that this drug lowers blood pressure by:

A. Promoting vasodilation
B. Reducing blood volume
C. Increasing heart rate
D. Increasing peripheral vascular resistance

Q22. The physician has prescribed diltiazem to a patient with unstable angina. The nurse knows that this drug is also used in the following conditions *except*:

A. Hypertension
B. Dysrhythmia
C. Chronic stable angina
D. Second degree heart block

Q23. The primary reason for peripheral arterial occlusive disease is:

A. Atherosclerosis
B. Embolism
C. Thrombosis
D. Vasospasm

Q24. The most significant risk factors for peripheral arterial disease include:

A. Family history, sedentary lifestyle and stress
B. Cigarette smoking, hypertension, and diabetes
C. Hyperlipidemia, sedentary lifestyle and family history
D. Advanced age, female sex and obesity

Q25. Intermittent claudication of the calf muscle is due to:

A. Inadequate muscle oxygenation
B. Inadequate venous return of the lower extremity
C. Inadequate muscular activity and exercise
D. Inadequate glucose uptake by the muscle

Q26. Which of the following symptoms indicate intermittent claudication?

A. Extensive discoloration
B. Dependent rubor
C. Rest pain
D. Pain associated with walking

Q27. The manifestations of arterial insufficiency are all of the following, *except*:

A. Warm skin temperature
B. Thin shiny hairless skin
C. Thick ridged toe nails
D. Pain with walking

Q28. A patient with history of smoking and occasional consumption of alcohol is diagnosed with intermittent claudication and is prescribed with Pentoxifylline (Trental) 400 mg three times daily with meals. The nurse should instruct the patient to:

A. Reduce cigarette smoking
B. Increase body weight
C. Practice meticulous feet care
D. Report when symptoms worsen

Q29. Patient with peripheral arterial disease should be encouraged for daily walking as walking helps these patients particularly in:

A. Loosing body weight
B. Reducing stress
C. Increasing high-density lipoprotein level
D. Promoting collateral circulation

Q30. A patient comes to the clinic with complain of frequent numbness of hands and feet. The physician suspects peripheral arterial disease and assesses the patient's arms and legs for the same. What is the most commonly used overall indicator of arm and leg circulation?

A. Allen's test
B. Buerger's sign
C. Ankle-brachial pressure index
D. Exercise testing

Q31. A patient comes to the emergency department complaining of sudden onset of the right lower leg pain. On examination it was found that popliteal pulse was absent, right foot looked mottled, cyanotic, cold and cadaverous. The physician suspects acute peripheral arterial occlusion. What is the most common cause of acute occlusion?

A. Hypertension
B. Thrombosis
C. Emboli
D. None of the above

Q32. A patient is admitted in the emergency ward with the diagnosis of acute arterial occlusion in one lower limb. Before any definitive therapy is arranged, which of the following the nurse should do?

A. Place the affected limb at level or slightly lower than the rest of the body
B. Elevate the affected leg at 30° angle
C. Provide a hot water bottle to the affected extremity
D. Provide an ice cap to the affected limb

Q33. The nurse is teaching a patient with thromboangiitis obliterans (Buerger's disease) regarding self-care. Which statement by the patient indicates the need for further teaching?

A. 'I know it is essential that I quit smoking'
B. 'It will be helpful if I get a job that allows me to sit most of the time'
C. 'I need to take meticulous care of my feet'
D. 'I need to avoid exposing myself to cold environment as much as possible'

Q34. A patient is diagnosed with Raynaud's phenomenon. When teaching the patient about activities of daily living the nurse should include which of the following in the teaching plan?

A. To reduce smoking as much as possible
B. Take pain medication 1–2 hours before exposure to cold
C. Wear woollen sweaters and gloves when exposed to cold and cold objects
D. All of the above

Q35. During a routine medical examination an asymptomatic abdominal aneurysm measuring 3 cm was detected in a patient. The nurse caring for the patient anticipates:

A. A severe gastrointestinal bleeding leading to a shock within a few days
B. A complain by the patient of severe back or flank pain and presence of a pulsating mass in the abdomen

C. Excision of the aneurysm and replacement with a synthetic graft
D. Administration of an antihypertensive drug

Q36. A patient diagnosed with abdominal aortic aneurysm is admitted for surgery. The nurse suspects rupture of the aneurysm when:

A. Patient complains of sudden severe back pain
B. Patient complains of dyspnea and palpitation
C. Patient develops a pulsatile mass in the periumbilical area
D. Patient develops hypotension and bradycardia

Q37. The nurse is caring for a patient after surgical repair of an abdominal aneurysm. Which of the following nursing diagnosis is most important for this patient on the first postoperative day?

A. Ineffective peripheral tissue perfusion
B. Risk for infection
C. Self-care deficit
D. Pain related to surgical incision

Q38. Which of the following nursing measures is most appropriate in caring for a patient after an abdominal aortic aneurysm repair?

A. Keeping the legs elevated to 30° angle
B. Monitoring urine output, BUN, and creatinine
C. Assess carotid, radial and temporal artery pulses
D. All of the above are appropriate

Q39. Three important factors in the etiology of venous thrombosis are called Virchow's triad. Which of the following factors is not included in Virchow's triad?

A. Venous stasis
B. Injury to venous wall
C. Hypercoagulability
D. Hypocoagulability

Q40. An elderly patient with generalized arteriosclerosis complains to the nurse about inability to sleep at night due to coldness of feet. What should the nurse advise?

A. To rub the feet gently to improve circulation before sleep
B. To place a light blanket over feet at night
C. To place a covered hot water bottle below the feet at night
D. To take a warm footbath before going to bed

Q41. The patient who is most likely to have the highest risk for deep vein thrombosis is a:

A. 25-year-old man with fractured leg
B. 45-year-old obese woman who smokes and is on hormone replacement therapy
C. 60-year-old man with vericose veins
D. 70-year-old man with IV infusion

Q42. The nurse is taking care of an elderly woman who has undergone hip replacement surgery. Which of the following assessment data would indicate that the patient has developed deep vein thrombosis?

A. Pain in the calf that occurs with exercise
B. Paresthesia and coolness of the leg
C. Generalized edema of the involved extremity
D. Pallor and cyanosis of the involved extremity

Q43. Which of the following terms is used to describe pain in the calf on forced dorsiflexion of the foot when the leg is raised?

A. Positive Babinski's reflex
B. Positive Homan's sign
C. Positive Kernig's sign
D. Positive Brudzinski's sign

Q44. Which of the following nursing measures is appropriate for a patient with acute lower extremity deep vein thrombosis?

A. Keeping the leg in a dependent position to promote arterial circulation
B. Applying elastic stockings to the affected extremity
C. Encouraging ambulation to promote venous return
D. Administering anticoagulant as prescribed

Q45. A patient on anticoagulant therapy for deep vein thrombosis is being prepared for discharge. Which of the following instructions the nurse should provide?

A. To continue the medication regularly, if a dose is missed, take the double dose next time
B. Get blood tests done for Hb% regularly as prescribed
C. Report to the physician if diarrhea
D. Be aware of and report sign and symptoms of bleeding

Q46. The nurse is teaching a patient who is on warfarin (Coumadin) before discharge. Which of the following statements by the patient indicate effective teaching?

A. 'This drug will dissolve clots I may still have'
B. 'I need to increase the intake of leafy vegetables like cabbage'
C. 'If I miss a dose I need to double the next dose'
D. 'I need to avoid taking over-the counter drug like aspirin on my own'

Q47. Which of the following statements by the patient indicates that he needs further teaching about prevention of thrombi?

A. 'I should massage my legs once a day.'
B. 'I should drink a lot of fluids'
C. 'I need to perform range of motion exercises'
D. 'I should wear elastic stockings when out of bed.'

Q48. The cause of varicose veins is:

A. Injury in the intimal layer of veins
B. Occlusion by atherosclerotic plaque in the veins
C. Incompetent venous valves
D. Vasospasm of the affected veins

Q49. Patients with varicose veins commonly complain of:

A. Muscle aches, cramps and fatigue
B. Sharp pain in leg during walking
C. Fatigue and cool feet
D. Pallor and numbness of feet

Q50. Common site of occurrence of varicose veins is:

A. Greater and lesser saphenous veins
B. Femoral vein
C. Cephalic vein
D. Popliteal vein

Q51. The nurse is teaching a patient with vericose veins. Which of the following statements by the patient indicates the need for further teaching?

A. 'I should walk 1-2 miles everyday'
B. 'I should walk up the stairs rather than use the elevator'
C. 'I should wear tight elastic stockings'
D. 'I should take rest by elevating the legs when they are hurt'

Q52. Curative management of varicose veins is:

A. Sclerotherapy
B. Laser therapy
C. Ligation and stripping
D. Percutaneous transluminal balloon angioplasty

Q53. The nurse is taking care of a patient who has undergone ligation and stripping for varicose veins. Which of the following interventions is not recommended?

A. Elevating the foot of the bed
B. Applying compression stockings
C. Encouraging deep breathing
D. Encouraging sitting beside the bed and dangling feet

Q54. The surgical treatment of thrombophlebitis is aimed at reducing pulmonary embolism by:

A. Inserting a filter into the aorta to filter the blood before it reaches the lungs

B. Inserting a filter into the hepatic artery to filter the blood before it reaches the lungs

C. Inserting a filter into the vena cava to filter the blood before it reaches the lungs

D. Inserting a filter into the femoral artery to filter the blood before it reaches the lungs

Q55. Which type of cardiomyopathy is characterized by a disproportionate thickening of the interventricular septum?

A. Dilated cardiomyopathy

B. Restrictive cardiomyopathy

C. Hypertrophic cardiomyopathy

D. Congestive cardiomyopathy

Q56. Which of the following is the most common manifestation of hypertrophic cardiomyopathy?

A. Palpitations

B. Peripheral edema

C. Weight loss

D. Dyspnea

Q57. Which of the following conditions commonly occur in a patient with most common form of cardiomyopathy?

A. Heart failure

B. Sudden death

C. Cardiac tamponade

D. Pericardial effusion

Q58. While planning care of a patient with dilated cardiomyopathy, the nurse takes into consideration of which of the following facts?

A. Potential risk of the family members due to infectious nature of the disease

B. Early treatment can cure the disease completely

C. Prognosis of the disease is poor and patient and family members require emotional support

D. The condition may be successfully treated with ventriculomyotomy and myectomy

Q59. A 65-year-old lady has been admitted with left sided chest pain and weakness developed after an attack of viral fever one month back. The physician suspects pericarditis. Which assessment finding is the most symptomatic of pericarditis?

A. Chest pain relieved by the rotation of the trunk

B. Crackles at the base of lungs

C. Systolic murmurs

D. Pericardial friction rub

Q60. A patient with history of blunt trauma to the chest complains of chest pain, which increases on movement. On auscultation a pericardial friction rub is heard and the patient is diagnosed as acute pericarditis. The nurse caring for the patient should instruct which of the following positions for the relief of chest pain?

A. Semi-Fowler's

B. Leaning forward while sitting

C. Supine

D. Prone

Q61. A patient with history of myocardial infarction comes to the emergency department complaining of chest pain that radiates to his neck, shoulders, back and arms and decreases when he sits up and leans forward. Based on this subjective data the nurse suspects that he has:

A. Developed another myocardial infarction

B. Endocarditis

C. Myocarditis

D. Pericarditis

Q62. Which of the following is the most accurate technique for evaluating pericardial effusion?

A. ECG
B. Echocardiograph
C. Blood count
D. Blood culture

Q63. Which of the following types of infective endocarditis develops over days or weeks with an erratic course and earlier development of complications commonly caused by *Staphylococcus aureus*?

A. Subacute bacterial endocarditis
B. Acute bacterial endocarditis
C. Native valve endocarditis
D. Nonbacterial thrombotic endocarditis

Q64. The primary diagnostic tool for the evaluation of infective endocarditis is:

A. ECG
B. Echocardiography
C. Blood cultures
D. Blood count

Q65. Prophylactic antibiotics are indicated to prevent infective endocarditis for the high-risk individuals who:

A. Are undergoing any dental procedures
B. Are undergoing normal vaginal delivery
C. Have acquired a viral respiratory tract infection
D. Are exposed to human immunodeficiency virus

Q66. The nurse is teaching the patient with rheumatic fever about the disease. Which of the following statements about rheumatic fever is appropriate?

A. Rheumatic fever is caused by *Streptococcus viridans* infection
B. Rheumatic fever is a sequela of beta-hemolytic *Streptococcus* infection
C. Incidence of streptococcus infection is more in the developed countries
D. Both B and C

Q67. Long-term penicillin therapy for the patient with rheumatic fever is indicated to:

A. Prevent chronic rheumatic carditis
B. To arrest the progress of migratory arthritis
C. To destroy the infective organism and cure the disease
D. To prevent recurrence of rheumatic fever

Q68. Which of the following is the most common cause of mitral valve stenosis in Indian patients?

A. Congenital heart disease
B. Rheumatic endocarditis
C. Rheumatic arthritis
D. Infective endocarditis

Q69. The nurse caring for a patient scheduled for a percutaneous transluminal balloon valvuloplasty understands that this procedure:

A. Is a method of treatment for both mitral stenosis and mitral regurgitation
B. Involves insertion of a transventricular balloon catheter into the opening of the valve
C. Is a treatment of choice for patients who are poor candidates for other valvular surgery
D. Is done as a last resort when other valvular repair operations have failed

Q70. A patient after mitral valve replacement surgery is being advised regarding self-care after discharge. Which statement by the patient indicates effective teaching?

A. 'I shall be able to lead a normal life and forget that I ever had heart disease.'
B. 'I shall need to take warfarin life long'
C. 'I shall need to take ecosprin daily'
D. 'I shall need to get my blood examined for Hb% every month'

Q71. The most common cause of coronary artery disease is:

A. Atherosclerosis
B. Hyperglycemia
C. Stress
D. Vasospasm of coronary artery

Q72. Among the following risk factors for coronary artery disease which one can be corrected?

A. Advanced age
B. Male sex
C. High blood pressure
D. Heredity

Q73. The risk of coronary artery disease increases when serum cholesterol level is more than:

A. 200 mg/dL
B. 150 mg/dL
C. 100 mg/dL
D. 175 mg/dL

Q74. Which of the following laboratory values found in an individual indicate high-risk of development of coronary artery disease?

A. A high-density lipoprotein of 70 mg/dL and a low-density lipoprotein of 120 mg/dL
B. A high-density lipoprotein of 35 mg/dl and a low-density lipoprotein of 120 mg/dL
C. A high-density lipoprotein of 30 mg/dL and a low-density lipoprotein of 160 mg/dL
D. A high-density lipoprotein of 70 mg/dL and a low-density lipoprotein of 110 mg/dL

Q75. The physician advises Lipitor to a patient attending outpatient department. The nurse explains to the patient that this drug has been advised to:

A. To reduce the low-density lipoprotein (LDL) level in the blood
B. To reduce the high-density lipoprotein (HDL) level in the blood
C. To increase phospholipids level in the blood
D. To increase triglycerides level in blood

Q76. The nurse is teaching self-care to a patient who is being treated with atrovastatin. Which of the following teaching is *not* appropriate?

A. You need not stay on a low fat diet as long as you take the medicine
B. You need to do periodical blood test for the liver enzyme studies
C. The drug will lower your blood cholesterol at a desired level after 6 weeks
D. Report immediately if you have weakness or muscle pain

Q77. The sensation of pain that is described most commonly by the patients with angina is:

A. Knife-like
B. Heaviness
C. Sharp
D. Tearing

Q78. Which of the following types of angina is associated with the chest pain or discomfort triggered by a predictable degree of exertion or emotion?

A. Stable angina
B. Unstable angina
C. Variant angina
D. Nocturnal angina

Q79. Which of the following types of angina is most likely to progress into MI?

A. Stable angina
B. Unstable angina
C. Prinzmetal's angina
D. Nocturnal angina

Q80. The nurse is assessing a 70-year-old patient who complains of recent chest pain. Which statement by the patient strongly indicates anginal pain?

A. 'The pain occurred when I was walking briskly in the morning'
B. 'The pain increased when I was taking deep breath'
C. 'The pain resolved after I drank a cup of cold milk'
D. 'The pain lasted about 50 minutes'

Q81. A patient with angina is getting propranolol 80 mg twice a day. Which of the following assessment findings should be reported to the physician?

A. Lethargy and fatigue
B. Joint pain
C. Night cough and dyspnea
D. Dry mouth and constipation

Q82. The nurse is teaching an elderly patient with angina regarding the administration of nitrates. Which of the following instructions the nurse should emphasize?

A. Keep your medication in refrigerator at all times
B. You may repeat the dose of sublingual nitroglycerin every 30 minutes for 3 doses if required
C. Lie down or sit in a chair for 5–10 minutes after taking the drug
D. Swallow your pill with a big glass of water not milk

Q83. A patient with chronic angina has been advised to apply transdermal nitroglycerin pad. The nurse teaches the patient regarding its application. Which of the following teaching is correct?

A. Apply pad to the site whenever chest pain
B. Apply pad daily and keep in place for 24 hours
C. Apply the pad before and during activity or exercise
D. Apply pad daily in morning and remove at bedtime

Q84. The nurse is teaching a patient with angina regarding side effect of nitrates. Which of the following is appropriate?

A. Flashing
B. Dry mouth
C. Photosensitivity
D. Bradycardia

Q85. The nurse is teaching a patient with angina pectoris regarding management of anginal pain and reduction of risk factors that exacerbate this condition. The teaching is effective when the patient verbalizes an understanding of:

A. The need to avoid exercise
B. The need to stop smoking
C. The need to seek medical care if acute pain persists for more than 2 hours
D. The need to restrict dietary fat, cholesterol, and fiber

Q86. A hospitalized patient with angina tells the nurse that he is having chest pain. The nurse understands that anginal pain:

A. Will be relieved by the rest and nitroglycerin
B. Is less severe than pain of a myocardial infarction
C. Indicates irreversible myocardial damage
D. May cause nausea and vomiting

Q87. The nurse is educating a group of young men and women regarding prevention of coronary heart disease. She tells them that CAD has many risk factors. Risk factors that can be modified or controlled include:

A. Sex, inactivity, obesity and smoking
B. Diet, family history, smoking and inactivity
C. Stress, obesity and sex
D. Obesity, diet, smoking and inactivity

Q88. Which of the following interventions restores blood supply and improves long-term patency of coronary artery?

A. Percutaneous transluminal coronary angioplasty
B. Directional coronary atherectomy
C. Intracoronary stents
D. Laser ablation

Q89. The most common cause of myocardial infarction is:

A. Aneurysm of coronary artery
B. Thrombus formation in a coronary artery

C. Occlusion of coronary artery by an embolus
D. Vasospasm of coronary artery

Q90. In myocardial infarction the area of the heart most frequently affected is:

A. Conduction system
B. Atrioventricular septum
C. Left ventricle
D. Right ventricle

Q91. Within 4–6 hours after an attack of myocardial infarction the laboratory finding that would be elevated is:

A. Lactic Dehydrogenase (LDH-1)
B. Eosinophil sedimentation rate (ESR)
C. Serum aspertate aminotransferase (AST)
D. Creatine phosphokinase-MB (CPK-MB)

Q92. The most common complication after acute myocardial infarction is:

A. Cardiac tamponade
B. Cardiac failure
C. Pulmonary embolism
D. Dysrhythmia

Q93. A patient with myocardial infarction (MI) is admitted to the CCU. The physician prescribes IV morphine and streptokinase. This thrombolytic agent streptokinase must be administered how soon after onset of MI symptoms?

A. Within 3–6 hours
B. Within 12–24 hours
C. Within 24–48 hours
D. Within 3–6 days

Q94. The physician is considering administering Inj Streptokinase to a patient with myocardial infarction. The nurse understands that this drug:

A. Keeps blood thin
B. Slows clotting of blood
C. Dissolves clot that is obstructing coronary artery
D. Shrinks clot thus facilitating better perfusion of myocardium

Q95. A patient admitted with myocardial infarction is being evaluated for thrombolytic therapy. Which statement made by the patient would indicate a possible contraindication to thrombolytic therapy?

A. 'I have been having chest pain for 2 hours'
B. 'I feel really nauseated right now'
C. 'I have been taking insulin for the last 5 years'
D. 'I am still taking medicine for my stomach ulcer'

Q96. The pain medication of choice in acute myocardial infarction is:

A. Pethidine hydrochloride
B. Diclofenac sodium
C. Codeine sulfate
D. Morphine sulfate

Q97. A patient 5 days after myocardial infarction (MI) is restless and apprehensive. The nurse can help by:

A. Providing all care by doing everything for the patient
B. Modifying the environment so that the patient can rest
C. Encouraging the family to provide for the patient's physical care and emotional support
D. Allowing the patient in planning and carrying out activities

Q98. A patient with myocardial infarction is receiving myovin (IV GTN). Which of the following the nurse should assess frequently?

A. Blood pressure
B. Blood glucose
C. Breath sounds
D. Urine output

Q99. The nurse is assessing a patient who is recovering from myocardial infarction. The outcome criteria which indicates that the patient is responding well to the treatment provided is:

A. Patient gets relief from the chest pain with sublingual nitroglycerin

B. Patient is tolerating increasing activity without chest pain
C. Patient is exhibiting a regular heart rate above 100 beats/minute
D. Patient is intending to make all necessary lifestyle changes except smoking

Q100. The nurse understands that left heart failure may develop in a patient with myocardial infarction as a complication. To detect the early signs of the left heart failure she should assess patient for:

A. Jugular venous distention
B. Dry hacking cough
C. Dependent bilateral edema
D. Right upper quadrant abdominal pain

Q101. Nurse is assessing a patient after an attack of anterior wall myocardial infarction. During auscultation of lungs crackles are heard. Nurse understands that this assessment finding is indicative of:

A. Left-sided heart failure
B. Pulmonary valve stenosis
C. Right sided heart failure
D. Tricuspid valve stenosis

Q102. Presence of distended neck veins is an important indicator of heart's performances. Distension of neck veins will be more prominent in which of the following disorders?

A. Hemorrhagic shock
B. Left ventricular failure
C. Right ventricular failure
D. Myocardial infarction

Q103. One of the compensatory mechanisms that occurs in the heart failure is increased sympathetic nervous system stimulation. Which of the following responses is seen in the increased sympathetic nervous system stimulation?

A. Tachycardia
B. Bradycardia
C. Hypotension
D. Polyuria

Q104. Which of the following compensatory mechanisms is involved in congestive heart failure that leads to inappropriate fluid retention and additional workload of the heart?

A. Ventricular dilation
B. Ventricular hypertrophy
C. Neurohormonal response
D. Sympathetic nervous system activation

Q105. Initial response of the body with decreased cardiac output will be:

A. Restlessness and disorientation
B. Bradycardia and hypotension
C. Low blood pressure and tachypnea
D. Increased blood pressure and fluid volume

Q106. The nurse is assessing a patient admitted with left-sided heart failure. Which of the following the nurse should expect to find?

A. Engorged neck veins
B. Dyspnea
C. Abdominal distention
D. Tremors of hand

Q107. A patient with a history of chronic heart failure attends outpatient department with the complaints of increase in symptoms of ankle edema, dyspnea on exertion, and orthopnea. Which of the following signs of fluid retention may also be evident in this patient?

A. Weak and thready pulse
B. Decrease in hematocrit concentration
C. Increase in hematocrit concentration
D. Orthostatic hypotension

Q108. The nurse is aware that before administering digoxin she should check all of the following parameters, *except*:

A. Apical pulse for 1 full minute
B. Recent serum electrolyte levels
C. Most recent serum digoxin levels
D. Respiratory rates for 1 full minute

Q109. The group of drugs used to improve cardiac function of a failing heart by increasing its pump performance is:

- **A.** Beta-adrenergic antagonists
- **B.** ACE inhibitors
- **C.** Inotropes
- **D.** Diuretics

Q110. Moderate doses of dopamine (4–8 μg/kg/min) stimulate which receptor site?

- **A.** Alpha
- **B.** Beta
- **C.** Dopaminergic
- **D.** Both alpha and beta

Q111. A patient with heart failure is being treated with digoxin. During digoxin therapy which of the following conditions could predispose the patient to digitalis toxicity?

- **A.** Pneumonia
- **B.** Hyperkalemia
- **C.** Hypothyroidism
- **D.** Hypocalcemia

Q112. A patient with chronic congestive heart failure is being treated with digoxin and lasix. To prevent possible complication from this combination of drugs, the nurse should:

- **A.** Maintain an accurate record of intake and output
- **B.** Monitor serum potassium level
- **C.** Teach patient to take low potassium diet
- **D.** Withhold drug and notify physician if patient experiences postural hypotension

Q113. A patient is being treated with tab digoxin for supraventricular tachycardia. What signs and symptoms are indicative of digoxin toxicity?

- **A.** Convulsions
- **B.** Yellow vision
- **C.** Vertigo
- **D.** Muscle cramping

Q114. The nurse is auscultating the breath sounds of a patient with cardiac failure. The breath sounds what the nurse is expected to hear are:

- **A.** Crackles
- **B.** Wheezes
- **C.** Friction rub
- **D.** Rhonchi

Q115. A patient who is hospitalized with the left sided heart failure is complaining of increasing breathlessness. He is anxious and restless, coughing up large amount of pink frothy sputum. The nurse suspects these as signs and symptoms of:

- **A.** Pulmonary embolism
- **B.** Pulmonary edema
- **C.** Right-sided heart failure
- **D.** Pneumonia

Q116. Which of the following symptoms is most commonly associated with the right-sided heart failure?

- **A.** Tachycardia
- **B.** Crackles
- **C.** Jugular vein distention
- **D.** Elevated blood urea nitrogen level

Q117. Sinus bradycardia is best described as:

- **A.** A regular rhythm of ventricular origin with a rate of less than 60 beats per minute
- **B.** An irregular slow ventricular rate with variable numbers of P waves between complexes
- **C.** A normal rhythm with a rate of less than 60 beats per minute
- **D.** A normal rhythm with a rate of more than 100 beats per minute

Q118. Which of the following characterizes sinus tachycardia?

- **A.** A regular rhythm at a rate of 60 to 100 beats/minute with a normal P wave and QRS complex
- **B.** A regular rhythm at a rate of 100 to 180 beats/minute with a normal P wave and QRS complex

C. A ventricular rapid rhythm that may or may not produce a palpable pulse
D. An irregular rhythm originating from sinus node with a rate of 60 to 100 beats per minute

Q119. A patient is admitted to the intensive coronary care unit with the complain of dizziness and fatigue and is diagnosed as supraventricular tachycardia. The nurse is aware that due to rapid heart rate the patient is at risk of developing:

A. Unstable angina
B. Myocardial infarction
C. Heart failure
D. Hypertension

Q120. A patient with supraventricular tachycardia is being treated with IV esmolol (miniblock). During esmolol therapy the nurse should monitor which of the following?

A. Heart rate and blood pressure
B. Body temperature and skin turgor
C. Urine output and peripheral edema
D. All of the above

Q121. A patient attends hospital emergency with dizziness and lightheadedness. On examination he is found to have a pulse rate of 40 beats per minute and blood pressure of 80/50 mm Hg. ECG shows sinus bradycardia. Which of the following medication will be used to treat his bradycardia?

A. Lidocaine
B. Esmolol
C. Atropine
D. Digoxin

Q122. A patient admitted in the hospital emergency is unresponsive and has a very faint pulse. ECG shows supraventricular tachycardia of 220 beats per minute. The nurse anticipates that the patient will be treated by cardioversion using an electrical voltage of:

A. 20 joules
B. 50 joules
C. 200 joules
D. 360 joules

Q123. A patient in the intensive coronary care unit has developed ventricular tachycardia. His heart rate is 160 beats / minute. He is hemodynamically stable. The nurse anticipates that the patient will be treated by:

A. Defibrillation
B. Administration of verapamil
C. Administration of lidocaine
D. Administration of digoxin

Q124. The nurse notices ventricular fibrillation in a monitor of a patient admitted in coronary care unit (CCU). The nurse should immediately prepare for:

A. An IV line for emergency medications
B. Synchronized cardioversion
C. Immediate defibrillation
D. Intubation

Q125. During preparation of a patient for electrical cardioversion the nurse is aware that cardioversion differs from defibrillation in that:

A. Cardioversion requires a higher dose of electrical current
B. Defibrillation is synchronized to countershock during the QRS complex
C. Cardioversion is indicated only for the treatment of atrial tachyarrhythmias
D. Cardioversion may be done on a nonemergency basis with sedation of the patient

Q126. A patient with ischemic heart disease has the following ECG characteristics: Atrial rate 80 and regular, ventricular rate 66 and irregular, P waves and QRS complexes are of normal contour. PR intervals progressively lengthen until a P wave is not followed by QRS complex. The patient is experiencing which of the following types of arrhythmia?

A. First degree AV heart block
B. Second degree AV heart block type I

C. Second degree AV heart block type II
D. Third degree AV heart block

Q127. A patient admitted in coronary care unit with acute myocardial infarction complains of fatigue and light-headedness. The nurse finds ventricular bigeminy in the patient's monitor. She anticipates that the patient will be treated by:

A. Defibrillation
B. IV lidocaine
C. Insertion of a temporary pacemaker
D. Cardioversion

Q128. When providing discharge instructions to a patient with newly implanted pacemaker the nurse teaches the patient to:

A. To take and record a daily pulse rate
B. Immobilize the arm and shoulder on the side of the pacemaker insertion for 6 weeks
C. Avoid microwaves ovens because they emit radiowaves that alter pacemaker function
D. Keep insertion site dry for 6 weeks after implantation

Q129. Shock is best defined as:

A. Cardiovascular collapse
B. Loss of sympathetic tone
C. Inadequate tissue perfusion
D. Blood pressure less than 90 mm Hg.

Q130. A patient has been admitted with spinal cord injury at T4 level. During assessment the nurse finds the patient's blood pressure as 80/60 mm Hg and pulse 40 beats per minute. The nurse understands that the patient is experiencing:

A. An absolute hypovolemia due to internal bleeding at the site of injury
B. Cardiogenic shock resulting from bradycardia
C. Neurogenic shock resulting from low blood flow
D. Neurogenic shock from a maldistribution of blood flow

Q131. A patient admitted with the bleeding peptic ulcer has developed hypovolemic shock. The nurse is aware that hypotension resulting from hypovolemic shock can seriously compromise perfusion to vital organs. Below what systolic blood pressure level is perfusion to vital organs markedly compromised in a usually normotensive person?

A. 100 mm Hg
B. 90 mm Hg
C. 80 mm Hg
D. 70 mm Hg

Q132. The effect that shock has on the body includes:

A. Sympathetic nervous system activation that results in an increase in heart rate, cardiac output, and rate and depth of respiration
B. Stimulation of parasympathetic nervous system resulting in slowing of heart rate and hypotension
C. Massive vasoconstriction in the heart and brain that stimulates renin-angiotensin system
D. Decreased tissue perfusion that causes aerobic metabolism resulting in lactic acidosis

Q133. Which of the treatment modalities is appropriate for the management of cardiogenic shock?

A. Inotropes, e.g. dopamine to improve contractility
B. ACE inhibitors to increase preload and decrease the afterload of the heart
C. Vasopressors to increase systemic vascular resistance
D. Beta-blockers to increase the heart rate and increase contractility

Q134. In a patient with shock several compensatory mechanisms take place to maintain homeostasis. One such compensatory mechanism is the activation

of renin-angiotensin system. Renin-angiotensin system is stimulated by:

A. Central nervous system response to low blood pressure
B. Cardiac response to catecholamines
C. Renal response to ischemia
D. Adrenal response to antidiuretic hormone

Q135. Which of the following mechanical device is indicated in a patient with cardiogenic shock to provide temporary circulatory assistance?

A. Temporary pacemaker
B. Ventricular assist device
C. Intra-aortic balloon pump
D. Defibrillator

Q136. The nurse needs to review the history of the patient to find out any factor which contraindicates the use of intra-aortic balloon pump (IABP). Which of the following conditions contraindicates use of the IABP?

A. Unstable angina pectoris
B. Peripheral atherosclerosis
C. Diabetes mellitus
D. Hypertension

Q137. The nurse is observing a patient for symptoms of postoperative shock. The earliest sign of postoperative shock would be obtained by monitoring the:

A. Pulse rate
B. Pulse pressure
C. Body temperature
D. Urine output

Q138. Adequacy of fluid replacement in a patient with shock is best determined by:

A. Systolic blood pressure above 100 mm Hg.
B. Systolic blood pressure above 90 mm Hg.
C. Urine output of 30 mL/hour
D. Urine output of 20 mL/hour

Q139. An elderly patient has been admitted to coronary care unit following an acute myocardial infarction. Shortly after admission the patient develops cardiogenic shock. A balloon tipped pulmonary artery catheter is inserted and the nurse finds that the patient's pulmonary artery wedge pressure to be 18 mm Hg. She knows that this pressure is:

A. Within normal limits
B. Elevated above normal
C. Less than normal
D. Life-threatening

ANSWERS AND RATIONALS OF CIRCULATORY SYSTEM

1. **D.** Bicuspid valve or the mitral valve is situated in left atrioventricular orifice and permits blood to flow from the left atrium to left ventricle. So, disorder of this valve will cause impairment of forward flow of blood from the left atrium to left ventricle. The orifices where superior and inferior vena cava are opened in the right atrium are not guarded by any valves. The orifice between right atrium and right ventricle is guarded by tricuspid valve and the orifice between right ventricle and pulmonary artery is guarded by semilunar valve.

2. **C.** Left anterior descending artery is mainly supplying the anterior wall of heart. Right coronary artery supplies the inferior wall of heart, circumflex the lateral wall and left internal mammary artery the left chest wall.

3. **D.** 75% of coronary blood flow occurs during diastole. There is no relationship between respiratory pattern and blood flow.

4. **D.** Right coronary artery supplies the right ventricle or the inferior portion of the heart. So, occlusion of the coronary artery will produce ischemia in the inferior portion of the heart. Other areas listed are not supplied by right coronary artery.

5. **C.** In 90% of people, atrioventricular node and Purkinje fibers, (part of the conduction system) receive blood supply from right coronary artery. So, obstruction of this artery often causes serious conduction disturbances.

6. **B.** Apical pulse is palpated at the fifth intercostal space in the midclavicular line, which is the point of maximum impulse and the mitral area. The left midclavicular line at the second intercostal space is the pulmonic area, where pulmonic sound is auscultated. Apical pulse is not palpated in the midaxillary line or at the level of seventh intercostal space.

7. **A.** Murmur due to aortic valve abnormalities are heard at the second intercostal space, to the right of sternum. Murmur due to abnormality of pulmonic valve is auscultated at the second intercostal space along the left sternal border. Mitral valve abnormalities are heard at fifth intercostal space along the midclavicular line and tricuspid valve abnormalities are heard at third or fourth intercostal space along the left sternal border.

8. **B.** CK-MB is cardiac muscle specific, elevated level indicates myocardial damage. CK-MM is skeletal muscle specific, CK-BB is elevated in brain damage. Of the 5 isoenzymes of LDH numbered 1-5 only LDH1 and LDH2 are cardiac specific.

9. **A.** P wave of an ECG represents impulse originating at SA node and depolarizing the atria. No wave due to atrial repolarization is seen in ECG waves. Because of small muscle mass of atria, the wave is small and buried in QRS complex. Impulses originating in AV node may move in retrograde fashion depolarize the atria and produce an abnormal P wave just before or after the QRS complex or that is hidden in QRS complex. Impulse originating at the AV node and spreading to the bundle of His is represented as PR interval.

10. **C.** The nurse will limit the motion of the affected extremity and assess the puncture site as the patient is

at risk for hemorrhage from the puncture site following the invasive diagnostic procedure, e.g. cardiac catheterization and angiocardiography. Patient should drink a lot of fluid to flush out the dye used in the procedure. He should lie in supine position with the affected leg straight and the head elevated no more than 30 degrees. Application of heat to the puncture site would facilitate hemorrhage as would passive exercise to the affected extremity. Ambulation is contraindicated due to the risk of hemorrhage from the puncture site.

11. D. Thalium scan is a radionuclear study also known as myocardial scintigraphy. The test involves intravenous injection of a radioactive isotope (Thalium 201 most common). As the isotope is absorbed by the blood cells of the heart muscle, photons are emitted, which are detected by an external gamma camera. In well perfused cells high concentration of 201 Tl will be present. Whereas infarcted or scarred myocardium does not extract any 201 Tl and shows up as cold spots. Action of heart valves, direction and flow of blood through the heart may be determined by echocardiography. Electrophysiological studies determine intracardiac electrical activity.

12. C. Trendelenburg's test is done to detect abnormal venous filling time and reveal valvular incompetence of the deep veins. Allen's test is used to assess the patency of the radial and ulnar arteries distal to the wrist. Test for elevation pallor is done when arterial insufficiency is suspected and Homan's test is done to detect deep vein thrombosis.

13. A. Systemic vascular resistance is the obstruction of blood flow by the arterioles that most predominantly affects diastolic pressure. Baroreceptors are nerve endings, located in the blood vessels and respond to the stretching of vessel walls. They do not directly affect diastolic blood pressure. Blood volume determines systolic blood pressure. Renal function helps control blood volume and indirectly affects diastolic blood pressure.

14. C. Kidneys respond to a rise in blood pressure by excreting sodium and water. This response affects blood volume and thus regulates blood pressure. Retention of either sodium or water will further increase blood pressure.

15. A. Primary hypertension accounts for 90 to 95% of all hypertensive cases. Exact cause is not known, thought to be due to several contributing factors. Secondary hypertension occurs secondary to a known correctible cause. Malignant hypertension is characterized by persistent severe hypertension and is rapidly progressive, uncontrollable. Isolated systolic hypertension occurs when the systolic blood pressure is 140 mmHg or higher, but the diastolic blood pressure remains normal.

16. B. Furosemide is a loop diuretic that inhibits sodium and water reabsorbtion in the loop of Henle and thus controls overall fluid volume and reduce blood pressure. Furosemide is not related to any other mechanism of actions mentioned in the question.

17. A. Lifestyle modifications are effective in lowering blood pressure and reducing cardiovascular risk factors. Lifestyle modifications are widely advocated to prevent high blood pressure. For some clients lifestyle modifications are suggested as definitive therapy for the first 6-12 months after initial diagnosis and as an adjunctive therapy for all patients with hypertension on pharmacologic therapy. It is difficult to reduce environmental stressors and thus it is not an effective means of controlling hypertension. Hypertensive patients need to reduce not increase dietary fats. Maintaining healthy lifestyle practices is helpful in lowering blood pressure, reducing the number and dosage of antihypertensive drugs.

18. B. Lisinopril is an angiotensin converting enzyme inhibitor used in mild to moderate hypertension. Hypotension may occur as a side effect. It does not treat palpitation and abdominal distention.

19. C. The expected outcome of angiotensin converting enzyme (ACE) inhibitor and loop diuretic therapy is lowering of blood pressure. ACE inhibitors prevent vasoconstriction and loop diuretics reduce circulating volume. Therefore by preventing vasoconstriction and reducing circulating volume blood pressure is decreased. Loop diuretics act by preventing sodium and water reabsorption, it does not cause calcium excretion. It does not cause increase in diastolic pressure. Hypotension is a side effect of ACE inhibitors and loop diuretics, not a therapeutic effect.

20. D. Lisinopril is an ACE inhibitor. Adverse effect of this drug is dry nonproductive cough. Cough disappears after the drug is discontinued. But the drug should not be discontinued abruptly. So the physician should be reported for a change in medication or its dose. The cough is not for respiratory infection so the options of avoiding chills and drafts; taking cough medication and increasing fluid intake are not correct.

21. A. Calcium channel blockers such as diltiazem decrease blood pressure by blocking entry of calcium into smooth muscle channels in arterioles thereby promoting vasodilation. Other effects of calcium channel blockers are decreased peripheral vascular resistance and decreased heart rate. It does not cause reduction of blood volume.

22. D. Diltiazem is a calcium channel blocker. Action of this drug is to inhibit calcium ion influx across the cell membrane of cardiac and vascular smooth muscle. The action produces relaxation of coronary vascular smooth muscle, dilates coronary arteries, slows SA/AV node conduction and dilates peripheral arteries. Calcium channel blockers are used for chronic-stable angina, unstable angina, dysrhythmias and hypertension. It is contraindicated in second or third degree AV block, sick sinus syndrome, hypotension, cardiogenic shock and Wolf-Parkinson-White syndrome.

23. A. The primary reason for peripheral arterial occlusive disease is atherosclerosis. Embolism, thrombosis and vasospasm also cause peripheral arterial occlusive disease but most of the pathologic changes that occur in this condition are caused by atherosclerosis.

24. B. The most significant risk factors for peripheral arterial disease are cigarette smoking. Other risk factors include family history, sedentary lifestyle, stress, hypertriglyceridemia and hyperuricemia. The disease occurs commonly in the sixth to eighth decades of life. Men in sixties have double the incidence than women, but as women age the incidence increases and equals as men.

25. A. Intermittent claudication results from muscular hypoxia causing anaerobic metabolism during exercise, resulting into angina like pain. Inadequate venous return of the extremity will give rise to edema, inadequate glucose uptake by the muscle will cause fatigue and inadequate muscular activity and exercise will give rise to diminished circulation due to venous stasis but not intermittent claudication.

26. D. Pain associated with walking that disappears on rest is characteristic of intermittent claudication. The pain is caused by inadequate arterial circulation to contracting muscle. Extensive discoloration, dependent rubor and rest pain do not indicate intermittent claudication.

27. A. In advanced arterial insufficiency skin will be deprived from adequate blood supply due to arterial steal. This phenomenon occurs when arterioles of the muscle steal from cutaneous and peripheral nerve vessels to meet muscular metabolic needs, resulting in coldness of skin, not warm skin and pins and needle sensation.

28. C. Intermittent claudication is ischemic pain of the leg precipitated by walking and relieved by rest. Ischemia in lower extremity predisposes the feet for poor healing. So the patient must practice meticulous foot care which will include bathing of feet, cutting the nail short and straight, avoiding injury by using proper fitting closed shoes, etc. The patient must stop smoking, exercise regularly and visit the physician frequently to evaluate the effectiveness of treatment, not just when symptoms worsen.

29. D. Regular exercise like walking is the best way to promote collateral circulation. A prescribed moderate program of exercise and rest helps increase collateral circulation. Regular exercise also aids in stress reduction and weight reduction and increases the formation of HDL. All these are helpful for a patient with peripheral arterial disease, but development of collateral circulation is more important for the patient.

30. C. The ankle brachial pressure index is the most commonly used overall indicator of arm and leg circulation. Allen test is used to evaluate blood flow in the arm. Buerger's sign is used to evaluate ischemia in lower limbs. Exercise testing is used to evaluate the severity of intermittent claudication in lower limb.

31. C. Acute occlusion of a limb's main artery most commonly is caused by emboli. The embolus most commonly arises from a thrombus within the heart. Conditions giving rise to emboli are: atrial fibrillation, myocardial infarction, prosthetic heart valves and rheumatic heart disease. Hypertension is not related with acute peripheral arterial occlusion. Thrombosis may also cause acute arterial occlusion but it is not as common as emboli.

32. A. Before any definitive therapy, e.g. surgery is arranged the nurse should put the patient in bed, placing the affected limb at level or slightly lower than the rest of the body and protecting it from pressure and trauma. Application of hot or cold will further compromise tissue perfusion. Elevation of limb will further cause tissue ischemia.

33. B. The patient with thromboangiitis obliterans should be taught to avoid sitting or standing in one position for a long time since this contributes to venous stasis. Patient with Buerger's disease must quit smoking since smoking promotes vasoconstriction and thrombus formation by promoting platelet adhesion. These patients should take meticulous skin care of their feet. As any cuts or injury in the extremity will take long time to heal when circulation is impaired. Patient also should avoid exposure to cold as cold causes vasoconstriction.

34. C. The patient with Raynaud's syndrome should be advised to stay warm by wearing woollen gloves and sweaters when exposed to cold weather or cold objects. The patients must stop smoking to control the disease not just reduce smoking. Pain medications do not relieve Raynaud's phenomenon. Calcium antagonists, e.g. nifedipine and verapamil, alpha adrenergic blockers and sympatholytic drugs may be taken prophylactically 1-2 hours before exposure to cold, by patients who rarely go out in the cold weather during the winter months.

35. D. The nurse will anticipate administering an antihypertensive drug and scheduling ultrasonographic study to determine any change in size of the aneurysm. Gastrointestinal bleeding leading to shock will be seen when an abdominal aortic aneurysm ruptures into the duodenum. In an asymptomatic abdominal aortic aneurysm, patients will not have any complain. Surgery is not generally performed when the size of the aneurysm is less than 4 to 5 cm in diameter.

36. A. If the abdominal aortic aneurysm ruptures posteriorly into the retroperitoneal space bleeding may be tamponated by surrounding structures preventing exanguination and death. In this case, the patient will have sudden severe back pain. Patient may also have back or flank ecchymosis. If the rupture occurs anteriorly, patient will have severe bleeding leading to hypovolemic shock. Pulsatile mass in the periumbilical area is the sign of abdominal aneurysm not the sign of ruptured aneurysm.

37. A. Ineffective peripheral tissue perfusion is a major concern in postoperative period following repair of abdominal aortic aneurysm related to graft thrombosis, embolism, prolonged aortic clamping, hypotension and blood loss. Peripheral pulses should be checked frequently during the first 24 hours. A weak or absent pulse accompanied by a pale, cold, mottled extremity may be a sign of embolization or graft closure. Infection is not a major concern on the first postoperative day. As 4 to 7 days time is usually required to develop an infection in the graft. Selfcare deficit and pain related to surgical incision occur in any patient after abdominal operation and is not specific.

38. B. Ineffective tissue perfusion: Renal related to hypotension, dehydration, prolonged aortic clamping or blood loss is a major postoperative concern after repair of abdominal aortic aneurysm. So, nurse must monitor urine output, BUN and creatinine to assess renal perfusion status. Legs should not be elevated as patients are at risk of ineffective peripheral tissue perfusion. Assessment of carotid, radial and temporal pulse is especially indicated when surgery of ascending aorta or aortic arch and in surgery of abdominal aorta assessment of femoral, popliteal, posterior tibial and dorsalis pedis is indicated.

39. D. The factor, which is not included in the Virchow's triad, is hypocoagulability. Venous stasis, injury to venous wall and hypercoagulability are included in the etiology of venous thrombosis called Virchow's triad.

40. B. The nurse should advise the patient to place a light blanket over the feet at night. This is the most effective and safest way to keep the feet warm. Since patient with arteriosclerosis is susceptible for thrombus formation, rubbing should be avoided, as it may release thrombi. Application of heat increases metabolic demand of tissue, which is already compromised, moreover patient with poor circulation may have paresthesia so application of heat by hot water bottle or warm foot bath would be unsafe.

41. B. Postmenopausal women who use hormone replacement therapy are at increased risk of venous thromboembolic disease. Women who smoke, use hormone replacement therapy, double their risk because of constricting effect of nicotine on blood vessel wall. Obesity is another risk factor of thrombosis. All other conditions also run the risk of thrombosis but less than obese woman who smokes and uses hormone replacement therapy.

42. C. The nurse would suspect deep vein thrombosis when there is unilateral leg edema. Other symptoms being extremity pain, warm skin, erythema and a systemic temperature more than 38°C. Pain in the calf that occurs with exercise, paresthesia and coolness of the leg and pallor and cyanosis of the involved extremity are the symptoms of peripheral arterial occlusive diseases, not venous disorders.

43. B. The pain in the calf associated with forced dorsiflexion of the foot when the leg is raised is positive Homan's sign. Positive Homan's sign when accompanied by other findings is diagnostic of deep vein thrombosis. Positive Babinski's sign is an extensor planter response. Positive Kernig's sign and Brudzinski's sign are for meningeal irritation.

44. D. The appropriate nursing measure for a patient with acute lower extremity deep vein thrombosis is administering anticoagulant as prescribed. The other treatment for deep vein thrombosis is keeping the leg elevated above the level of the heart, not keeping in a dependent position, and bed rest, not encouraging ambulation. The patient is ambulated when therapeutic level of anticoagulation is achieved and edema is resolving. Elastic compression stockings are recommended when the patient starts ambulating and should be continued at least 3–6 months.

45. D. The patient on anticoagulant therapy should be taught to be aware of sign and symptoms of bleeding, e.g. hematuria, gum bleeding, heavy menstrual bleeding, etc. and report to the physician immediately. The patient should continue with the drugs regularly, taking it at the same time of the day. If a dose is missed he should not compensate by taking the double dose next time. Regular blood tests for activated partial thromboplastine time (APTT) and international normalized ratio (INR) not Hb%, should be done to determine the therapeutic level of the drug and regulate the doses. Patient should report any adverse effects of the drug, e.g. headache, stomach pains, weakness, dizziness or mental changes. Diarrhea is not associated with anticoagulant therapy.

46. D. Patient should be cautioned about various drugs that interact with warfarin and must be instructed to avoid self-medication. Aspirin decreases platelet aggregation and interferes with clotting. So simultaneous use of aspirin and warfarin will increase the anticoagulation action and may lead to bleeding. Warfarin does not dissolve clots already formed but interrupts the normal clotting cycle preventing clot formation. Patient does not need any marked changes in dietary habits. He needs to take the medicine exactly as prescribed to maintain the desired level of anticoagulation.

47. If a thrombus is developing massaging of legs would be unsafe as this would dislodge the thrombus and form emboli. Fluids decreases blood viscosity and thus chances of thrombus formation. Range of motion exercises improves muscle strength and promotes venous return. Elastic stockings compress veins and thus prevent venous stasis and thrombus formation.

48. C. Varicose veins are dilated tortuous subcutaneous veins due to increased venous pressure resulting from congenital weakness of the vein structure, obesity, pregnancy, obstruction by thrombosis, etc. As the veins enlarge, the valves are stretched and become incompetent. Other conditions listed are not the cause of varicose veins.

49. A. The most common symptoms of varicose veins are muscle aches, cramps and increased fatigue. Other symptoms listed are the symptoms of peripheral arterial disease.

50. A. The greater and lesser saphenous veins and perforator vein in the ankle are common sites of varicose veins. They do not develop in the veins listed above.

51. C. Wearing tight elastic stockings or any other tight clothing beneath the waist would cause venous stasis. Walking 1–2 miles every day, walking the stair case, and elevating the legs while resting promote circulation.

52. C. Ligation and stripping of vein is done as a curative measure. Sclerotherapy and laser therapy is done for superficial varicosities. Percutaneous transluminal angioplasty is not for varicose veins.

53. D. Sitting beside the bed and dangling feet is not recommended after ligation and stripping for varicose veins. Postoperatively bed rest is maintained for 24 hours. Thereafter patient should walk every 2 hours for 5–10 minutes. Standing still and sitting is discouraged. Other nursing interventions promote venous return.

54. C. Surgical treatment of thrombophlebitis is aimed at preventing pulmonary embolism by filtering blood flow from the lower extremities and pelvis through a filter inserted into the inferior vena cava. Thrombus originated in a vein travels upwards in the larger vein to right heart and then to pulmonary artery to cause pulmonary embolism. So, the filter has to be placed in the inferior vena cava. Filter placed in aorta, hepatic artery or femoral artery may prevent systemic embolism not pulmonary embolism.

55. C. Hypertrophic cardiomyopathy is characterized by disproportionate thickening of the interventricular septum, compared with the free wall of the ventricle. Hypertrophic cardiomyopathy sometimes called asymmetrical septal hypertrophy. Dilated cardiomyopathy is characterized by dilatation of both left and right ventricles, degeneration of myocardial fibers and replacement of the same with fibrotic tissue. Restrictive cardiomyopathy is characterized by excessively rigid ventricular walls impairing filling during diastole. Congestive cardiomyopathy is another name of dilated cardiomyopathy.

56. D. The most common manifestation of hypertrophic cardiomyopathy is dyspnoea. Dyspnea is due to the high pulmonary pressures produced by the elevated left ventricular end-diastolic pressure. Palpitations may be present, but it is not most common symptoms in this disease. Peripheral edema is a sign of right ventricular failure, which is less common occurrence of this disease. Weight loss is not associated with hypertrophic cardiomyopathy.

57. A. The most common form of cardiomyopathy is dilated cardiomyopathy. Severe dilatation of the heart leading to decreased stroke volume, low cardiac output and a compensatory increase in heart rate eventually results in heart failure. Sudden death is mostly associated with hypertrophic cardiomyopathy. Cardiac tamponade and pericardial effusion are not associated with dilated cardiomyopathy.

58. C. Patients with dilated cardiomyopathy are very ill people with a grave prognosis so providing emotional support to the patient and family members is a priority. Though dilated cardiomyopathy may follow infectious myocarditis, the disease cannot be transmitted to the family members. Family members may be at risk because of genetic or familial predisposition. Whatever may be the initial cause, dilated cardiomyopathy rapidly progresses to heart failure by diffuse inflammation and rapid degeneration of myocardial fibers, so treatment is palliative in nature. Ventriculomyotomy and myectomy may be helpful for patients with hypertrophic cardiomyopathy but not for patients with dilated cardiomyopathy.

59. D. Pericardial friction rub is a classic objective manifestation of acute pericarditis. The rub is produced by inflamed, roughened pericardial layers that create friction as their surfaces rub together during heart movement. The chest pain of pericarditis is exacerbated and not relieved by rotation of the trunk. Crackles at the base of the lungs signal left heart failure. Systolic murmurs also called benign murmurs are often found in children, young adults and pregnant women and are not related to pericarditis.

60. B. The nurse should instruct the patient to sit up and lean forward on a padded overboard table to reduce the pain. When the patient leans forward the heart is pulled away from the diaphragmatic pleura. Other positions do not cause this pulling action and therefore do not relieve chest pain of pericarditis.

61. D. The nature of pain of pericarditis varies with the patient. The nature of pain may be similar to myocardial infarction or pleurisy. But the most suggestive history of pericarditis is relief of pain while sitting or leaning forward. Leaning forward while sitting upright pulls the heart away from diaphragmatic pleura resulting in relief of pain. Pain of myocardial infarction is unrelieved by change of position. Symptoms of endocarditis are intermittent fever and malaise resulting from infection of the endocardium. Chest pain of myocarditis is felt as a mild continuous pressure or soreness of the chest.

62. B. Echocardiography is the most accurate technique for evaluating pericardial effusion. The test is sensitive enough to detect as little as 20 mL of pericardial fluid. Other tests are not diagnostic of pericardial effusion.

63. B. Acute bacterial endocarditis develops over days or weeks with an erratic course and earlier development of complications, commonly caused by *Staphylococcus aureus*. Subacute bacterial endocarditis develops gradually over several weeks or months, usually caused by organism of low virulence, e.g. *Streptococcus viridans*. Native valve endocarditis is an infection of a normal or previously damaged valve and non-bacterial thrombotic endocarditis caused by sterile thrombotic lesions which may develop in people with cancer or other chronic diseases.

64. C. Blood cultures are the primary diagnostic tool for the evaluation of infective endocarditis. Positive blood cultures are found in 90 to 95% of patients with infective endocarditis. ECG and echocardiography are all important in the diagnostic work up for a patient with infective endocarditis but cannot conclude about the infectious origin. A mild leukocytosis indicates infective nature of the disease.

65. A. Individuals at high-risk of infective endocarditis, e.g. patients with prosthetic valve, previous endocarditis, acquired valvular disease, mitral valve prolapse, surgically constructed systemic pulmonary shunts, etc. should take prophylactic antibiotics before any dental work or surgical procedures. The other conditions do not require prophylactic antibiotic coverage.

66. B. Rheumatic fever is a sequela of beta-hemolytic *Streptococcus* infection. It is not due to the infection of Streptococcus viridans. The incidence of rheumatic fever is more in the developing countries among the people of lower socioeconomic group and who live in the crowded places. The incidence of the disease has dramatically declined in the developed countries like UK and USA due to an emphasis on prevention.

67. D. Once a patient acquires rheumatic fever, the person becomes more susceptible for recurrent infection. Long-term penicillin therapy is recommended to eradicate the infection and prevent recurrent rheumatic fever. Antibiotic therapy does not modify the course of the acute disease or the development of carditis. Salicylates and corticosteroids, not antibiotics are effective in controlling fever and arthritis. Antibiotic will prevent recurrence by destroying the infective organisms, but it does not cure rheumatic fever.

68. B. The most common cause of mitral valve stenosis in Indian patients is rheumatic endocarditis. Congenital heart disease, rheumatic arthritis and infective endocarditis are the less common causes of mitral stenosis.

69. C. Percutaneous transluminal balloon valvuloplasty is a treatment of choice for the patients who are poor candidates for other extensive valvular surgery. The procedure is done to treat any stenotic valve and not a regurgitant valve. In this procedure, the balloon catheter is inserted through the femoral artery or femoral vein and not through the apex of the ventricle. The procedure is an alternative treatment method for some people with heart disease. If not successful more extensive surgery, e.g. open valvuloplasty may be carried out.

70. B. Patient's statement about anticoagulation therapy reflects effective teaching. The patient after mitral valve replacement surgery needs to take anticoagulant, e.g. warfarin lifelong and must have the international normalized ratio (INR) checked every month, not Hb%. Patient must realize that valve surgery is not a cure and regular follow-up examinations by the healthcare provider will be required. Patient should avoid aspirin containing drug and they should also avoid taking over-the counter drug without the advice of the physician.

71. A. Atherosclerosis, a disorder of lipid metabolism resulting in an abnormal accumulation of lipid or fatty substances and fibrous tissue in the vessel wall is the main cause of coronary artery disease (CAD). CAD due to vasospasm of coronary artery is a less frequent cause. Stress and hyperglycemia are the risk factors of CAD.

72. C. High blood pressure can be corrected by altering one's diet, exercise and medication. Age, sex and heredity canot be changed.

73. A. Person with cholesterol level above 200 mg/dL is considered to be high-risk. Other levels are below the accepted level and considered as low risk

74. C. Laboratory values with the high-risk for coronary artery disease would be high-density lipoprotein (HDL) of 30 mg/dL and low-density lipoprotein of 160 mg/dL. HDL levels below 35 mg/dL and LDL levels above 130 mg/dL are major risk factors. All other values are within desirable levels.

75. A. Lipitor (atrovastatin) is a lipid lowering drug. This drug and other statin drugs inhibit the synthesis of cholesterol in the liver by blocking hydroxylmethylglutaryl coenzyme A (HMG-CoA) reductase. Inhibition of cholesterol synthesis results in an increase of LDL receptors. So the liver is able to remove more LDLs from the blood resulting in decrease of LDL level.

76. A. The patient must be taught to adhere to other prescribed regimen for lowering blood cholesterol, e.g. low fat diet, exercise and smoking cessation. Liver dysfunction is an adverse effect of the drug so baseline and periodical evaluation of liver enzymes should be done. The desired therapeutic effect is usually observed after 6 weeks. Rhabdomyolysis is an another adverse effect of the drug. So physician must be notified if weakness or muscle pain is noticed.

77. B. Patients with angina usually describe chest pain as tightness, heaviness, pressing and squeezing or burning. Knife-like and sharp pain is usually associated with the pericarditis and pleuritis. Patients with dissecting aortic aneurysm describe the chest pain as knife-like tearing sensation.

78. A. The pain of stable angina is predictable in nature having a stable pattern of onset, duration and relieving factor. Unstable angina is triggered by an unpredictable degree of exertion or emotion. Variant angina occurs at rest and not due to exertion or stress. Nocturnal angina is believed to be associated with rapid eye movement (REM) sleep during dreaming.

79. B. Unstable angina is often due to rupture of a stable atherosclerotic plaque. This unstable lesion is at increased risk of complete thrombosis of the lumen with progression to myocardial infarction (MI). The other types listed are less likely to progress into MI.

80. A. Anginal pain occurs when there is a decrease oxygen supply compared to the heart's need for oxygen. Brisk walking increases workload of the heart which in turn increases the heart's need for oxygen precipitating anginal pain. Deep breathing has no effect on anginal pain. Food and fluid intake does not relieve this pain; it may relieve pain due to peptic ulcer. Anginal pain is self-limiting and lasts for 10-15 minutes.

81. C. Propranolol is a beta-adrenergic blocker. The drug is used for the treatment of angina, hypertension, dysrhythmia, migraine and many other conditions. In patient with heart disease, the drug may cause congestive heart failure (CHF). Signs and symptoms of CHF are dyspnea on exertion, orthopnea, peripheral edema, distended neck veins, dry persistent cough etc. So physician should be informed if any of these is noticed in patient. Lethargy, fatigue, joint pain, dry mouth, and constipation are the side effects of this drug and do not require physician information.

82. C. Nitrates relax coronary smooth muscle and produce vasodilatation relieving anginal pain. Nitrates are also peripheral vasodilators. Vasodilatation results in hypotension making the patient feel dizzy due to postural hypotension. So, the patient should sit or lie down after taking the drug and not to rise quickly to a standing position. Nitroglycerine should be kept with the patient who experiences angina and should be accessible. Protecting the medication from extreme temperatures is adequate. Patient may repeat the dose at 5 minutes interval for maximum 3 doses if required. If pain persists patient should seek medical attention. Nitroglycerin is to be taken via the sublingual route, not swallowed.

83. D. Nitroglycerine transdermal pad to be applied daily and should be removed at bedtime to provide 10-12 hours nitrate free interval to avoid tolerance. As it provides slow sustained action it is not effective for immediate pain relief.

84. A. Common side effects of nitrates are headache, flashing, postural hypotension, dizziness, nausea, vomiting, pallor, sweating and rash. Dry mouth, photosensitivity and bradycardia are not the side effects of nitrates. They may occur with beta-blocker drugs.

85. B. Patient with angina must stop smoking. Smoking increases carboxyhemoglobin level in the blood, which will reduce the oxygen supply in the heart and may induce angina. The patient should exercise to promote collateral circulation. The patient must seek medical care if pain persists for more than 15 minutes and not wait for 2 hours. The patient should avoid dietary fat and cholesterol but consume foods containing fibers, since fibers help excreting cholesterol.

86. A. Anginal pain is self-limiting and may be relieved on cessation of activity or rest, or by taking nitroglycerine tablets or both. Anginal pain also may be severe particularly in patient with unstable angina. Anginal pain does not cause irreversible tissue damage. It is not usually associated with nausea and vomiting.

87. D. The risk factors of CAD that could be modified or controlled include: Diet, smoking, stress and inactivity. Sex, family history are the risk factors that cannot be controlled.

88. C. Intracoronary stents are designed to reduce restenosis and abrupt closure of coronary vessels resulting from the complications of coronary angioplasty. They are now used instead of PTCA to eliminate the risk of acute closure and to improve long-term patency. Directional atherectomy and laser ablation also cause acute vessel occlusion as complication.

89. B. Myocardial infarction is almost always due to the formation of occlusive thrombus at the site of rupture or erosion of an atheromatous plaque in a coronary artery. Aneurysm is an outpouching of a vessel and does not cause MI. Occlusion of coronary artery by an embolus and vasospasm of coronary artery may occur but less commonly.

90. C. The left ventricle of the heart which contributes most to contraction, is most frequently affected by myocardial infarction.

91. D. CPK-MB is an isoenzyme found only in cardiac muscle. Its level starts rising 4-6 hours after the onset of chest pain and reaches its peak after 12 hours. LDH-1 is elevated after 12 hours of chest pain. Elevated level of ESR is nonspecific. It indicates presence of inflammation or infection. Serum AST level rises only after 12 hours. So CPK-MB is the only early indicator of the myocardial infarction.

92. D. Dysrhythmia caused by ischemic and damaged myocardium are the major causes of death after acute MI (40 to 50% of deaths). Cardiac tamponade is the complication of acute pericarditis and heart surgery. Heart failure is responsible for 1/3rd of deaths after an acute MI. Pulmonary embolism is mostly secondary to phlebitis and occurs in 10 to 20% of patients.

93. A. A thrombolytic agent must be administered within 3-6 hours after the onset of symptoms of MI, as the first 6 hours is the crucial time for the salvage of the myocardium. Other options are not ideal for administration of thrombolytic agent.

94. C. Inj streptokinase is a thrombolytic agent. It lyses clot by activating conversion of plasminogen to plasmin (fibrinolysin). Plasmin breaks down clots. Inj Streptokinase when administered in a patient with myocardial infarction, it dissolves clot that is obstructing the artery, allowing reperfusion of the myocardium.

95. D. Patient with stomach ulcer may not receive thrombolytic therapy. Bleeding ulcers, recent surgeries, blood dyscrasias and aneurysms are the examples of disorders that are possible contraindication of thrombolytic therapy. Thrombolytic therapy has been found to be very successful if administered early in the course of the disease. Nausea is an expected symptom of myocardial infarction and is not a contraindication of thrombolytic therapy. Treatment with insulin is also not a contraindication of thrombolytic therapy.

96. D. Morphine sulphate is the drug of choice in acute myocardial infarction because it is potent, has a rapid action, relieves anxiety, has a diuretic effect and results in slight coronary vasodilatation which are particularly beneficial for a patient with a myocardial infarction.

97. D. The activity level of the patient after MI is gradually increased so that by the time of discharge the patient can tolerate moderate energy activities of daily living. Allowing the patient in the planning of activities and carrying out the same will relieve anxiety and apprehension of the patient. Providing all care and doing everything for the patient will result in dependence. Conducive environment for rest is important but prolonged rest is also not desired. Patient must maintain balance between the activity and rest. Family member should provide assistance in physical care whenever required and not provide all the care needed.

98. A. The nurse should assess the blood pressure of the patient who is receiving IV glyceryl trinitrate (Myovin). Myovin is the intravenous form of nitroglycerin. Because of its vasodilating effects the blood pressure should be monitored frequently for the frequent side effect of hypotension. Administration of myovin does not affect blood glucose. Respiratory system and urinary system are not directly affected by the administration of myovin.

99. B. The ability to tolerate increasing activity without chest pain indicates that the patient who is being treated for MI is responding favorably to the therapy. Patient who is responding well to the treatment should not have, chest pain and should exhibit a regular heartbeat of 60 to100 beats/minute and have a normal ECG. Patient who had an effective teaching program which is a part of therapy would be intending to stop smoking.

100. B. In left heart failure, impaired blood flow from the left ventricle causes blood to back up into the left atrium and into the pulmonary veins. Increased pulmonary pressure and fluid accumulation in the lung tissues gives rise to pulmonary congestion and edema which are manifested as persistent, dry cough unrelieved by cough suppressants and bilateral crackles.

101. A. Anterior wall MI may result in decrease in the left ventricular function and subsequently left- sided heart failure. Left ventricular failure causes pulmonary congestion, so fluid accumulates in the interstitial and alveolar spaces of the lungs and heard as crackles during auscultation. In right sided failure congestion occurs in the great veins giving rise to peripheral edema and venous congestion of the organs. Pulmonic valve stenosis and tricuspid valve stenosis causes right-sided heart failure.

102. C. Distention of neck veins is the result of elevated central venous pressure which indicates a failure of right heart to pump giving rise to venous congestion. In hemorrhagic shock, the neck veins are collapsed due to volume depletion. Left ventricular failure does not give rise to systemic venous congestion. Myocardial infarction may progress to heart failure but myocardial infarction in itself will not cause neck vein distention.

103. A. Increase sympathetic activity produces vasoconstriction, tachycardia and increased myocardial contractility. In addition sympathetic activity reduces renal blood flow and stimulates renin-angiotensin system causing oliguria. Bradycardia and hypotension is due to parasympathetic activity.

104. C. Neurohormonal responses, e.g. renin-angiotensin system and increased secretion of antidiuretic hormone causes sodium and water retention resulting in an increased blood volume and additional workload of the heart. The other compensatory mechanisms do not cause inappropriate fluid retention.

105. D. Initial response of low cardiac output is activation of the sympathetic nervous system resulting in the increased heart rate, venous and arteriolar constriction, reduction of renal blood flow and stimulation of rennin-angiotensin system. So the patient will experience tachycardia, increased blood pressure and increased fluid volume.

106. B. Left sided heart failure causes pulmonary congestion which precipitates respiratory distress or dyspnea. An engorged neck vein is due to systemic venous congestion occurring in right sided heart failure. Abdominal distention is also secondary to venous congestion of the gastrointestinal tract occurring in right sided heart failure. Tremors of hand are not related to the heart failure.

107. B. Fluid retention leading to increase in the extracellular fluid volume can cause an apparent decrease in hematocrit concentration is due to dilution of the blood. In fluid volume excess there is a full and bounding pulse and not weak and thready. Orthostatic hypotension occurs in the fluid volume deficit.

108. D. Digoxin has no effect on the respiratory rate and status. All other observation parameters are essential. Digoxin should be withheld if the pulse rate is less than 60 or newly irregular. Disturbances in the electrolyte level, e.g. hypokalemia may potentiate digoxin toxicity. Serum Digoxin level must be below or within therapeutic level (0.8 2.0 ng/mL).

109. C. Inotropic agents, e.g. dopamine, dobutamine and amrinone facilitate myocardial contractility and enhance stroke volume. Beta-adrenergic antagonists decrease the heart rate and blood pressure and thus reduce the workload of the heart. Diuretics decrease overall circulating volume, reduce blood pressure and thus workload of the heart.

110. D. Dopamine is a naturally occurring catecholamine with alpha adrenergic, beta-adrenergic and dopaminergic activity. When given in moderate doses (4-8 μg/kg/min) it stimulates both alpha adrenergic and beta-adrenergic receptors in the vasculature and myocardium and results in increase in the heart rate, stroke volume and cardiac output. If given in the larger doses than 10 μg/kg/min alpha-adrenergic stimulation predominates and results in the intense vasoconstriction. In low doses, i.e. <4 μg/kg/min dopamine stimulates the dopaminergic receptors in the renal, mesenteric, cerebral and coronary vascular beds and causes vasodilation.

111. C. Hypothyroidism affects the body's ability to metabolize digoxin and predisposes the patient to digitalis toxicity. Pneumonia does not affect metabolism of digoxin. Hypokalemia not hyperkalemia predisposes a patient to digitalis toxicity and hypercalcemia not hypocalcemia predisposes a patient to digitalis toxicity.

112. B. The nurse should monitor serum potassium level as lasix, a loop diuretic promotes potassium excretion and hypokalemia. The risk of digoxin toxicity increases in the presence of hypokalemia. Maintenance of intake output chart is important to maintain the fluid balance in this patient. The nurse should teach the patient to take potassium rich diet to prevent hypokalemia. Postural hypotension is not related to the digoxin toxicity.

113. B. Signs and symptoms of digoxin toxicity include headache, yellow vision, blurred vision, drowsiness, restlessness, muscle weakness, anorexia, nausea, vomiting, diarrhea and cardiac dysrhythmias. Convulsions, vertigo and muscle cramping are not among the side effects of digoxin toxicity.

114. A. Crackles are due to the presence of fluid in the alveoli and commonly occur in patients with heart failure.

Wheezes are due to bronchial obstruction or bronchospasm which occur in asthma, tumor, etc. Friction rub occurs with pericarditis. Rhonchi occurs from the obstruction of large airways with secretion, e.g. COPD, bronchiectasis, pneumonia, etc.

115. B. Increasing dyspnea, anxiety, restlessness and expectoration of the large amount of pink frothy sputum characteristic of pulmonary edema. Manifestations of pulmonary embolism include tachypnea, dyspnea, anxiety and chest pain. In right-sided heart failure patient will experience dyspnea, anxiety, depression, peripheral edema and jugular vein distention and in pneumonia patient will exhibit fever, chills, chest pain, cough with rusty sputum and dyspnea.

116. C. Jugular venous distention is very specific sign of right heart failure resulting from increased venous pressure. Tachycardia is the early sign of left heart failure that is the result of a compensatory effort to increase cardiac output. Crackles in the lungs are classic sign of the left heart failure. Elevated blood urea nitrogen is due to reduced perfusion in the kidney as a result of low cardiac output.

117. C. Sinus bradycardia is best described as a normal rhythm with a rate of less than 60 beats/minute. In sinus bradycardia, the impulse originates from sinus node follows the regular conduction pathways through the ventricles and does not originate from the ventricles. In sinus bradycardia, P waves and QRS complexes are normal. An irregular slow ventricular rate with variable P waves between complexes describes a heart block. A normal rhythm with a rate of more than 100 beats per minute is sinus tachycardia.

118. B. Sinus tachycardia is characterized by a regular rhythm at a rate of 100 to 180 beats/minute with a normal P wave and QRS complex. Impulse originates from sinus node and follows normal conduction pathways. A regular rhythm at a rate of 60 to 100 beats per minute is considered as normal sinus rhythm in an adult patient. A ventricular rapid rhythm that may or may not produce a palpable pulse is ventricular tachycardia and an irregular rhythm originating from sinus node with a rate of 60 to 100 beats/minute is sinus dysrhythmia.

119. C. In supraventricular tachycardia the heart rate may be 100 to 300 beats per minute. An increase heart rate will result in low cardiac output and myocardial ischemia. If the condition persists the patient will develop heart failure. Unstable angina and myocardial infarction is not due to rapid heart rate. Rapid heart rate will result in low cardiac output with hypotension, not hypertension.

120. A. Esmolol a class II antidysrhythmic drug blocks sympathetic stimulation at the sinus node resulting in bradycardia. Hypotension with IV administration may also occur. It does not affect the body temperature and urine output. However, esmolol can cause bronchospasm and it is contraindicated in bronchial asthma.

121. C. IV push atropine is used to treat symptomatic bradycardia. Lidocaine is used to treat ventricular tachycardia. Esmolol is used to treat supraventricular tachycardia and digoxin is used to treat atrial fibrillation.

122. B. Patient with symptomatic supraventricular tachycardia who is hemodynamically unstable is treated with emergency cardioversion.

Cardioversion using an electrical voltage of 50 joules is appropriate. 20 joules is pediatric dose. 200 joules is the dose of defibrillation for pulseless ventricular tachycardia or ventricular fibrillation. If needed defibrillation may be repeated up to three times using 200, 300, and 360 joules to treat pulseless ventricular tachycardia and ventricular fibrillation.

123. C. Patients with ventricular tachycardia who are hemodynamically stable usually treated with IV lidocaine. Defibrillation is used for pulseless ventricular tachycardia. Verapamil is administered for the treatment of supraventricular tachycardia. Digoxin is the treatment of choice in atrial fibrillation.

124. C. Immediate intervention for ventricular fibrillation is defibrillation. It is the only intervention that can terminate the dangerous arrhythmia. Synchronized cardioversion is done on R wave but there is no R wave in ventricular fibrillation. Intubation cannot terminate ventricular fibrillation.

125. D. Cardioversion may be done as a nonemergency basis on a patient who is awake and hemodynamically stable. But before the procedure the patient should be sedated with IV diazepam. Cardioversion requires a low voltage electrical current, not a higher dose of electrical current. Defibrillation is asynchronized, whereas cardioversion is synchronized to countershock during the QRS complex. Cardioversion is indicated for the treatment of atrial tachyarrhythmia as well as ventricular tachycardia.

126. B. The patient is experiencing dysrhythmia of second degree AV heart block, type I. This dysrhythmia is characterized by the PR interval that progressively lengthens until a P wave is not followed by a QRS complex. First degree AV block is characterized by a PR interval greater than .20 seconds. Second degree AV block, type II is characterized by the non-conducted sinus impulses despite constant PR intervals and in third degree AV block, all the sinus or atrial impulses are blocked and the atria and ventricles are forced to beat independently.

127. C. Ventricular bigeminy occurs in the second degree AV block, type II. In this type of cardiac rhythm every third impulse from the SA node is not conducted to the ventricles resulting in bradycardia. This type of dysrhythmia often progresses to third degree AV block and is associated with a poor prognosis. Treatment involves insertion of a temporary pacemaker until a permanent pacemaker is inserted. Defibrillation and cardioversion are not indicated in this type of arrhythmia. IV push atropine may be tried as temporary measure to increase the heart rate until the pacemaker therapy is available but not IV lidocaine which is used for ventricular tachycardia.

128. A. The patient should be taught to take his pulse daily and record it. If the pulse rate is slower than the set rate of the pacemaker he should notify the physician. The patient should restrict movement of the arm and shoulder on the operative side above the shoulder level for 1 week and not keeping it immobilized for 6 weeks. Patient can safely use ordinary household electrical equipments like microwave ovens, television and office equipments, e.g. computers, copying machine, etc. Insertion site should be kept dry for 1 week only and not for 6 weeks.

129. C. Shock is a syndrome characterized by the decreased tissue perfusion and impaired cellular metabolism. This results in an imbalance between the supply of and demand for oxygen and nutrients. Cardiovascular collapse may be the cause of shock. Loss of sympathetic tone and activation of parasympathetic system gives rise to massive vasodilatation resulting in pooling of blood in the blood vessels and impairing perfusion in the tissue producing shock. So loss of sympathetic tone is a step in the development of shock. Blood pressure less than 90 mm Hg is a manifestation of shock.

130. D. Neurogenic shock is a hemodynamic phenomenon often seen in the spinal cord injury at T5 and above. The injury results in a massive vasodilatation without compensation as a consequence of the loss of sympathetic nervous system vasoconstrictor tone. The massive vasodilatation leads to a pooling of blood in the blood vessels, manifested as hypotension. Unopposed activation of parasympathetic nervous system leads to bradycardia. So neurogenic shock is from maldistribution of blood flow due to massive vasodilatation and not from low blood flow. Spinal cord injury is unlikely to cause severe internal hemorrhage resulting into absolute hypovolemia. Cardiogenic shock results from conditions where heart fails to act as a pump.

131. C. In a normotensive person a drop in systolic blood pressure is below 80 mm Hg would markedly compromise perfusion to vital organs.

132. A. The initial effect that shock has on the body includes activation of sympathetic nervous system resulting in an increase in heart rate, cardiac output, rate and depth of respiration. Stimulation of parasympathetic nervous system resulting in slowing of heart rate and hypotension occurs during development of shock and not after effect of shock. Renal vasoconstriction leading to decreased blood flow to kidneys stimulates rennin- angiotensin system. It is not due to vasoconstriction of heart and brain. Decreased tissue perfusion causes anaerobic metabolism not aerobic metabolism.

133. A. Hemodynamic management of a patient in the cardiogenic shock is aimed towards reducing the workload of the heart. Dopamine is an adrenergic agonist increases myocardial contractility, cardiac output and blood flow to the renal artery, coronary artery and brain and are extremely useful in the treatment of cardiogenic shock. ACE inhibitors prevent vasoconstriction so reduces both preload and afterload of the heart and do not increase preload. Vasopressor are usually not indicated in the patients with shock since these patients show remarkable vasoconstriction and poor tissue perfusion, so increase in the systemic vascular resistance will increase the workload of the heart. Beta-blockers reduce the contractility and heart rate thus decreasing the workload of the heart. They do not increase the heart rate and contractility.

134. C. Reduced blood flow to kidneys stimulates release of renin into the blood which in turn causes production of angiotensin I. Angiotensin I is converted to angiotensin II. Low cardiac output giving rise to low blood pressure stimulates parasympathetic nervous system not central nervous system. Cardiac response in shock occurs due to the effect of activation of parasympathetic nervous system which in turn releases catecholamines, e.g. epinephrine and norepinephrine. Adrenal response to release increased amount of aldosterone is due to stimulation by angiotensin II and not due to the action of antidiuretic hormone.

135. C. Intra-aortic balloon pump provides temporary circulatory assistance by increasing the coronary perfusion and cardiac output but decreasing the myocardial oxygen consumption and workload in a patient with cardiogenic shock. Pacemaker maintains the heart rate at a predetermined rate. Ventricular assist device also provides circulatory assistance like IABP. But it is used for longer term for support of the failing heart, usually months. Defibrillation is used to treat life-threatening ventricular arrhythmias.

136. B. A history of peripheral atherosclerosis contraindicates the use of the IABP. Other contraindications for use of this therapy include aortic insufficiency, aortic aneurysm, chronic end stage heart disease, multisystem failure, chronic debilitating disease, bleeding disorders and history of embolism. Unstable angina pectoris that does not respond to drug therapy is an indication for IABP. Hypertension and diabetes are not contraindication to IABP.

137. A. The nurse should monitor patient's pulse rate for signs of postoperative shock. The earliest sign of shock is a pulse rate that steadily increases over time. An increase in the heart rate is an attempt to compensate for a decrease in the circulatory volume. Pulse pressure is the difference between systolic and diastolic pressure. In a patient with shock pulse pressure would drop, but it would not be the earliest sign as blood pressure might remain normal in the earlier phases of shock. A drop in the body temperature is also a late sign of shock. The rate and depth of respiration increases in shock but this is also not the earliest sign of shock.

138. C. An urine output of at least 30 mL/hour indicates that there is an adequate kidney perfusion. Elevation of systemic blood pressure, increase in urinary volume both are indication of on adequate fluid replacement. But sometimes a systolic blood pressure over 90 or 100 mm Hg does not ensure adequate kidney perfusion.

139. B. The nurse recognizes this pulmonary artery wedge pressure to be elevated than normal. The normal pulmonary artery wedge pressure is 5–12 mm Hg. Elevated pressure is above 18 to 20 mm Hg indicates increased left ventricular pressure which occurs in the left ventricular failure and signals the onset of pulmonary congestion. Pressure elevated to 30 mm Hg or above indicates the pulmonary edema which is life-threatening. Less than normal pulmonary artery wedge pressure suggests insufficient volume and pressure in the left ventricle as seen in the hypovolemic shock.

3 CHAPTER

Respiratory System

Q1. The nurse is assessing a 40-year-old male patient complaining of cough and dyspnea for a long time and found that anteroposterior diameter of the chest is increased and equals the transverse diameter. Which of the following conditions describes the finding?

A. Normal chest wall configuration
B. Barrel chest
C. Pigeon chest
D. Funnel chest

Q2. The nurse during auscultation of a patient's lungs detects wheezes. Which statement about wheeze is true?

A. Rumbling, snoring or rattling sound usually heard on expiration and may clear on coughing
B. Hissing or musical sound heard during inspiration or expiration or both, if severe may be audible without stethoscope
C. High pitched sound produced on inspiration heard over the trachea
D. Creaking and grating sound heard over the problem area on both inspiration and expiration

Q3. During respiratory assessment of a patient diagnosed as cerebrovascular accident, the patient was found to exhibit alternating periods of deep and shallow breathing and apnea lasting for 15-16 secs. The nurse understands that the patient is exhibiting:

A. Kussmaul breathing
B. Cheyne-Stokes respiration
C. Biot's breathing (ataxia)
D. Hypoventilation

Q4. A patient has undergone bronchoscopy for collection of tissue specimen. After the procedure which of the following the nurse should observe in order to detect possible complication?

A. Difficulty in breathing
B. Hoarseness of voice
C. Difficulty in swallowing
D. Blood tinged sputum

Q5. Patient admitted with chronic obstructive pulmonary disease is experiencing shortness of breath, nausea and dizziness. To assess the patient's level of hypoxia, the nurse will:

A. Prepare the patient for pulmonary function test
B. Send blood sample for arterial blood gas analysis

C. Utilize a pulse oxymetry
D. Check hemoglobin level of the patient with a hemoglobinometer

Q6. Asthma is characterized by:

A. An inflammatory disease
B. Irreversible bronchospasms resulting from inflammation of airways
C. Obstruction of airways by mucous plugs
D. Obstructive disease caused by destruction of alveolar walls

Q7. Medications to treat asthma are categorized to which of the two major classes?

A. Long-term control medications and short-term control medications
B. Long-term control medications and quick-relief medications
C. Short-term control medications and quick relief medications
D. Short-term relief medications and quick control

Q8. A patient who was admitted in the hospital with severe asthma is discharged home with the prescription–beclomethasone dipropionate 2 puffs QID. The nurse understands that the drug acts by:

A. Stimulating beta-adrenergic receptors to produce bronchodilation
B. Antinflammatory and immunosuppressive effects
C. Blocks action of acetylcholine resulting in bronchodilation
D. Relaxation of bronchial smooth muscle resulting in bronchodilation

Q9. A patient with asthma has been ordered theophylline100 mg TDS. When asked by the patient regarding the action of the drug, the nurse explains that the drug is given to:

A. Relieve bronchospasm
B. Decrease sputum production
C. Suppress coughing
D. Treat respiratory infection

Q10. The nurse is teaching a patient with asthma during discharge regarding home care. Which of the following teaching points has the highest priority?

A. Learn what causes asthma (asthma triggers) and try to avoid it
B. Take prescribed medications as scheduled
C. Maintain good nutrition and drink 8-10 glasses of water
D. Breath through pursed lips during asthma episodes

Q11. A patient with acute asthma is admitted to the emergency department. Patient is anxious, has a respiratory rate of 44/minute and inspiratory and expiratory wheeze audible. Which of the following medications should be administered to give immediate relief to the patient?

A. Propranolol
B. Morphine
C. Oral steroids
D. Salbutamol inhalation

Q12. Emergency management of a patient in status asthmaticus includes which of the following medications?

A. Inhaled beta 2-agonists
B. Inhaled corticosteroids
C. IV beta 2-agonists
D. Oral corticosteroids

Q13. The nurse is teaching a patient with asthma regarding self-care. Which of the following statement by the patient indicates the need for further teaching?

A. 'I should see my physician if I have an upper respiratory infection'
B. 'I should practice meditation to reduce my stress level'
C. 'I should use my corticosteroid inhaler when I feel short of breath'
D. 'I should schedule my bronchodilator inhaler before my morning exercise'

Q14. Physician has prescribed azithromycin 500 mg daily for 5 days to a patient

with upper respiratory tract infection. The nurse teaches the patient to take the medicine.

A. With meal
B. With antacid
C. With milk
D. 1 hour before or 2 hours after meal

Q15. Chronic obstructive lung disease (COPD) is a disease state characterized by airflow obstruction caused by:

A. Increased airway resistance secondary to bronchial mucosal edema
B. Increased airway resistance due is to smooth muscle contraction
C. Decreased elastic recoil
D. All of the above

Q16. The nurse is assessing a patient with pulmonary disorder. Assessment findings include history of smoking for 30 years, chronic cough with thick sputum, peripheral edema and bluish red color of the skin. Based on this data, the patient most likely has which of the following conditions?

A. Asthma
B. Chronic bronchitis
C. Emphysema
D. Pulmonary tuberculosis

Q17. The most common early manifestation of chronic bronchitis is:

A. A daily productive cough
B. Dyspnea
C. Cyanosis
D. Right ventricular failure

Q18. Physician has prescribed tablet deriphyllin daily to a patient with chronic bronchitis. The nurse explains to the patient regarding the drug. Which of the following is not appropriate?

A. Take the medicine as prescribed in morning daily.
B. Take lot of fluids to keep bronchial secretions thin and prevent dehydration.
C. Avoid taking coffee, cola and chocolate.
D. Take the medicine at bed time for uninterrupted sleep.

Q19. An important component in the collaborative care for a patient with COPD would include:

A. Long-term use of oral corticosteroids
B. Treatment of respiratory infections
C. Restriction of fluid to 1500 mL/day
D. A planned program of vigorous exercise

Q20. A patient with chronic obstructive pulmonary disease admitted in the hospital experiencing shortness of breath. Which of the following nursing actions best promotes adequate gas exchange and should be done by the nurse first?

A. Keeping the patient in semi-Fowler's position
B. Delivering oxygen with a high flow Device system and venturi mask
C. Administering a bronchodilator by nebulizer
D. Giving a sedative as prescribed

Q21. A patient with COPD who cannot use an (MDI) metered-dose inhaler effectively is ordered oral theophyllin. When asked by the patient about the action of the drug, the nurse explains that the drug treats COPD by:

A. Stimulation of respiratory drive
B. Relaxing bronchial smooth muscle
C. Only B
D. Both A and B

Q22. The nurse is teaching a patient with emphysem a. Which of the following she should include in her teaching?

A. Strategies to lose weight
B. Postural drainage
C. Early detection of respiratory infections
D. Moving to a place of high altitude

Q23. A patient with emphysema is admitted in the medical-surgical unit of a hospital with resting hypoxemi. The nurse anticipates that the patient will be treated with:

A. Theophyllin
B. Aminophyllin
C. Corticosteroids
D. Oxygen

Q24. A patient with COPD is receiving oxygen inhalation 2 liters per minute via a nasal cannula. The nurse closely monitors oxygen flow and patient's respiratory status, anticipating which of the following complications?

A. Apnea
B. Hyperventilation
C. Metabolic alkalosis
D. Respiratory alkalosis

Q25. The nurse prepares to perform postural drainage for a patient with COPD. To determine the best postural drainage position the nurse should perform:

A. Palpation
B. Auscultation
C. ABG analysis
D. Chest X-ray

Q26. A nurse is teaching a patient with chronic obstructive pulmonary disease regarding exercise. Which of the following she should emphasize?

A. Have established rest periods
B. Exercise strenuously when possible
C. Use medications during exercise
D. Avoid exercise

Q27. For a patient admitted with advanced COPD which nursing diagnosis is most important?

A. Imbalanced nutrition: Less than body requirements related to the shortness of breath
B. Disturbed sleep pattern related to anxiety, dyspnea, hypoxemia
C. Risk for infection related to retained secretions
D. Ineffective airway clearance related to airflow obstruction

Q28. Which of the following oxygen administration devices has the advantage of providing high oxygen concentration?

A. Nasal catheter
B. Partial rebreathing mask
C. Simple face mask
D. Venturi mask

Q29. Which of the following is the major advantage of a venturi mask?

A. It can deliver up to 100% oxygen
B. It is comfortable
C. It can deliver precise high flow rates of oxygen
D. Patient can eat and talk with the mask in place

Q30. The pathological process that occurs in lung parenchyma in order to develop pneumonia is:

A. Occlusion of a few terminal bronchioles with effusion
B. Collapse of alveoli due to inadequate surfactant
C. Development of ischemia due to block in one of the branches of bronchial artery
D. Inflammation of the lung parenchyma

Q31. Which of the following organisms is mostly implicated in causing community acquired pneumonia?

A. *Staphylococcus aureus*
B. *Pseudomonas aeruginosa*
C. *Streptococcus pneumoniae*
D. *Mycoplasma pneumoniae*

Q32. The nurse is taking care of a patient at high-risk of aspiration pneumonia. Which of the following nursing interventions will help to prevent aspiration pneumonia?

A. Performing mouth care with the patient in supine position

B. Elevating the head of the patient in at least 45° angle after enteral feeding

C. Providing pulmonary toilet after feeding the patient

D. Both B and C

Q33. The clinical manifestations which a person with pneumococcal pneumonia would frequently exhibit include:

A. Low-grade fever, mucopurulent cough and night sweat

B. Fever, chills and a productive cough with rust-colored sputum

C. Fever, myalgia and nonproductive cough

D. Fever, cough with foul smelling sputum

Q34. Which of the following symptoms may be an early indication of pneumonia in an elderly patient?

A. Fever and chills

B. Pleuritic chest pain and cough

C. Productive cough and dyspnea

D. Altered mental status and dehydration

Q35. The nurse is assessing a patient admitted with community acquired pneumonia. During auscultation, which of the following sounds, she is expected to hear?

A. Bronchial breath sounds

B. Bronchovesicular sounds

C. Wheeze

D. Vesicular breath sounds

Q36. Which of the following diagnostic tests help to confirm the diagnosis of pneumonia?

A. Chest X-ray

B. Sputum culture

C. Blood culture

D. ABG analysis

Q37. A patient admitted with pneumonia develops dyspnea with a respiratory rate of 30/minute and cough with thick tenacious sputum. On auscultation, bronchial sounds are heard in the right lower lobe and pulse oxymetry revealed oxygen saturation of 75 percent. Which of the following treatment the nurse should carry out first?

A. Administering broad spectrum antibiotics

B. Administering bronchodilator

C. Providing oxygen

D. Providing oral fluids 3 liters/day

Q38. A 70-year-old patient has been admitted to the medical unit with a diagnosis of pneumonia. He has a persistent cough and complains of chest pain on coughing. In order to decrease the patient's chest pain, the nurse would:

A. Instruct the patient to hold cough as much as possible

B. Teach the patient to increase the depth of respirations

C. Support the patient's rib cage with a pillow during coughing

D. Restrict fluids help to decrease the amount of sputum

Q39. An elderly patient with left lower lobe pneumonia has been treated with antibiotic therapy and is evaluated before discharge. Which outcome indicates an improvement in the patient's condition and readiness for discharge?

A. Bronchial breath sounds over the affected area

B. Oxygen saturation >92 percent

C. Restless and confusion

D. Respiratory rate of 28 breath/minute

Q40. The nurse while caring for a patient with pneumonia formulates a nursing diagnosis of ineffective airway clearance related to thick secretions and fatigue. Which of the following nursing interventions is appropriate for the stated nursing diagnosis?

A. Provide rest to the patient by keeping him in an isolated room

B. Teach patient to perform postural drainage

C. Teach patient how to cough effectively to bring secretions to the mouth

D. Administer oxygen as prescribed to maintain optimal oxygen level

Q41. Pulmonary tuberculosis (TB) very commonly occurs in which of the following people?

A. People who smokes
B. People living in village and engaged in agricultural farming
C. Elderly people with asthma
D. People with HIV infection

Q42. A patient with suspected pulmonary tuberculosis has undergone a Mantoux test. When should he return to the hospital to have the test read (examined)?

A. 12 hours after the intradermal injection
B. 24 hours after the intradermal injection
C. 48 hours after the intradermal injection
D. 1 week after the intradermal injection

Q43. A positive reaction to Mantoux test indicates that:

A. The individual has active tuberculosis
B. The individual has developed immunity to tuberculosis
C. The individual has been exposed to tuberculosis
D. The individual will develop active tuberculosis in near future

Q44. Which of the following sign and symptoms are usually found in a patient with pulmonary tuberculosis?

A. Dyspnea, chest pain, and fever with chills
B. Fever, headache, vomiting and photophobia
C. High fever, upper respiratory tract infections, and headache
D. Low-grade fever, fatigue, night sweat, and haemoptysis

Q45. Which of the following diagnostic tests confirms pulmonary tuberculosis?

A. Chest X-ray
B. Sputum for AFB
C. Mantoux test
D. Blood culture

Q46. A patient is being treated with pyrazinamide for a chronic infection. To evaluate the effectiveness of the therapy, the physician will order for culture of which of the following?

A. Blood
B. Sputum
C. CSF
D. Urine

Q47. A patient with multidrug resistant tuberculosis is under multiple antibiotic therapy. The patient will be considered as non-infectious when the patient must:

A. Remain afebrile for 5 days
B. Show a negative blood culture
C. Show a white blood cell count that is within normal limits
D. Show negative daily sputum cultures for 3 consecutive days

Q48. A patient with multidrug resistant tuberculosis is being treated with multiple antibiotics. Which of the following evaluation criteria would indicate that the patient is not responding to the treatment?

A. Patient is afebrile for a week
B. Patient has non-productive cough
C. Increasing infiltrates or cavity formation on X-ray
D. Negative AFB in sputum

Q49. The nurse is teaching a patient diagnosed with pulmonary tuberculosis regarding medications. Which of the following she should emphasize in her teaching?

A. To continue medicines as prescribed until feeling better
B. If a dose is missed one day, take double dose on the next day

C. To stop taking medicine if adverse reactions to a drug occur and report to the physician
D. To comply with the treatment regimen for complete recovery

Q50. A patient is undergoing treatment for pulmonary tuberculosis. The physician prescribed isoniazid preventive therapy for his adolescent boy of 14 years. The isoniazid preventive therapy consists of:

A. 300 mg of the drug weekly for 9 months
B. 300 mg of the drug twice a week for 6-12 months
C. 300 mg of the drug daily for 6-12 months
D. 300 mg of the drug daily for 2-4 months

Q51. Treatment for patient with uncomplicated pulmonary tuberculosis is started with which of the following combinations of pharmacologic agents?

A. Rifampicin, isoniazide, pyrazinamid and either ethambutol or streptomycin
B. Rifampicin, isoniazide and pyrazinamide
C. Rifampicin, isoniazide, thioacetazone
D. Isoniazid, pyrazinamide, streptomycin, para-aminosalicylic acid

Q52. A patient is being treated with an antitubercular regimen containing ethambutol. On follow-up visit the nurse teaches the patient to report to the physician which of the following have adverse effects of the medicine?

A. Red-orange colored urine
B. Visual changes
C. Tinnitus
D. Fever

Q53. The nurse teaches a patient with pulmonary tuberculosis being treated with rifampicin. Which of the following teaching is appropriate?

A. Avoid coffee and cola
B. Avoid using contact lenses
C. Report tingling sensation in extremities
D. Take the drug after breakfast

Q54. A patient with pulmonary tuberculosis has been advised a combination of rifampicin and isoniazid. Which of the following instructions by the nurse is correct?

A. Take both the medications together in empty stomach.
B. Report to the physician if red-orange urine.
C. Take both the medicines together after food
D. If a dose is missed, double dose should be taken next.

Q55. The physician prescribes vitamin B_6 to a patient with tuberculosis who is on treatment with a combination of isoniazid and rifampicin. The nurse understands that vitamin B_6 is added to the treatment regimen to:

A. Improve nutritional status of the patient
B. Enhance bacteriocidal effect of isoniazid
C. Enhance bacteriostatic effect of rifampicin
D. Prevent and treat peripheral neuropathy that is caused by treatment with isoniazid.

Q56. A primary tubercular infection which remains dormant for a long time is due to body's immune response may progress to active disease for which of the following factors?

A. HIV infection
B. Substance abuse
C. Malabsorption syndrome
D. All of the above

Q57. The nurse formulates a nursing diagnosis of noncompliance for a patient with pulmonary tuberculosis. The most common causative factor for this diagnosis is:

A. Lack of knowledge regarding disease transmission
B. Fatigue and lack of energy to manage self-care

C. Lack of motivation to adhere to a long-term drug regimen
D. Feelings of shame and response to the social stigma associated with TB

Q58. Which of the followings is the most important risk factor for lung cancer?

A. Cigarette smoking
B. Working in asbestos industry
C. Genetic predisposition
D. Exposure to the low level radiation

Q59. Which of the following types of lung cancers are considered to have a better prognosis because it is resectable?

A. Squamous cell carcinoma
B. Adenocarcinoma
C. Large cell carcinoma
D. Small cell carcinoma

Q60. Which of the following is the warning signal of lung cancer?

A. Persistent cough
B. Sputum streaked with blood
C. Unexplained dyspnea
D. All of the above

Q61. Which of the following is one of the earliest manifestations of lung cancer?

A. Hemoptysis
B. Persistent pneumonitis
C. Weight loss
D. Hoarseness

Q62. Which of the following diagnostic procedures most accurately confirms the diagnosis of lung cancer?

A. Chest X-ray
B. Bronchoscopy
C. Cytologic studies of early morning sputum specimen
D. Surgical biopsy

Q63. Physician is planning a wedge resection for a patient with lung cancer. The nurse explains to the patient that a wedge resection means removal of:

A. A small localized area containing the tumor near the surface of the lung
B. One segment of the lung including a bronchiole and its alveoli
C. A lobe of the lung
D. One entire lung

Q64. Following removal of an entire lung in pneumonectomy the empty side of the thoracic cavity:

A. Remains empty
B. Fills with serous fluid which eventually consolidates the region
C. The space is filled with a synthetic gel
D. The mediastinum, heart, remaining lung and the diaphragm shifts to the affected side to fill the space

Q65. A nurse is taking care of a patient after pneumonectomy. Which of the following nursing interventions she should carry out?

A. Auscultation of the lung sounds on the affected side frequently
B. Monitoring chest-tube drainage and its functioning
C. Positioning the patient on the unaffected side
D. Performing passive range of motion exercises of the arm and shoulder on the affected side

Q66. A patient with lung cancer returns to the postoperative ward after lobectomy with a chest tube attached to water-seal drainage. Which of the following nursing measures is most important in preventing respiratory complications?

A. Securing the tubing above the level of the incision
B. Reinforcing the dressing over the incision site
C. Observing intermittent bubbling in the water-seal compartment
D. Keeping the water-seal drainage system on the floor

Q67. A patient is scheduled to undergo chest surgery and insertion of a chest tube attached to the water-seal drainage. During preoperative teaching, the nurse

explains to the patient that the purpose of chest tube is to:

A. Allow for the removal of fluid and air
B. Make deep breathing and coughing easier
C. Prevent rapid expansion of the lung
D. Control internal hemorrhage

Q68. A patient with chest tube attached to the water-seal drainage needs to be transported to X-ray department for the investigation. Which of the following nursing actions is appropriate to provide safety during transport?

A. Clamp the chest tube and transport the patient with the water-seal drainage
B. Clamp the chest tube, disconnect the tube from the water-seal drainage unit and transport
C. Attach a pair of forceps to the patient's gown and transport the patient with the tube and water-seal unit
D. Instruct the patient to take deep breaths should the chest tube become dislodged

Q69. A nurse taking care of a patient with closed chest drainage observes constant bubbling in the water-seal compartment during both inspiration and expiration. What the nurse should conclude?

A. The system is functioning normally
B. The patient has developed pneumothorax
C. The chest tube is obstructed
D. The system has an air leak

Q70. While caring for a patient with closed chest drainage the nurse observes tidaling of the water level in the tube submerged in water seal chamber. Which of the following the nurse should do?

A. Check all the connections for leak in the system
B. Lower the water seal chamber further from chest level
C. Clamp the tubing to stop tidaling
D. Consider the finding as normal and continue monitoring the patient as required

Q71. A patient after resection of the right lung is attached with closed chest drainage. In addition to administering the prescribed analgesic, which of the following actions should the nurse take that would provide the most comfort for the patient while coughing and deep breathing?

A. Splinting the chest with a pillow
B. Lowering the head of the bed
C. Clamping the chest tube
D. Removing oxygen catheter temporarily

Q72. A patient with pneumothorax is being treated with a chest tube attached to the water-seal drainage. The nurse is assessing the bubbling in the water seal compartment. Which of the following observations by the nurse indicates that the system is normal and accomplishing its purpose?

A. Intermittent bubbling in the water seal chamber
B. Continuous bubbling in the water seal chamber
C. Rapid bubbling in the water seal chamber
D. No bubbling in the water seal chamber

Q73. Which of the following observations will indicate that the patient with thoracic surgery will no longer need the chest tube?

A. The drainage from the chest tube for the last 24 hours equals 60 mL only
B. Cessation of intermittent bubbling in the water seal chamber
C. Cessation of fluctuation in the water seal chamber
D. Arterial blood gas levels confirms adequate oxygenation

Q74. The nurse is taking care of a patient with bronchiectasis. Which of the following goals of care she should try to achieve while caring for the patient?

A. Patient will have no recurrence of disease
B. Patient will avoid environmental agents that precipitate inflammation

C. Patient will maintain normal pulmonary function
D. Patient will maintain removal of bronchial secretions

Q75. The pathophysiologic characteristic of different types of pneumoconiosis is:

A. Diffuse airway obstruction
B. Diffuse pulmonary fibrosis
C. Necrosis of lung tissue
D. Hyperplasia of lung parenchyma

Q76. A patient who has met with an automobile accident is admitted in the trauma unit. During assessment the nurse identifies flail chest. Which of the following observations helped to identify the problem?

A. Chest X-ray reveals multiple rib fracture
B. Crepitus of the ribs
C. Paradoxical movement of the chest wall during respiration
D. Arterial blood gas analysis reveals hypercapnia and hypoxia

Q77. Pleural effusion is defined as:

A. The collapse of alveoli
B. The inflammation of pleura
C. The accumulation of fluid in the alveoli
D. The accumulation of fluid in the pleural space

Q78. Which of the following method is employed for removal of pleural fluid in pleural effusion?

A. Insertion of a chest tube in the pleural space
B. Perform paracentesis
C. Perform thoracentesis
D. Diuretic therapy

Q79. The physician has prescribed antibiotics, bronchodilators and an expectorant to a patient with bronchiectasis. In evaluating the effects of the prescribed expectorant, the nurse will anticipate:

A. Cough suppression
B. Bronchial dilation
C. Reduced viscosity of respiratory secretions
D. Decreased production of respiratory secretions

Q80. A patient attends hospital emergency after a motor vehicle accident. He complains of dyspnea and chest pain. On auscultation the nurse finds absent breath sounds over the right upper lobe of the lung. The nurse anticipates the patient may have which of the following conditions?

A. Chronic bronchitis
B. Pneumonia
C. Rib fracture
D. Pneumothorax

Q81. Which of the following symptoms would suggest a tension pneumothorax?

A. Hemoptysis
B. Sucking sounds made on inspiration
C. Collapsed neck veins
D. Deviation of the trachea

Q82. Which of the following treatments would the nurse expect for a patient with spontaneous pneumothorax?

A. Antibiotic
B. Thoracentesis
C. Insertion of chest tube
D. Mechanical ventilation

Q83. Which of the following statements best describes pulmonary embolism?

A. It is a thrombus originating from arterial circulation that has occluded a bronchiole
B. It is a thrombus originating from venous circulation that has occluded a pulmonary vessel
C. It is a thrombus originating from arterial circulation that has occluded a pulmonary vessel
D. It is a blood clot that has developed in the pulmonary vessel

Q84. Which of the following persons are at greater risk of developing pulmonary embolism?

A. A 30-year-old lady on oral contraceptive
B. A 50-year-old lady with pneumonia
C. A 40-year-old lady on hormonal replacement therapy
D. A 50-year-old patient with pelvic exenteration

Q85. The nurse is taking care of a patient after vaginal hysterectomy for prolapse uterus. Which of the following nursing interventions by the nurse would best minimise the risk of pulmonary embolism in this patient?

A. Positioning the patient at high Fowler's position
B. Providing a small pillow under the knees for comfort
C. Assessing lower extremities for warmth and swelling
D. Early ambulation

Q86. Which of the following statements best describes the pathophysiological changes that occur in pulmonary embolism?

A. A blood clot blocks ventilation, but perfusion continues, so ventilation–perfusion mismatch occurs
B. A blood clot blocks both ventilation and perfusion in the affected area resulting in hypoxia
C. A blood clot blocks perfusion but ventilation continues in the affected area, so ventilation-perfusion mismatch occurs resulting in hypoxemia
D. A blood clot blocks a pulmonary vessel, the affected area of the lung collapses results in severe hypoxia

Q87. The nurse is assessing a patient who has undergone hip replacement surgery 2 days ago. Which of the following assessment findings would indicate pulmonary embolism?

A. Nonproductive cough and fever
B. Bradypnea, bradycardia and hypotension
C. Mucopurulent sputum, dyspnea and depression
D. Tachypnea, chest pain and anxiety

Q88. Which of the following diagnostic tests is the definitive means of diagnosis of pulmonary embolism?

A. Chest X-ray
B. CT scan
C. Ventilation-perfusion scan
D. Pulmonary angiography

Q89. The nurse understands that the patient diagnosed with pulmonary embolism will be treated by:

A. Streptokinase
B. Tissue plasminogen activator
C. IV Heparin sodium
D. Sodium warfarin

Q90. The nurse is taking care of a patient who is undergoing the treatment for pulmonary embolism. Which of the following nursing actions is most important?

A. Monitoring patient for hypoxemia and respiratory compromise
B. Be with patient as much as possible to relieve his anxiety
C. Monitoring for effects of anticoagulation
D. Elevate lower legs to promote venous return

Q91. Vena cava interruption with the insertion of filter is one of the surgical interventions for which of the following disorders?

A. Pulmonary hypertension
B. Pulmonary embolism
C. Chronic bronchitis
D. COPD

Q92. Atelectasis is a common complication after abdominal and thoracic surgery. Which of the following nursing inter-

ventions can prevent or reduce the risk of atelectasis in a postoperative patient?

A. Frequent turning
B. Steam inhalation
C. Use of an incentive spirometer
D. Coughing exercise

Q93. Which of the following arterial blood gas values defines acute respiratory failure?

A. PaO_2 equal or less than 50 mm Hg, $PaCO_2$ equal or more than 50 mm Hg
B. PaO_2 equal or less than 60 mm Hg, $PaCO_2$ equal or more than 40 mm Hg
C. PaO_2 equal or less than 70 mm Hg, $PaCO_2$ equal or more than 30 mm Hg
D. PaO_2 equal or less than 80 mm Hg, $PaCO_2$ equal or more than 20 mm Hg

Q94. A patient admitted with status asthmaticus is experiencing restlessness, air hunger and tachycardia. The nurse suspects possible acute respiratory failure and obtains arterial blood gas reports. Which of the following blood gas results would be most indicative of possible respiratory failure?

A. PaO_2 - 95 mm Hg
B. $PaCO_2$ - 60 mm Hg
C. pH - 7.35
D. O_2 saturation –95%

Q95. The nurse is caring for a patient with respiratory disorder. In assessing oxygenation, the nurse is aware that when the PaO_2 drops below 60 mm Hg, the patient will exhibit:

A. Wheezing and hypotension
B. Diminished breath sounds and cyanosis
C. Bradypnea and bradycardia
D. Restlessness and tachycardia

Q96. Which of the following arterial blood gas values is consistent with metabolic acidosis?

A. pH- 7.35
B. $PaCO_2$–46 mm Hg
C. HCO_3–15 Eq/L
D. PaO_2–95 mm Hg

Q97. A patient has following arterial blood gas values: pH-7.48, $PaCO_2$- 40 mm Hg, HCO_3 –34 mEq/L. Which of the following is the correct interpretation?

A. Respiratory acidosis
B. Respiratory alkalosis
C. Metabolic acidosis
D. Metabolic alkalosis

Q98. A patient has following arterial blood gas values: pH-7.35, $PaCO_2$– 42 mm Hg, PaO_2– 60 mm Hg. The nurse is aware that the patient is exhibiting:

A. Hypercapnia
B. Hypoxemia
C. Alkalosis
D. Acidosis

Q99. The normal pH value ranges from:

A. 7.20-7.34
B. 7.35-7.45
C. 7.46-7.55
D. 7.56-7.65

Q100. Patients at high-risk for respiratory failure include those with which of the following diagnoses?

A. Pulmonary edema
B. Pulmonary tuberculosis
C. Thoracic spinal cord injuries
D. Hyperthyroidism

Q101. A patient admitted in the hospital with smoke inhalation from house fire developed severe hypoxia 12 hours after the incident and was placed on mechanical ventilation. He most likely had developed which of the following conditions?

A. Acute respiratory failure
B. Acute respiratory distress syndrome
C. Bronchial asthma
D. Atelectasis

Q102. A patient after a motor vehicle accident was brought to hospital with multiple

injuries. The nurse anticipates that the patient may develop acute respiratory distress syndrome. What early manifestations of acute respiratory distress syndrome she should assess at this time?

A. Dyspnea and tachypnea
B. Cyanosis and restlessness
C. Hemoptysis
D. Diffuse crackles and rhonchi

Q103. The nurse has formulated a nursing diagnosis, activity intolerance related to decreased oxygenation for a patient with pneumonia. To promote activity tolerance in the patient, the nurse will plan to:

A. Ask the patient to decide which activities will be performed for the day
B. Complete all care at one time to avoid disturbing the patient later
C. Space nursing activities to allow the patient frequent rest periods
D. Suggest ways in which the patient can participate in performing care

Q104. A patient is experiencing metabolic acidosis. Which of the following compensatory mechanism will be seen in this patient?

A. A deep gasping type of respiration
B. A marked sustained inspiratory effort
C. Several short breaths followed by long irregular periods of apnea
D. Periods of apnea followed by gradually increasing depth and frequency of respirations

Q105. Pancuronium bromide (pavulon) has been ordered for a patient who is on a mechanical ventilator. The nurse understands that this drug:

A. May cause marked bradycardia
B. May be given when the patient is off from the ventilator
C. Is an analgesic with hypnotic effect
D. Should be given with sedation or analgesia

Q106. A patient on mechanical ventilation is receiving pancuronium bromide .01 mg/kg IV as needed. Which of the following assessment findings indicates that the patient requires another dose?

A. Leg movement
B. Arm movement
C. Tachycardia
D. Fighting the ventilator

Q107. When a patient is on mechanical ventilation which of the following equipments should be kept ready at bedside?

A. Water-seal chest drainage setup
B. Manual resuscitation bag
C. Oxygen analyzer
D. Trachestomy cleaning kit

Q108. Which of the following nursing actions is most essential for a patient with an endotracheal (ET) tube?

A. Monitoring proper placement of the tube every 2 hours
B. Suctioning endotracheal tube every 1 hour
C. Monitoring arterial blood gas every 4 hours
D. Provide frequent oral care

Q109. The nurse is assessing respiratory status of a patient. Which of the following observations indicates that patient is experiencing difficulty in breathing?

A. Rapid breathing
B. Pursed lip breathing
C. Diaphragmatic breathing
D. Use of accessory muscles

Q110. The chest X-ray of a patient with refractory hypoxemia shows diffuse and extensive bilateral interstitial and alveolar infiltrates (white lung) indicating acute respiratory distress syndrome. The fluid filled alveoli in acute respiratory distress syndrome arises from:

A. Administration of large volume of intravenous fluid within a short time
B. Acute left ventricular failure

C. Acute renal failure
D. Increased pulmonary capillary permeability

Q111. The nurse is assessing a dark-skinned patient for cyanosis. Inspection of which of the following areas is more reliable?

A. Lips
B. Mucous membrane
C. Nail beds
D. Ear lobes

Q112. The nurse hyperventilates and hyper-oxygenates a patient before endotracheal suctioning. Which of the following complications is prevented by this intervention?

A. Atelectasis
B. Tracheal mucosal damage
C. Pneumothorax
D. Cardiac arrythmias

Q113. While taking care of a patient with endotracheal intubation and mechanical ventilation, the nurse measures and monitors endotracheal cuff pressure. The cuff pressure that prevents tracheal injury is:

A. 10-15 mm Hg B. 15-20 mm Hg
C. 20-25 mm Hg D. 25-30 mm Hg

Q114. A patient is scheduled for septoplasty for deviated nasal septum. Preoperative preparation for septoplasty involves teaching the patient to:

A. Withheld aspirin containing drugs or nonsteroidal anti-inflammatory drugs 2 weeks prior surgery
B. Take nonsteroidal anti-inflammatory drugs as prescribed 3 days prior surgery
C. Withheld food and fluids 8 hours prior surgery
D. A and C

Q115. A patient attending hospital clinic with epistaxis was treated by an anterior nasal packing. During discharge teaching the nurse instructs the patient to:

A. Remove the packing after 24 hours
B. Take aspirin if pain
C. Avoid vigorous nose blowing and strenuous activity
D. All of the above

Q116. A patient with allergic rhinitis reports severe nasal congestion, sneezing, watery, itchy eyes and nose and profuse thin nasal discharge. To control these symptoms the nurse teaches the patient:

A. To use corticosteroid nasal spray before exposure to allergen
B. To use decongestant nasal spray prescribed regularly for a period of 10 days
C. To avoid oral antihistamines
D. To keep a diary of when the allergic reaction occurs and what precipitates it

Q117. The nurse is teaching a patient with sinusitis regarding nasal cleaning techniques. Which of the following instructions she should include in the teaching?

A. To take hot shower in the morning and evening followed by blowing the nose thoroughly
B. To irrigate nose with saline
C. To take steam inhalations 2-3 times a day
D. Any of the above

Q118. Chronic pharyngitis commonly occurs in which of the following individuals?

A. Individuals who work or live in dusty environment
B. Individuals who use their voices excessively
C. People who habitually use tobacco and alcohol
D. All of the above

Q119. Which of the following types of chronic pharyngitis is also known as clergyman's sore throat?

A. Hypertrophic

B. Atrophic
C. Chronic granular
D. None of the above

Q120. Which of the following types of sleep apnea is characterized by the lack of airflow due to pharyngeal occlusion?

A. Simple
B. Obstructive
C. Central
D. Mixed

Q121. The patients with obstructive sleep apnea are at risk of which of the following complications?

A. Hypotension
B. Dysrhythmia
C. Respiratory alkalosis
D. Pulmonary edema

Q122. Which of the following diagnostic tests may make the diagnosis of sleep apnea?

A. Barium swallow
B. Electrocardiography
C. Electroencephalography
D. Polysomnography

Q123. Which of the following measures may help a patient with obstructive sleep apnea to get relief from the symptoms?

A. Reducing excess body weight
B. Take a nap during the day
C. Eat a high protein diet at bedtime
D. Use mild sedatives or alcohol at bedtime

Q124. The type of tracheostomy tube that is sometimes indicated during weaning as an intermediate measure between a standard tracheostomy tube and extubation is the:

A. Metal tracheostomy tube
B. Fenestrated tracheostomy tube
C. Communi-Trach tube
D. Tracheostomy button

Q125. How often should a tracheostomy tube be changed?

A. 1-2 weeks
B. 2-3 weeks
C. 3-4 weeks
D. 3-4 days

Q126. The nurse is caring for a patient who recently underwent a tracheostomy. Which of the following nursing goal is most important?

A. Prevention of infection
B. Relief of pain
C. Maintenance of patent airway
D. Helping him to communicate

Q127. The nurse is taking care of the tracheostomy of a patient. She should:

A. Place the patient in recumbent position
B. Maintain sterile technique in performing tracheostomy care
C. Monitor the client's temperature after the procedure.
D. Remove inner canula and clean with betadine.

Q128. While caring for a patient with tracheostomy, the nurse finds mild air leak from tracheostomy cuff. What should the nurse do?

A. Inform the physician
B. Remove malfunctioning cuff
C. Add more air into the cuff
D. Withdraw residual air, then reinflate the cuff

Q129. Which of the following types of tracheostomy tube prevents speech?

A. A cuffless tracheostomy tube
B. A cuffed tube with the cuff deflated
C. A fenestrated tracheostomy tube
D. A tube with an inflated foam cuff

Q130. To prevent excessive pressure on tracheal capillaries the pressure in the cuff of a tracheostomy tube should be:

A. Less than 15 mm Hg or 20 cm H_2O
B. Less than 20 mm Hg or 25 cm H_2O
C. Less than 25 mm Hg or 30 cm H_2O
D. Monitored every 2-3 days

Q131. The primary etiologic agent in laryngeal cancer is:

A. Nutritional deficiencies
B. Cigarette smoking
C. Upper respiratory infection
D. Familial predisposition

Q132. The most widely used techniques of a laryngeal communication is:

A. Esophageal speech
B. Electric larynx
C. Tracheoesophageal puncture
D. All of the above

Q133. A patient who has undergone a laryngectomy suffers wound breakdown. The nurse monitors him carefully as the patient is at high-risk for developing which of the following complications?

A. Pulmonary embolism
B. Pneumonia
C. Carotid artery rupture
D. Hypoxia

Q134. The nurse is teaching the family member and the patient with total laryngectomy during discharge. Which of the following teaching is appropriate?

A. To restrict fluid to 1.5 liter per day
B. To consume a high protein diet
C. To clean the tracheostomy wound with absolute alcohol daily
D. Family members to continue to talk with the patient

Q135. Treatment of choice in a patient with chronic tonsillitis is:

A. Antibiotics
B. Surgery
C. Steroids
D. Saline throat irrigations

Q136. A patient with tonsillectomy is prepared for discharge. Which of the following instructions is appropriate?

A. To take hot saline throat irrigations thrice a day
B. To take aspirin tablet as prescribed for pain
C. To report if difficulty in talking
D. To report if bleeding occurs after discharge

ANSWERS AND RATIONALS OF RESPIRATORY SYSTEM

1. **B.** Barrel chest is present when the anteroposterior diameter is increased and equals the transverse diameter. It is a characteristic finding where ventilation is impaired for a long time. In normal chest configuration transverse diameter is usually twice the antero-posterior (AP) diameter. In pigeon chest AP diameter is increased and the sternum juts forward. Funnel chest is the opposite of pigeon chest. In this deformity the sternum is depressed and the organ lie below it is compressed.

2. **B.** Hissing or musical sound heard during inspiration or expiration or both is a wheeze. In rhonchi there is rumbling, snoring or rattling sound usually heard on expiration and may clear on coughing. High pitched sound produced on inspiration heard over the trachea is a stridor and pleural friction rub is heard as creaking and grating sound over the problem area on both inspiration or expiration.

3. **B.** The patient is exhibiting Cheyne-Stokes breathing which is characterized by alternating periods of deep breathing and shallow breathing and apnea which lasts only for 15-16 secs. This type of breathing is a common finding in heart failure, anemia, and brain damage. Kussmaul breathing is characterized by slightly increased respiratory rate, often occurs with strenuous exercise and metabolic acidosis. Biot's breathing is characterized by unpredictable irregularity, breaths may be shallow, deep and stop for short periods of time associated with respiratory, depression and brain damage. In hypoventilation, there is inadequate alveolar ventilation in an relation to metabolic demands.

4. **A.** Difficulty in breathing would indicate a possible complication associated with a bronchoscopy. A serious complication following a bronchoscopy would be swelling due to the trauma and the initial symptom the patient would experience is the difficulty in breathing. Other complications associated with bronchoscopy include reaction to the local anaesthetic, infection, aspiration, bronchospasm, hypoxemia, pneumothorax, bleeding and perforation. Hoarseness of voice, difficulty in swallowing and coughing and blood tinged sputum may occur due to the irritation of the mucous membrane during the procedure and passing off the instrument through larynx, trachea and should not be considered as complications.

5. **C.** To assess the patient's level of hypoxia, the nurse will use a pulse oxymetry. A pulse oxymetry is a safe, simple, non-invasive device that measures patient's arterial blood oxygen saturation. Being a non-invasive device it does not require order of the physician. Pulmonary function tests provide respiratory function by measuring lung volumes, and not oxygenation of blood. Arterial blood gas analysis is a superior tool for measuring of pH, arterial oxygen and carbon dioxide but it is an invasive procedure and requires an arterial puncture. Being an invasive procedure requires order of physician and is usually done for more serious patients. Estimation of hemoglobin level cannot assess for hypoxia.

6. A. Asthma is a chronic inflammatory disorder of the airways in which inflammation causes varying degrees of obstruction in the airways. This inflammation causes recurrent episodes of wheezing, breathlessness, chest tightness and cough, and is associated with an increase in existing hyperresponsiveness to a variety of stimuli. Hyperresponsiveness of airways gives rise to a period of reversible, not irreversible bronchospasms which may reverse spontaneously or with treatment. Mucous production is increased in asthma but blocking of airways due to mucous plug is not the only cause of asthma. Obstruction of airways caused by destruction of alveolar walls occurs in emphysema, not in asthma.

7. B. Drug therapy for the treatment of asthma depends on the severity of the disease. Persistent asthma requires daily long-term therapy in addition to the appropriate medications to manage acute asthma exacerbation. Accordingly asthma medications are categorized into two general classifications: (1) Long-term control medications to achieve and maintain control of persistent asthma and (2) quick-relief medications to treat the symptoms and exacerbation.

8. B. Beclomethasone dipropionate is a corticosteroid administered by a metered-dose inhaler and is used in the long-term control of asthma. It acts by anti-inflammatory and immunosuppressive effects locally in the respiratory tract with relatively little systemic effects. Beta-adrenergic agonists stimulate beta-adrenergic receptors and produces bronchodilation. Anticholinergics block action of acetylcholine and produces bronchodilation. Methylxanthine derivatives cause bronchodilation by relaxing smooth muscles of bronchial wall.

9. A. Theophylline and other methylxanthine derivatives relieve bronchospasm by relaxing smooth muscle of bronchial wall. Theophylline does not decrease sputum production, suppress coughing and treat respiratory infection.

10. B. The nurse should teach the patient to take prescribed medications as scheduled. Taking medications regularly and correctly as prescribed is the most important measure in preventing acute attacks of asthma. All other teachings are appropriate for patients with asthma, but taking medications regularly and correctly as prescribed has the highest priority.

11. D. The patient is in respiratory distress because of bronchoconstriction as evidenced by wheezing. His greatest need is bronchodilation, which can be achieved by administering salbutamol, a beta 2-agonist by nebulization or by metered-dose inhalation. Inhaled salbutamol produces bronchodilation within 5 minutes and is the drug of choice in acute attacks of asthma. Propranolol, a beta-blocker is contraindicated in patients with asthma, since it can cause severe asthmatic attack. Morphine is a central nervous system depressant and it can also precipitate further asthmatic attack by its histamine releasing action. Steroids in inhaled or oral form are usually given to the patients with asthma to reduce inflammation but are not appropriate for immediate relief of respiratory distress.

12. A. Inhaled beta 2-agonists help to promote bronchodilation which improves oxygenation. IV beta 2-agonists can be used when inhaled beta 2-agonists do not work. Status asthmaticus is treated with IV corticosteroids, not oral or inhaled corticosteroids.

13. C. Regular use of corticosteroid inhalation helps to reduce inflammation of airways in asthma. It does not cause bronchodilation hence, does not give immediate relief. To get relief from shortness of breath patient has to use bronchodilator inhaler. So patient needs further instructions regarding the use of corticosteroid inhaler. All other statements regarding treatment of upper respiratory infections, reduction of stress by meditation and scheduling bronchodilator inhaler before exercise are appropriate and indicate adequate teaching.

14. D. Azithromycin is a macrolid antibiotic with long duration of action. So once daily dose is prescribed. It should be taken with water 1 hour before meal or 2 hours after meal. Taking the drug with milk, food or antacid especially aluminium and magnesium containing antacid reduces its absorption.

15. D. Chronic obstructive pulmonary disease (COPD) is a disease characterized by the presence of airflow obstruction by chronic bronchitis or emphysema. In chronic bronchitis, inflamed edematous bronchi give rise to increased mucous production, and obstruction of airways. Decreased elastic recoil occurs in emphysema. Airway resistance due to smooth muscle contraction occurs in asthma. Although asthma is now being defined separately, patients with COPD may have asthma and some patients with asthma may go on to develop fixed or irreversible airflow obstruction. So all these disorders, e.g. chronic bronchitis, asthma and emphysema are present to some degree in patients with COPD.

16. B. The assessment data most likely suggests chronic bronchitis with complication of cor pulmonale. Patients with asthma and emphysema usually do not have chronic cough or peripheral edema. Patients with tuberculosis complain of cough with sputum, hemoptysis, fever, night sweat, fatigue, and loss of body weight, etc. history of smoking may or may not be there.

17. A. The most common early manifestation of chronic bronchitis is a daily productive cough lasting for 3 months in each of two successive years in a patient in whom other causes of chronic cough have been excluded. Patient with chronic bronchitis progresses to develop dyspnea, cyanosis and right ventricular failure in the later course of disease.

18. D Deriphyllin (theophyllin) is a xanthine derivative relaxes smooth muscle of respiratory tract. The dose should be taken in the morning in order to have maximum benefits from it during day time activities. It should not be taken at bed time as it causes insomnia. Patient should take a lot of fluids to keep respiratory secretions thin and also to prevent dehydration as it causes diuresis. Coffee, cola and chocolate contain xanthine and should be avoided by the patient as additional xanthine may potentiate side effects.

19. B An important component in the collaborative care for a patient with COPD is treating respiratory infections as soon as possible. Other components of care include: Cessation of smoking, bronchodilator therapy, low flow oxygen if indicated, oral corticosteroids therapy in only a small percentage of patients for short duration, not long-term, optimum hydration by 3 liters of fluid per day, not restricted, chest physiotherapy and postural drainage, breathing exercises, planned progressive exercise program, not vigorous exercise, etc.

20. B The patient with COPD retains carbon dioxide. Due to long-standing hypercapnia, low oxygen levels rather than increased carbon dioxide levels trigger the respiratory drive in these patients. So oxygen should be given cautiously with a venturi mask which can maintain oxygen flow accurately and consistently. The desired oxygen flow should be 1 to 3 liters. Unspecified and uncontrolled amount of oxygen may depress ventilation. The patient also requires bronchodilators, which should be administered by the nurse later by nebulizer as prescribed by the doctor. The patient should be placed on high Fowler's position, not semi-Fowler's to ease breathing. Sedative depresses respiratory center and use of the same should be avoided.

21. D. Theophyllin benefits by causing bronchodilation and stimulating respiratory drive and by augmenting diaphragmatic contractility. In asthma, theophyllin decreases nonspecific airway reactivity by decreasing release of inflammatory mediators. The drug also directly stimulates the myocardium causes diuresis and increase Na^+ and Cl^- excretion.

22. C. Recurring respiratory tract infections are a major contributing factor to the aggravation and progression of emphysema. Recurring infections impair normal defence mechanisms making the alveoli more susceptible to injury or destruction resulting in more inflammation, more edema and exudate formation. So the patient must be taught to avoid respiratory tract infections, detect early symptoms of infections if any, e.g. increasing quantity, viscosity and purulence of sputum and start antibiotic therapy as prescribed at the earliest. Patients with emphysema are usually malnourished, so they need to learn measures to gain weight, not to lose weight. These patients usually have scanty amount of sputum, so postural drainage is usually not indicated. They should be discouraged to move into a place of high altitude where partial pressure of oxygen is less.

23. D. Oxygen therapy is the only therapy for patients with emphysema or COPD that has been demonstrated to be life preserving. Severe hypoxemia is treated with low concentrations of oxygen to raise the PaO_2 to 65 to 80 mm Hg. In severe emphysema oxygen is administered at least 16 hours per day, 24 hours preferable. Oxygen therapy alleviates patient's symptoms and improves the quality of life. Theophyllin and aminophyllin as bronchodilators are less frequently used because of their narrow margin of safety. Instead beta 2-adrenergic agonist and anticholinergic agents are preferred and administered via MDI to reverse bronchospasm. Corticosteroids are not helpful to give immediate relief in hypoxemia. It is used as long-term anti-inflammatory agent in a very small percentage of patients with emphysema or COPD.

24. A. Hypoxia is the main breathing stimulus for a patient with COPD, not carbon dioxide since they develop a tolerance for high carbon dioxide levels overtime. For these patients 'O_2 drive' to breath is hypoxemia. So high oxygen concentration reduces the ventilatory drive leading to apnea, or hypoventilation not hyperventilation. Hypoventilation will cause respiratory acidosis not respiratory alkalosis. Metabolic alkalosis is not caused from respiratory etiology.

25. B. Postural drainage positions are determined by the areas of involved

lung, which are assessed by chest X-rays, percussion, palpation and auscultation. But the most convenient technique of assessment for a nurse is auscultation. ABG analysis gives information about respiratory functions but does not give information about the lung areas requiring postural drainage.

26. A. Mild exercise such as walking is the best for COPD patients. Patient should be taught to walk at slow pace with rest periods when necessary to conserve energy. Patient with COPD must avoid strenuous exercise to prevent hypoxia. Use of medications may help to tolerate exercise but the medications should be given 10 minutes before exercise and not during exercise. Some exercise is beneficial for patient, but the extent or type depends on the general condition of the patient.

27. D. A patent airway and adequate breathing pattern is vital and top priority for any individual. So the diagnosis of ineffective airway clearance related to airflow obstruction is the most important nursing diagnosis. Other diagnoses are also appropriate but less important.

28. B. In a partial rebreathing mask 40-60% oxygen can be delivered using a flow rate of 6–10 liter/minute. Nasal catheter can deliver oxygen up to 30% with a flow rate of 5-6 liter/minute. A simple facemask can provide 35–50% of oxygen concentration with a flow rate of 6–12 liter/minute, and venturi mask can provide up to 50% of oxygen.

29. C. The major advantage of a venturi mask is that it can deliver precise, high flow rates of oxygen. This is especially helpful for administering low, constant oxygen concentrations to patients with COPD. Venturi mask is available for delivery of 24%, 28%, 31%, 35%, 40% and 50% oxygen. It does not deliver up to 100% oxygen. The mask is uncomfortable and must be removed when patient eats. Patient can talk but voice may be muffled.

30. D. Pneumonia is an acute inflammation of the lung parenchyma is caused by a microbial agent. It is not due to occlusion of a few bronchioles with effusion or due to block of a branch in bronchial artery. Collapse of alveoli is due to inadequate surfactant is atelectasis.

31. C. Streptococcal or pneumococcal pneumonia caused by streptococcal pneumoniae is the most common cause of community acquired pneumonia. Other organisms are mostly involved in hospital acquired pneumonia.

32. B. Elevating the head of the patient in at least 45° angle reduces the risk of regurgitation and aspiration of stomach content into the lungs. Mouth care should be performed with the patient in lateral position not in a supine position to prevent aspiration. Providing pulmonary toilet after feeding may cause vomiting and aspiration of vomitus in the lungs.

33. B. Fever, chills, productive cough with rust colored sputum, chest pain are the common manifestations of pneumococcal pneumonia. Low-grade fever with mucopurulent cough and night sweats indicate pulmonary tuberculosis. Fever, myalgia and nonproductive cough are common symptoms of influenza, and in lung abscess, patients experience fever, cough with foul smelling sputum.

34. D. The common symptoms of pneumonia are fever, chills, sweat, pleuritic chest pain, cough, sputum production, hemoptysis, dyspnea, headache and fatigue. Elderly patients may present with altered mental status and dehydration without fever or respiratory manifestations.

35. A. In pneumonia chest auscultation reveals bronchial breath sounds over areas of consolidation, as consolidated lung tissue transmits bronchial sound waves to outer lung fields. Bronchovesicular sounds are normal, heard over the central, large airways. Wheeze is adventitious breath sound heard as a continuous, musical or hissing noise commonly associated with bronchial asthma. Vesicular breath sounds are normal, heard throughout the chest and heard best towards the bases of lungs.

36. B. Definitive diagnosis of pneumonia is usually determined through the sputum culture or serologic testing. Chest X-ray examination provides information about the extent and location of pneumonia. Blood culture will determine whether the infection is systemic. ABG analysis will determine the extent of hypoxia.

37. C. The patient is dyspnoeic and is hypoxic. So the nurse should first provide with oxygen. Patient probably requires treatment with antibiotic and bronchodilator. But this requires physician's decision and order. As an emergency measure nurse can provide with oxygen without waiting for a physician's order. Patients require 3 liters of fluid per day, as he is having fever and thick tenacious sputum, but dyspnea must be relieved before the patient is encouraged to take oral fluids.

38. C. Supporting the rib cage during coughing will diminish pain. Holding in cough will only increase his pain. Increasing depth of respiration will help to treat pneumonia by improving oxygenation but will not relieve chest pain. Patient should be encouraged to increase fluid intake to liquefy cough so that the sputum is expelled easily.

39. B. Oxygen saturation is 92 percent or more indicate an improvement in the patient's condition. Restlessness and confusion means that the patient is still having pneumonia. Respiratory rate of 28 breaths/minute indicate dyspnea, which means that the patient still has pneumonia.

40. C. The patient has to be taught practicing effective coughing technique in order to promote effective coughing and raising of thick tenacious sputum out of lungs. Providing rest by placing the patient in an isolated room is done to prevent disease transmission. Postural drainage is helpful in bringing secretions from terminal bronchioles to larger, more central airways, e.g. chronic bronchitis and emphysema. Administration of oxygen helps in maintaining oxygen level. It does not help in expectoration of secretions. Optimum hydration is useful in liquefying secretions.

41. D. People with HIV infection are particularly susceptible to TB because mycobacterium tuberculosis, the organism causing TB is an extremely opportunistic pathogen. Individual with HIV infection are at greater risk for acquiring a new infection with rapid progression to active disease or for experiencing reinfection from dormant lesion. Smoking, agricultural farming and asthma are not associated with tuberculosis. Although advanced age may be a factor in the development of active disease from a dormant infection, HIV infection poses a much greater chance of developing the disease.

42. C. In Mantoux test, a purified protein derivative (PPD) tuberculin is injected intradermally to form a wheal in the lower left forearm. The wheal must be examined (read) in 48 to 72 hours. Reading it too early or too late will give a false result.

43. C. Mantoux skin test is based on antigen-antibody reaction. Person who has been exposed to tuberculosis, possesses antibodies against the tuberculosis bacteria and show positive reaction towards the Mantoux test is due to antigen-antibody reaction. So positive test indicates exposure to tuberculosis, but it does not indicate the presence of active disease, nor it indicates the possibility of developing the disease in near future. Exposure does not confer immunity as it has been seen that some of the individuals with primary infection develop disease later in life. So positive Mantoux test does not indicate immunity towards the disease.

44. D. Most patients with pulmonary tuberculosis have a low-grade fever, fatigue, night sweat and hemoptysis. Symptoms are usually insidious. Dyspnea, chest pain and fever with chills are usually seen in community acquired pneumonia. Fever, headache, vomiting and photophobia are seen in meningitis. High fever, upper respiratory tract infections and headache are usually found in the seasonal viral fever.

45. B. A more definitive diagnosis of pulmonary tuberculosis is made from AFB smear. Sputum specimens are collected on three consecutive mornings and presence of AFB in any of the smear confirms active disease. Lesion in the lung may not be big enough to be seen on X-ray. Mantoux test is only a screening test, not a definitive test for pulmonary tuberculosis. Sputum culture, not a blood culture is a more definitive test for tuberculosis. But results are available after 2-12 weeks; hence this test is usually not used for diagnosis.

46. B. Pyrazinamide is an antitubercular agent used in tuberculosis with other antitubercular drugs. The effectiveness of its therapeutic response is evaluated by decreased symptoms of tuberculosis and negative culture report of sputum for mycobacterium tuberculosis.

47. D. Sputum cultures on three consecutive mornings must be negative for the tubercular bacillus, for a patient to be declared as no longer infectious. Remaining afebrile for 5 days showing a negative blood culture and showing a white blood cell count that is within normal limits are not tests that determine whether the patient with multidrug resistant tuberculosis is no longer infectious.

48. C. If the medication regimen does not seem effective, the patient would exhibit worsening manifestation of the disease, continued presence of AFB in sputum and increasing infiltrates or cavity formation on the chest X-ray. Remaining afebrile for a week or having nonproductive cough or negative AFB in sputum indicate patient's response towards the treatment.

49. D. Treatment of TB is a long-term process, and completion of treatment is critical for the arrest of the disease. Incomplete treatment or irregular treatment leads to reactivation of TB and the development of drug resistant strains of TB.

50. C. Chemoprophylaxis with isoniazid or isoniazid preventive therapy IPT consists of 300 mg of isoniazide daily for a period of 6-12 months. IPT stops the growth of bacilli, thus preventing active pulmonary or extrapulmonary TB.

51. A. Treatment for patient with uncomplicated pulmonary tuberculosis is started with four drugs regimen consisting of rifampicin, isoniazide, pyrazinamid and either ethambutol or streptomycin. Therapy may be given daily or 2-3 times weekly if DOT. Ethambutol or streptomycin may be discontinued if susceptibility to rifampicin or isoniazide is documented. Pyrazinamide should be discontinued after 8 weeks. The total duration of the therapy should be at least 6 months and at least 3 months after sputum cultures convert to negative.

52. B. The most important adverse effect of ethambutol is optic neuritis leading to deterioration of visual acuity and color vision. So vision should be tested before the initiation of therapy and at regular intervals. Red-orange colored urine occurs with rifampicin. Tinnitus is due to ototoxicity occurs with streptomycin. Low-grade fever is a symptom of tuberculosis which should disappear with the treatment.

53. B. Rifampicin turns the urine, feces, saliva, sputum, sweat and tears red-orange colored. Contact lenses may be stained permanently with red-orange color. Patient should avoid alcohol. Tingling sensation of the extremities is not associated with rifampicin and the drug should be taken in empty stomach.

54. A. Antitubercular drugs are given in combination and all the drugs are to be taken at a time. The drugs are absorbed better if taken in empty stomach at least 1 hour before meal or 2 hours after meal. Red-orange coloration of urine is normal and need not be reported. Compliance with the therapeutic regimen should be strictly adhered to but patient should not take double dose for a missed dose.

55. D. One of the most common side effect of isoniazid is peripheral neuropathy that may occur due to vitamin B_6 deficiency caused by this drug. So adding vitamin B_6 in the treatment regimen will prevent and treat this problem. To improve nutritional status patient should be given a well balanced diet not only vitamin B_6. Vitamin B_6 does not enhance the therapeutic effects of antitubercular drugs mentioned above.

56. D. Why a primary tubercular infection which remain dormant for some time due to body's immune response may progress to active disease is poorly understood. However, some factors, e.g. HIV infection, substance abuse, malabsorption syndromes play a role in the progression from a dormant TB infection to active disease. Other factors are advanced age, immunosupression, prolonged corticosteroid therapy, low body weight, presence of other disease, e.g. diabetes, end-stage renal disease or malignancy and genetic predisposition.

57. D. Noncompliance with therapeutic regimen is a major problem regarding control of TB in the community. Various factors play a role for noncompliance. The most important being – feelings of shame and response to the social stigma associated with TB. Other factors for noncompliance are: Lack of knowledge regarding disease process and therapeutic regimen, not regarding disease transmission, lack of motivation to remain healthy, and long-term nature of treatment. Fatigue is not the cause of noncompliance, since compliance to therapeutic regimen does not require much energy. An individual motivated to get well will adhere to long-term treatment regimen.

58. A. Cigarette smoking is the most important risk factor for the lung cancer. 90 percent of the patients with lung cancer are or have been smokers. Other risk factors are exposure to industrial pollutant, e.g. asbestos, arsenic, genetic predisposition, advanced age, exposure to low level radiation and tuberculosis.

59. A. Squamous cell carcinoma is associated with better prognosis in the terms of survival rate because this type of carcinoma produces earlier symptoms, slow growing, metastasis not common, surgical excision is often attempted. Adenocarcinoma has no clinical manifestations until widespread metastasis occurs. Does not respond well to chemotherapy. Large cell carcinoma is highly metastatic. Metastasizes via lymphatics and blood. Tumor may be radiosensitive but often recurs. Small cell carcinoma is the most malignant form, spreads early via lymphatics and bloodstream, has poorest prognosis.

60. D. The warning signals of the lung cancer include persistent cough, sputum streaked with blood, unexplained dyspnea. Other warning signals include frank hemoptysis, rust colored or purulent sputum, unexplained weight loss, pain in arm, shoulder, chest or back and recurrent pleural effusion.

61. B. Clinical manifestations of the lung cancer are nonspecific and appear late in the disease process. Persistent pneumonitis that is a result of obstructed bronchi may be one of the earliest manifestations. Hemoptysis is not a common early manifestation. Weight loss and hoarseness appear late in the disease process.

62. D. A biopsy is the best method for establishing the presence of a malignant tumor. Biopsy specimen may be obtained by the fine needle aspiration (FNA), bronchoscopy and surgery. FNA is useful in peripheral lesion, bronchoscopy is useful in endobronchial lesion only. So surgical biopsy only can confirm with 100 percent accuracy. Cytologic studies of early morning sputum also provide accurate results. However, malignant cells may not be obtained even in the presence of a malignant tumor. X-ray can identify the location of the tumor, extent of metastasis to the ribs or vertebra, presence of pleural effusion, etc. but cannot diagnose type of tumor, i.e. malignant or non-malignant.

63. A. Removal of a small, localized area containing the tumor near the surface of the lung is wedge resection. In segmental resection one segment or more segments (a bronchiole and its alveoli) is or are removed. A lobe of the lung is removed in lobectomy and an entire lung is removed in pneumonectomy.

64. B. Serous fluid accumulates in the empty thoracic cavity which eventually consolidates and prevents extensive shifts of the mediastinum, heart and remaining lung. The space is not filled with any synthetic gel. A temporary shift of mediastinum and other structures occurs until the area is filled as stated above.

65. D. Passive range of motion exercises of the arm and shoulder on the affected side should begin 4 hours after recovery from anesthesia. Range of motion exercises help prevent adhesion formation in the operative area giving rise to frozen shoulder. In pneumonectomy, the entire lung is removed so nurse need not auscultate for lung sounds on the affected side. Chest drainage is usually not given after pneumonectomy as the empty space is allowed to fill with serous fluid collection. Patient should be positioned on the affected side not on unaffected side to allow expansion of remaining lung.

66. D. Keeping the water-seal drainage system on the floor is the most important nursing measure the nurse can take to prevent respiratory complication, as maintaining the drainage system on the floor below the patient's chest will prevent back flow of fluid and air into the patient's pleural cavity. The tube has to be secured below the level of the incision and not above to prevent back flow of fluid and air into the pleural cavity. There is no need to reinforce the dressing around the incision site unless there is a leak at the insertion site. Observing intermittent bubbling in the water-seal compartment is also an important nursing activity but maintaining the drainage system below the patient's chest level is more important and should be done first.

67. A. The nurse should explain to the patient that the purpose of chest tubes is to allow for the drainage of fluid and air and to re-establish negative pressure. Deep breathing and coughing will be easy only when the pleural space is free from fluid and air and having negative pressure. Removal of fluid and air from pleural space will cause re-expansion of the lung and is a desired outcome. Chest tubes do not have any impact on internal haemorrhage. However, increased chest tube drainage together with other symptoms, e.g. tachycardia, hypotension, etc. may indicate hemorrhage.

68. C. During transport, a pair of forceps to be attached with patient's gown, so that the pair of forceps is readily available if the chest tube become dislodged during the transport. Chest tube should never be clamped for prolonged periods of time, unless necessary. Neither should it be disconnected from the water seal unit. Deep breaths will not prevent complications following the chest tube dislodgement.

69. D. Continuous bubbling during both inspiration and expiration indicates that air is leaking into the drainage system or pleural cavity, which must be corrected. A normally functioning system will have intermittent bubbling and is caused by air passing out of the pleural space into the fluid in the chamber. Patient with pneumothorax is treated with closed chest drainage. Chest drainage does not cause pneumothorax. If the chest tube is obstructed the nurse should notice tidaling (fluctuation of fluid) to stop, not continuous bubbling in the water seal chamber.

70. D. Fluid in the water seal compartment rises with inspiration and falls with expiration. This is called tidaling. When tidaling is occurring, the drainage tube is patent and the apparatus is functioning properly. So nurse should continue monitoring patient as required and need not intervene to check air leak, adjust height of the drainage bottle or clamp tubing. Tidaling will stop if the drainage tube is kinked or obstructed, or lung re-expanded. Tidaling may not occur or may be minimal in systems using suction.

71. A. Administering analgesics and splinting the chest with a pillow will provide most comfort for the patient while coughing and deep breathing. Head of the bed should be elevated not lowered to facilitate breathing and help in easy expectoration. Chest tube should not be clamped, unless it is really needed to prevent tension pneumothorax. Oxygen catheter should not be removed as coughing and deep breathing can deplete a patient's oxygen reserve.

72. A. Air from the pleural space can be removed by inserting a chest tube attached to a water seal compartment. A normal functioning drainage system will remove air or fluid during expiration which will be evident by intermittent bubbling. Continuous bubbling or rapid bubbling during both inspiration and expiration indicates an air leak which should be immediately corrected. No bubbling indicates that the system is not serving its purpose, as the tube may not be positioned properly.

73. C. The chest tube is removed after chest surgery when the lung is re-expanded. The indication that the lung has re-expanded is cessation of fluctuations in the water seal chamber. Chest auscultation, chest percussion and chest X-ray also can confirm lung expansion. Chest tube is usually not removed when the chest drainage exceeds 50 mL per day. Cessation of intermittent bubbling indicates that the air in the pleural space has been removed, but it does not indicate complete removal of fluid. Arterial blood gas analysis is not necessary to find out re-expansion of lung.

74. D. The most important goal in caring for a patient with bronchiectasis is to promote drainage and removal of bronchial mucopurulent secretions. This is achieved by teaching the patient effective deep breathing and coughing exercises, and performing chest physiotherapy and postural drainage. The other goals are not appropriate, as bronchiectasis is a chronic disease with permanent dilatation of one or more bronchi that is difficult to treat. So recurrent flare-ups are common. The disease is not due to environmental agents producing inflammation but due to bacterial infections weakening bronchial walls. Repeated flare-ups cause decline in the lung function. So the goal of maintaining normal pulmonary function is difficult.

75. B. Pneumoconiosis is a general term for lung diseases caused by inhalation and retention of dust particles. The pathophysiological response to the inhaled substances is diffuse parenchymal infiltration with phagocytic cells. This eventually results in diffuse pulmonary fibrosis, as fibrosis is the result of tissue repair after inflammation. The other pathophysiological changes mentioned are not seen in pneumoconiosis.

76. C. A flail chest consists of fractures of two or more adjacent ribs on the same side of chest. Since the affected area of the chest cannot provide the bony structures necessary to maintain bellows action and ventilation, moves paradoxically to the intact portion of the chest during respiration. This paradoxical movement of the chest wall during respiration is usually apparent on visual examination of the unconscious patient and is diagnostic of flail chest. Chest X-ray and arterial blood gas analysis will determine the management strategies. Palpation to find out crepitus of the ribs is not performed by the nurses.

77. D. Pleural effusion is an accumulation of fluid in the pleural space. The collapse of alveoli/lung tissue is atelectasis. Inflammation of pleura is pleurisy/pleuritis. Accumulation of fluid in the alveoli is pulmonary edema.

78. C. Thoracentesis is done to remove pleural fluid developed in pleural effusion. Paracentesis is done to remove ascitic fluid from peritoneal cavity. Insertion of chest tube is usually not indicated in pleural effusion. Diuretic therapy does not remove fluid from pleural cavity. Pleural fluid to be removed from pleural cavity as early as possible by thoracentesis in order to re-expand the lung.

79. C. The nurse will anticipate an expectorant to improve the removal of respiratory secretions by thinning and decreasing the viscosity of the secretions in the patient with bronchiectasis. Antitussives provide symptomatic relief of coughing by suppressing cough reflex. Bronchodilators reverse airway obstruction by bronchial dilation and anticholinergics decrease production of respiratory as well as oral secretions.

80. D. History of injury, sign and symptoms suggest closed or spontaneous pneumothorax, which may arise from fractured ribs. Chronic bronchitis would have rhonchi, pneumonia would have bronchial breath sounds over the area of consolidation, and not absent breath sounds. Patient with uncomplicated rib fracture will have shallow breathing due to pain but not absent breath sounds.

81. D. Deviation of the trachea would suggest tension pneumothorax. Tension pneumothorax is caused by injury that perforates the chest wall resulting in air to enter into pleural space. Air gets trapped in the pleural space and builds up pressure which causes lung on the injured side to collapse and mediastinal contents to shift to the unaffected side. Hemoptysis suggests pulmonary embolism. Sucking sounds on inspiration may be due to open pneumothorax. Collapsed neck veins indicate dehydration or hypotension.

82. C. Management of pneumothorax involves inserting a chest tube in the pleural space via the fourth intercostal space and then connecting the chest tube to closed chest drainage. Chest tube permits continuous escape of air thus helping lung re-expand by establishing negative pressure in the pleural space. Antibiotic has no role in lung re-expansion. Thoracentesis is done as a life saving measure in tension pneumothorax when delay is anticipated in inserting a chest tube. Mechanical ventilation is indicated in patients with more severe disorder, e.g. hemopneumothorax accompanied by flail chest.

83. B. Pulmonary embolism is an occlusion of a portion of the pulmonary blood vessels by an embolus. An embolus is a blood clot or other materials, e.g. air, fat, amniotic fluid, etc. that is carried by the bloodstream from its point of origin. Most of the pulmonary embolisms develop from thrombi originating in the deep calf, femoral, popliteal or iliac veins and not in arteries and pulmonary vessels. The embolism remains in the bloodstream and lodges in one of the pulmonary vessels and not in bronchioles. The blood clot in pulmonary embolism does not develop in pulmonary circulation.

84. D. Major operations especially hip, knee, abdominal and extensive pelvic procedures predispose the patient to thrombus formation because of the reduced flow of blood through the pelvis. Persons with other conditions are not at increased risk for pulmonary embolism.

85. D. Early ambulation helps to reduce stasis and pooling of blood which reduces the risk of venous thrombosis that may then dislodge. Positioning the patient at high Fowler's position and providing pillow under the knees favors venous stasis and pooling of blood and subsequent thrombus formation. Assessing lower extremities for warmth and swelling helps in detection of deep vein thrombosis but does not prevent the risk of pulmonary embolism.

86. C. The blood clot blocks a branch of pulmonary artery leading to decreased perfusion of the section of the lung supplied by the vessel. The patient continues to ventilate the area of the lung, but the perfusion is obstructed, so ventilation- perfusion mismatch occurs resulting in hypoxemia. Ventilation is usually not affected initially unless a large vessel is obstructed causing atelectasis.

87. D. Manifestations of pulmonary embolism are nonspecific and may not appear until late in the event. The most common manifestations of pulmonary embolism are tachypnea, dyspnea, chest pain and anxiety. The other symptoms are not suggestive of pulmonary embolism.

88. D. Pulmonary angiography remains the definitive means of diagnosis of pulmonary embolism. A radiopaque contrast agent is injected and visualization of any filling defects of the pulmonary artery is achieved by serial X-rays. Thus the test can locate the clot and extent of the perfusion defect. Chest X-ray cannot diagnose pulmonary embolism but is done to rule out other pulmonary abnormalities. CT scan is a non-invasive test effective for identifying the location of infarcted or ischemic tissue. Ventilation-perfusion scan gives an indication of ventilation - perfusion mismatch present and define the amount of tissue involved, but none are definitive test than pulmonary angiography.

89. C. Treatment with pulmonary embolism begins with IV standard heparin sodium to reduce the risk of further clots and to prevent existing clots to extend. Heparin is administered until a therapeutic partial thromboplastin time (PTT) is achieved. Sodium warfarin is administered 3-5 days before heparin is stopped to provide a transition to oral anticoagulation. Use of thrombolytics like tPA has been tried in hemodynamically unstable patient to lyse the clot, but mortality rate is not improved. Hence, their use in pulmonary embolism is not clear.

90. A. Maintenance of cardiopulmonary stability is the first priority. So patient should be monitored for hypoxemia and respiratory compromise. Staying with patient reduces patient's anxiety and apprehension but monitoring for hypoxemia, respiratory compromise and instituting appropriate measure to maintain oxygenation is more important. Monitoring for anticoagulation is necessary later in the course of the disease when therapeutic anticoagulation is achieved. Lower legs should be elevated with caution as elevation may cause severe flexure of the hips and eventual thrombus formation.

91. B. One of the surgical interventions for the treatment of pulmonary embolism is vena cava interruption with the insertion of a filter. The other surgical procedure is pulmonary embolectomy. There is no known cure for pulmonary hypertension. Chronic bronchitis is treated with pharmacologic agents. Surgical intervention for COPD is relatively uncommon. Bullectomy and lung volume reduction surgery may benefit patients with recurrent spontaneous pneumothorax.

92. C. Use of an incentive spirometer requires the patient to take deep breaths which promotes lung expansion, thus prevents atelectasis. Frequent turning, steam inhalation and coughing exercises help to mobilize secretions but would not prevent atelectasis.

93. A. Acute respiratory failure is defined as a fall in arterial oxygen tension (PaO_2) to 50 mm Hg or less and a rise in arterial carbon dioxide tension ($PaCO_2$) to 50 mm Hg or more.

94. B. $PaCO_2$ of 60 mm Hg is indicative of acute respiratory failure. The normal $PaCO_2$ is 35-45 mm Hg. $PaCO_2$ is greater than 50 mm Hg (hypercapnia) suggests hypoventilation and acidosis due to retention of carbon dioxide in the blood. Normal PaO_2 is 95-100 mm Hg, normal pH is 7.35-7.45 and normal oxygen saturation is 94-100%. So these values are in normal range.

95. D. In hypoxemia, heart rate is elevated as a compensatory mechanism. By increasing heart rate body tries to compensate inadequate oxygen in the blood. Restlessness results from inadequate oxygenation to the brain. Wheezing and hypotension are not associated with low oxygen level. Cyanosis is associated with the low oxygenation but diminished breath sounds are not always connected to low oxygenation. Tachypnea and tachycardia are related to low oxygenation, not bradypnea and bradycardia.

96. C. In metabolic acidosis pH will be low, $PaCO_2$ will be normal, HCO_3 and base excess will be low. Here HCO_3 value is below normal, which is consistent with metabolic acidosis. Other values are within normal range.

97. D. The patient's pH value is high (7.48), indicating alkalosis. The HCO_3 value is also high, which suggests alkalosis. The $PaCO_2$ value is normal (40 mm Hg), indicating absence of respiratory compensation. These ABG values eliminate other options.

98. B. Low oxygen level in the blood (hypoxemia) is evident from the extremely low blood gas value. pH value of 7.35 is normal, so this value does not suggest alkalosis or acidosis. $PaCO_2$ value is also normal (42 mm Hg), so hypercapnia is also not present.

99. B. The normal pH value of arterial blood ranges from 7.35-7.45. A pH of less than 7.35 is considered to be acidosis and a pH of more than 7.45 indicates alkalosis.

100. A. Dysfunction of lung parenchyma, e.g. pulmonary edema, pulmonary embolism, pneumonia, etc. may lead to acute respiratory failure by interfering with ventilation. Pulmonary tuberculosis, a chronic disease usually not associated with acute respiratory failure. Cervical spinal cord injury, not thoracic spinal cord injury can affect respiratory muscles and cause respiratory failure. Metabolic disorder, e.g. hypothyroidism, not hyperthyroidism decreases respiratory drive and may cause acute respiratory failure.

101. B. Severe hypoxia after smoke inhalation is typically related to acute respiratory distress syndrome. The other conditions are not typically associated with smoke inhalation.

102. A. Early manifestations of acute respiratory distress syndrome are dyspnea and tachypnea. Other manifestations include cough and restlessness. Cyanosis, diffuse crackles and rhonchi are later

manifestations of acute respiratory distress syndrome.

103. C. To promote activity tolerance in the patient, the nurse should space nursing activities. Spacing activities will diminish the amount of oxygen needed at any one time and allows the oxygen reserves to be built up during periods of rest. Asking the patient decide which activities will be performed for the day will not affect oxygen reserves. Completing all care at one time will deplete oxygen reserves. There are energy - efficient methods that could be helpful for patients to learn in performing their care. However, it is the spacing of activities that is most helpful as it allows to build up of oxygen.

104. A. Compensatory mechanism seen in clients experiencing metabolic acidosis is a deep, gasping type of respiration called Kussmaul breathing. A marked sustained inspiratory effort associated with central nervous system disorder is known as apneustic breathing. Several short breaths with apnea, seen in patients with increased intracranial pressure is known as Biot's respiration. Periods of apnea followed by gradually increasing depth of respiration is Cheyne-Stokes respiration. This type of respiration in adults is pathological, but normal in children.

105. D. Pancuronium should be given with sedation or analgesia. This paralytic agent does not affect pain sensation or anxiety levels and is very stressful to the patient if given alone. Pancuronium bromide causes tachycardia not bradycardia. The drug causes paralysis by blocking neuromuscular junction. Pancuronium bromide does not affect pain sensation or consciousness.

106. D. Pancuronium bromide is a neuromuscular blocking agent, is used for muscle relaxation and paralysis to provide more effective synchrony with the ventilator and increased oxygenation. Fighting is a sign that the patient requires another dose. Movement of arms and legs has no effect on ventilation and therefore it is not used to determine the need for another dose. Tachycardia occurs as a side effect, if given rapid IV injection. So it is not an indication for another dose.

107. B. Manual resuscitation bag should be ready at bedside, in case there is any mechanical failure with the ventilator. Since the patient does not have a chest tube or a tracheostomy, keeping water-seal drainage setup or tracheostomy cleaning kit is not necessary. Although the oxygen analyzer (pulse oximeter) may be kept to analyze the effectiveness of ventilation this equipment is less important than the manual resuscitation bag.

108. A. Most essential nursing action for a patient with endotracheal tube is to monitor proper placement of the tube every 2-4 hours, as accidental extubation is a major complication of an endotracheal tube. Nurse maintains proper tube position by confirming the exit mark on the tube which remains constant, observing symmetrical chest wall movement and auscultating bilateral breath sounds. Suctioning should not be done on a routine basis, but should be done as and when required. Other options are important but secondary.

109. D. Use of accessory muscles of respiration during breathing indicates dyspnea or difficulty in breathing. Rapid breathing indicates increased need of oxygen. Pursed lip breathing and diaphragmatic breathing are two controlled breathing by which patients conserve energy.

110. D. Acute respiratory distress syndrome results from increased pulmonary capillary permeability leading to a noncardiogenic pulmonary edema. ARDS does not result from rapid administration of intravenous fluid within a short time, left heart failure or acute renal failure.

111. B. Inspection of mucous membrane for the detection of cyanosis is more reliable for a dark-skinned individual, since skin color does not affect the mucous membrane. The lips, nail beds and ear lobes are less reliable indicator of cyanosis since they are affected by skin color.

112. D. Endotracheal suctioning removes oxygen lowering the partial pressure of arterial oxygen causing hypoxemia. Hypoxemia results in myocardial hypoxia. Myocardial hypoxia; vagal stimulation caused by tracheal irritation; and increased sympathetic nervous stimulation caused by anxiety, discomfort or pain gives rise to arrhythmia. Hyperventilation and hyperoxygenation prevents this condition. Atelectasis is not caused due to endotracheal suctioning. Tracheal mucosal damage may be prevented by avoiding excessive suction pressure, gentle catheter insertion and not by hyperventilation and hyperoxygenation. Pneumothorax is not associated with endotracheal suctioning.

113. C. Normal capillary perfusion is estimated at 30 mm Hg to ensure adequate tracheal perfusion, cuff pressure is maintained at 20-25 mm Hg.

114. A. The patient should withheld aspirin containing drugs or nonsteroidal anti-inflammatory drugs to reduce the risk of bleeding during and after surgery. Patient need not withheld food and fluids 8 hours prior operation as the surgery is usually done by using local anesthesia combined with mild sedation.

115. C. Patient with epistaxis should be instructed to avoid vigorous nose blowing and strenuous activity. Patient should also avoid aspirin containing products or NSAIDs. Anterior packing should remain in place for 48-72 hours and should not be removed by the patient after 24 hours.

116. D. The most important action in managing allergic rhinitis involves identifying and avoiding triggers of allergic reactions. In order to do so the patient should be instructed to keep a diary of times when the allergic episode occurs and the activities those precipitate it, so that steps can then be taken to prevent it. Corticosteroid nasal spray should be taken on a regular basis and not just for prophylactic purpose. Decongestant nasal sprays should not be used for more than 3 days. Patient need to take oral antihistamine as prescribed for the relief of symptoms together with regular use of corticosteroid spray.

117. D. The patient may be instructed to adopt any or all of the options for the cleaning of nasal passages and promotion of drainage. Other interventions which may promote drainage are optimum hydration and use of drugs, e.g. decongestant and mucolytics as prescribed.

118. D. Chronic pharyngitis is common in adults, who work or live in dusty environment, use the voice to excess, habitually use tobacco and alcohol and suffer from chronic cough.

119. C. Chronic granular pharyngitis is also known as clergyman's sore throat. This type of pharyngitis is characterized by numerous swollen lymph follicles on the pharyngeal wall. Hypertrophic pharyngitis is characterized by general thickening and congestion of the pharyngeal mucous membrane and atrophic pharyngitis is characterized by a membrane that is thin, whitish, glistening and at times wrinkled.

120. B. Obstructive sleep apnea is characterized by the lack of airflow due to pharyngeal occlusion. Types of sleep apnea do not include a simple characterization. Central sleep apnea is characterized by simultaneous cessation of both airflow and respiratory movements and mixed sleep apnea is characterized by a combination of central and obstructive sleep apnea within one apneic episode.

121. B. Patients with obstructive sleep apnea are at increased risk of developing dysrhythmia. The other complications that may occur are myocardial infarction, stroke and systemic hypertension not hypotention. Respiratory alkalosis which may occur due to hyperventilation is not associated with sleep apnea. Patient with sleep apnea develop hypercapnia (increased partial pressure of carbon dioxide). Pulmonary hypertension not pulmonary edema may develop in sleep apnea.

122. D. The diagnostic test carried out to diagnose obstructive sleep apnea is polysomnography or sleep test. The test is conducted in a sleep disorder clinic where overnight electroencephalography (EEG), electro-oculography (EOG) and electromyography (EMG) with surface electrodes are taken. The test may also include recording of arterial oxygen saturation, airflow measurement and status of heart by ECG. So the test detects the status of cardiopulmonary system of the patient during an episode of sleep. Barium swallow cannot visualize the obstruction which occurs during sleep. Electrocardiography and electroencephalography as a part of polysomnography is diagnostic not when the patient is awake.

123. A. Patient with mild obstructive sleep apnea may respond to simple measures, e.g. reducing extra weight, avoiding sedatives and alcoholic beverages for 3-4 hours before sleep. High protein diet before sleep has sedative action, so need to avoid it. Taking a nap during daytime does not help, as obstructive sleep apnea may occur during daytime also.

124. D. Tracheostomy button is used during weaning as an intermediate measure between using a standard tracheostomy tube and extubation. A button is a short, straight tracheostomy tube that fits into the stoma of a tracheostomy but is not deep enough to enter the tracheal lumen. It has a removable cap with a one-way flap inside that permits inhalation but not exhalation. When the cap is on, the patient can talk. Metal tracheostomy tubes are reusable after sterilization. It does not help in weaning. Fenestrated tracheostomy tubes have an inner cannula that has large opening or several small ones. Used during weaning of a mechanically ventilated patient. Communi-Trach tube allows speech by coordination of phonation efforts.

125. C. Tracheostomy tube should be changed 3-4 weeks or once a month.

If the patient is at risk of recurrent tracheobronchial infection the tube may be changed more frequently.

126. C. The most important nursing goal in caring for a patient who has recently undergone a tracheostomy is to maintain a patent airway. Pain is not a major problem after tracheostomy. Other options are also important but have low priority than keeping the airway patent.

127. B. Tracheal site is a portal of entry for microorganisms. Sterile technique must be used while performing tracheostomy care. High Fowler's position promotes maximum ventilation of the lungs. The canula is generally cleaned with hydrogen peroxixde and saline.

128. D. After discovering an air leak nurse should check for insufficient air in the cuff which is the most common cause of air leak. Physician should not be called first until the nurse checks and correct the problem. The cuff cannot be changed or removed. If required the total tube has to be changed. Adding more air in the leaking cuff may lead to problems of more cuff pressure.

129. D. A tracheostomy tube with an inflated foam cuff does not allow speech in patient using it. The tracheostomy tubes in other options allow speech.

130. B. Cuff pressure which would prevent excessive pressure on tracheal capillaries is less than 20 mm Hg or 25 cm H_2O. Less than this would cause aspiration and more than this would cause tracheal damage. Cuff pressure must be monitored every 8 hourly not every 2-3 days.

131. B. The primary etiologic agent in laryngeal cancer is cigarette smoking. 3 out of 4 patients who develop laryngeal cancer have smoked or currently smoke. Other risk factors of laryngeal cancer include occupational exposure to asbestos, mustard gas, wood dust, tar products, etc. Nutritional deficiencies especially riboflavin deficiency, chronic laryngitis and familial predisposition may also play a part, but are not considered to be primary etiological agent.

132. C. Tracheoesophageal puncture is the most widely used procedure for alaryngeal communication. The reason for its wide use is that the speech associated with this procedure resembles normal speech and is easily learned. Esophageal speech is difficult to learn, takes a long time to be proficient, and the success rate is low. The electric larynx is used as temporary measure when esophageal speech is not successful or until the technique is not mastered.

133. C. Wound breakdown is due to infection, poor wound healing or development of a fistula, or as a result of radiation therapy, can create a serious life-threatening emergency. The carotid artery, which is close to the stoma, may rupture from erosion if the wound does not heal properly. Pulmonary embolism is a complication of immobility. Pneumonia may occur in any postoperative patient. Hypoxia may occur as complication after laryngectomy which may require immediate intervention but not life-threatening.

134. D. Family members are reluctant to talk with the patient as the patient cannot speak. To promote a supportive environment the nurse should encourage family members to continue normal communication. Patient should be encouraged to drink at least 3 liters of fluid daily to keep the secretion liquid. Patient should take a well balanced diet. Cleaning of tracheostomy wound should be done by hydrogen peroxide, followed by rinsing with normal saline. Tracheostomy wound should not be cleaned with absolute alcohol which will cause tissue irritation and breakdown.

135. B. In chronic tonsillitis patient suffers from recurrent sore throat. Tonsils are enlarged and infected. Treatment of choice is surgical removal of tonsils. Surgery is contraindicated during acute tonsillar infection. Antibiotics are used to subside acute infection. Patient with chronic tonsillitis needs repeated antibiotic therapy, and in order to avoid repeated antibiotic therapy and suffering of the patient surgery should be done. Steroids are not used, as they will flare-up the infection. Saline throat irrigations give temporary relief from pain and discomfort. It is not a curative treatment.

136. D. The patient and the family members must be taught the sign and symptoms of bleeding and they should be instructed to report any bleeding to the physician. Patients are instructed to take alkaline mouthwashes or warm saline mouthwashes, not hot throat irrigations to combat halitosis that may occur after tonsillectomy. Aspirin is contraindicated because of risk of bleeding. Mild analgesic, e.g. acetaminophen with/without codeine may be taken. Generalized throat pain, sore throat giving rise to difficulty in talking may occur 7-10 days postoperatively.

4 CHAPTER

Gastrointestinal System and Nutrition

Q1. All of the following methods may be employed to determine the proper placement of an enteral tube *except*:

A. Observing the fluid that is removed through aspiration
B. Visualizing the gastric area by X-ray
C. Injecting air into the feeding tube and listening with stethoscope for the sound
D. Palpating over the epigastric region following the injection of 100 mL of air into the tube

Q2. The most accurate assessment for correct placement of the nasogastric tube tip is:

A. pH paper test of the fluid removed from the feeding tube
B. Visualizing the gastric area by radiography
C. Observing the gastric aspirate
D. Auscultation over the gastric area for the sound of air after injecting air into the feeding tube

Q3. Enteral feeds can be delivered into the:

A. Stomach only
B. Small intestine only
C. Stomach and small intestine
D. Anywhere in the gastrointestinal tract

Q4. Which of the following is the recommended enteral access placement for a patient with high-risk of aspiration during enteral feeding?

A. Esophageal
B. Gastric
C. Postpyloric
D. Any of the above

Q5. Gastric acid stimulation test has been conducted for a patient. The results of the test showed a markedly increased level of gastric secretion. The nurse anticipates that the patient may be suffering from:

A. Pernicious anemia
B. Gastric cancer
C. Gastric ulcer
D. Zollinger-Ellison syndrome

Q6. All of the following factors may influence obesity *except*:

A. Genetics
B. Socioeconomics
C. Gender
D. Sedentary lifestyle

Q7. Obesity is commonly determined by measuring:

A. Body weight
B. Circumference measurement
C. Frame size
D. Body mass index

Q8. Which of the following categories of drugs is used in the treatment of obesity?

A. Appetite suppressing drugs
B. Satiety inhibiting drugs
C. Nutrient absorption – blocking drugs
D. A and C only

Q9. A woman with morbid obesity has been prescribed orlistat one tablet twice before meal. The nurse understands that the drug reduces obesity by:

A. Decreasing absorption of simple sugars in the intestine
B. Decreasing starch breakdown and absorption in the intestine
C. Decreasing fat breakdown and absorption in the intestine
D. A and B only

Q10. The nurse is teaching a 40-year-old obese woman who has been prescribed orlistat by the physician. Which of the following statements indicates the need for further teaching?

A. 'I should not modify the dose of the drug on my own'
B. 'I need to take vitamin supplements regularly as prescribed by the physician'
C. 'I may experience flatulence during the course of treatment by this drug'
D. 'I feel relieved because I do not need to exercise any more'

Q11. Which of the following symptoms is not a characteristic manifestation of anorexia nervosa?

A. Menorrhagia
B. Hypotension
C. Pallor
D. Constipation

Q12. Which of the clinical manifestations is a characteristic feature of bulimia nervosa?

A. Episodes of binge eating and purging (vomiting)
B. Loss of body weight
C. Common among middle aged woman
D. Sensitivity to cold

Q13. Which of the following methods of administration is used in gastric feeding?

A. Bolus
B. Continuous
C. Intermittent
D. All of the above

Q14. Which of the following methods of administration is the desired choice for intestinal feeding?

A. Bolus
B. Intermittent
C. Continuous
D. Any of the above

Q15. Which of the following methods is the best way to prevent dental caries?

A. To brush and floss regularly
B. Eat a diet high in simple carbohydrates
C. Regular visits to dentist for examination, cleaning and treatment of dental caries
D. A and C only

Q16. A nurse is teaching a patient who had a tooth extraction regarding postoperative care. Which of the following statements by the patient indicates further teaching?

A. 'I need to report to the dentist if the bleeding continues for more than an hour'
B. 'I need to take soft foods and avoid hot and cold foods'
C. 'I need to brush my teeth after each meal'
D. 'I need to gently rinse my mouth with normal saline several times a day for a few days'

Q17. Which of the following conditions is less likely to cause stomatitis?

A. Nutritional disorders
B. Chemotherapy
C. Heart failure
D. Allergies

Q18. Which of the following is the major risk factor of candidiasis of oral cavity?

A. Poor oral hygiene
B. Long-term use of antibiotics
C. Malnutrition
D. Smoking

Q19. Which of the following conditions is caused by an acute bacterial infection of the gingiva?

A. Aphthous stomatitis
B. Herpes simplex stomatitis
C. Vincent's angina
D. Oral candidiasis

Q20. The nurse explains to a patient with Vincent's angina that the treatment of the condition will include:

A. Viscous lidocaine rinses
B. Application of topical antibiotics
C. Consuming lot of fibrous foods
D. All of the above

Q21. Which of the following etiological factors is responsible for the occurrence of leukoplakia in oral cavity?

A. Malnutrition
B. Smoking and chewing tobacco
C. Broken teeth
D. All of the above

Q22. The nurse is teaching a group of young men regarding prevention of oral cancer. Which of the following she should include in her teaching?

A. Avoid use of tobacco in any form
B. Avoid drinking carbonated beverages
C. Avoid too much of fibrous foods
D. Avoid commercial mouthwashes

Q23. Which of the following is the most common type of oral cancer?

A. Basal cell carcinoma
B. Squamous cell carcinoma
C. Adenocarcinoma
D. None of the above

Q24. Teletherapy is a common method of treatment of oral cancer. In teletherapy:

A. An external beam of radiation passes through the skin or mucous membrane to the tumor
B. An internal beam of radiation passes through the skin or mucous membrane to the tumor
C. Light waves passes through the skin or mucous membrane to the tumor
D. Laser waves passes through the skin or mucous membrane to the tumor

Q25. The nurse is taking care of a patient with oral cancer scheduled for surgery. Which of the following nursing diagnosis is appropriate?

A. Ineffective airway clearance related to obstruction by the tumor
B. Activity intolerance due to weakness and fatigue
C. Social isolation related to disease or change in appearance
D. All of the above

Q26. The nurse is taking care of a patient who has undergone surgery for oral cancer. Which of the following nursing intervention is most important?

A. Providing wound care
B. Monitoring for bleeding
C. Maintaining the airway
D. Providing adequate nutrition

Q27. Inflammation of the parotid gland (parotitis) is a frequent complication in postoperative patients. Which of the following interventions is not appropriate to prevent parotitis?

A. Administering frequent oral hygiene
B. Administering a lot of fluid

C. Ask the patient to chew sugarless gum to stimulate saliva secretion
D. Ask the patient to chew hard sugar candy on frequent interval

Q28. Which of the following is not a common symptom of esophageal disorders?

A. Dysphagia
B. Nausea
C. Pain
D. Heartburn

Q29. The nurse is taking care of a patient who has undergone endoscopy for upper gastrointestinal tract. Which of the following nursing interventions for this patient is appropriate?

A. Instructing the patient to lie on his right side
B. Auscultating abdomen for the presence of bowel sounds
C. Administering analgesics for pain
D. Withholding food and fluids until gag reflex returns

Q30. Physician has advised barium swallow to a patient. The nurse should:

A. Ask the patient about allergies to sea food
B. Administer only clear liquid diet 8-12 hours before the test
C. Ensure a laxative is ordered after the test
D. Tell patient that the stool may be black up to 72 hours after the test

Q31. The nurse is teaching a family member of the patient with gastrostomy about the technique of feeding. Which of the following instructions is appropriate?

A. Instill water before administering feed in order to ensure that the tube is in proper place
B. Instill water after administering feed.
C. Place the patient in supine position during entire feeding
D. Warm the feed 10°F above the room temperature

Q32. Which of the following conditions is characterized by impaired motility of distal esophagus accompanied by failure of the lower esophageal sphincter to relax?

A. Diffuse spasm
B. Achalasia
C. Gastroesophageal reflux disease
D. Barrett's esophagus

Q33. A patient with achalasia has undergone a pneumatic dilation. Which of the following the nurse should monitor?

A. Pulse and blood pressure
B. Fever and abdominal tenderness
C. Persistent pain and dysphagia
D. All of the above

Q34. The occurrence of reflux in gastroesophageal reflux disease is due to:

A. Altered nerve innervation in the region of the gastroesophageal junction resulting in low pressure in the region
B. Displacement of the angle of the gastroesophageal junction
C. An incompetent lower esophageal sphincter
D. All of the above

Q35. Physician has prescribed metoclopramide (reglan) to a patient with gastroesophageal reflux disease (GERD). The nurse teaches the patient about this medication. Which one is not appropriate?

A. This will increase peristalsis of upper gastrointestinal tract
B. This increases gastrointestinal secretions and thus promotes digestion
C. The medicine to be taken half hour before meals and at bedtime
D. Avoid driving or other hazardous activities

Q36. Which of the following surgical procedures is done for the treatment of gastroesophageal reflux disease that

is unrelieved by conservative management?

A. Esophagomyotomy
B. Fundoplication
C. Pneumatic dilation of lower end of esophagus
D. None of the above

Q37. The nurse is teaching a patient who had undergone fundoplication for gastroesophageal reflux disease during discharge. Which of the following teaching is not appropriate?

A. To stop all anti-reflux medication
B. To avoid being overweight
C. To limit smoking, caffeine, chocolate and high fat foods
D. To avoid lifting, straining, bending and tight and constricting clothing

Q38. Which of the following is the most common type of hiatal hernia?

A. Sliding or rolling
B. Sliding or axial
C. Rolling or paraesophageal
D. Axial or paraesophageal

Q39. Which of the following factors is responsible for the development of hiatal hernia?

A. Weakness and dilation of the cardiac end of stomach
B. Muscular weakness of the diaphragm around the esophagogastric opening
C. Increase in intrathoracic pressure
D. Dilation of gastroesophageal sphincter

Q40. Which of the following health promotion behavior may prevent or delay the development of hiatal hernia?

A. Consuming adequate fibrous diet to prevent constipation
B. Avoiding extremely hot or cold foods
C. Avoiding wearing constricting clothing around the waist
D. All of the above

Q41. The most common symptom of a sliding hiatal hernia is:

A. Feeling of fullness
B. Difficulty in breathing
C. Gastroesophageal reflux
D. All of the above

Q42. In order to reduce the discomfort associated with hiatal hernia the patient should be taught to:

A. Lie down in bed for 30 minutes after meals
B. Drink a glass of water after meals
C. Drink a glass of water before meals
D. Rest in a sitting position for at least 30 minutes after meals.

Q43. Which is the most common surgical procedure for patient with hiatal hernia who does not respond with conservative management?

A. Nissen fundoplication
B. Hill operation
C. Belsey operation
D. Insertion of angelchik prosthesis

Q44. Regurgitation, halitosis and sour taste in the mouth are manifestations of which of the following conditions?

A. Achalasia
B. Gastroesophageal reflux
C. Hiatal hernia
D. Esophageal diverticula

Q45. All of the following conditions can stimulate the emetic center *except*:

A. Distention of stomach
B. Action of chlorpromazine
C. Pain
D. Increased intracranial pressure

Q46. Which of the following forms of chronic gastritis is associated with pernicious anemia?

A. Superficial gastritis
B. Atrophic gastritis
C. Hypertrophic gastritis
D. All of the above

Q47. A patient's gastric analysis test reveals excess secretion of gastric acid. The nurse would suspect which of the following diagnosis?

A. Duodenal ulcer
B. Gastric ulcer
C. Gastric cancer
D. Chronic atrophic gastritis

Q48. A nurse is assessing a patient with duodenal ulcer. Which of the following findings she is not expected to find?

A. Pain 2-3 hours after eating
B. Melena
C. Weight loss
D. Epigastric tenderness

Q49. Which of the following symptoms indicate gastric ulcer?

A. Patient experiences abdominal pain at night
B. Vomiting may relieve abdominal pain
C. Abdominal pain may lessen with eating
D. Pain occurs when the stomach is empty

Q50. Which of the following persons is more likely to develop chronic gastritis?

A. A 25-year-old lady teacher
B. A middle aged man with *Helicobacter pylori* infection
C. A college student on metronidazole therapy for amoebiasis
D. A 40-year-old lady with gallbladder disease

Q51. The nurse is assessing nutritional status of a patient with chronic gastritis. Which of the following findings she should expect?

A. Weight gain
B. Dry scaly skin
C. Macrocytic anemia
D. Bleeding tendencies

Q52. A patient has been admitted with acute gastritis. Which of the following assessment findings will indicate that the patient is bleeding from the stomach?

A. Clay colored stool
B. Black tarry stools
C. Stool with frank bleeding
D. Coffee ground like stool

Q53. A patient diagnosed with peptic ulcer has been prescribed with a therapeutic regimen that includes cessation of smoking, small frequent diets, antacids and famotidine. The patient asks the nurse how famotidine helps. The nurse's best response is:

A. It helps in formation of a protective covering on the ulcer and thus promotes healing
B. It helps in neutralizing the excessive gastric acid produced in this disorder
C. It reduces hydrochloric acid secretion by blocking vagal stimulation
D. It reduces hydrochloric acid secretion by blocking the action of histamine on the H_2 receptors and decreases conversion of pepsinogen to pepsin

Q54. Physician has prescribed tablet ranitidine (rantac) to a patient with erosive esophagitis. Nurse teaches patient to take the medicine:

A. Before breakfast
B. Before lunch
C. Before dinner
D. At bedtime

Q55. The nurse is teaching a patient with peptic ulcer regarding self-care. Which of the following instructions she should include?

A. Limit smoking and caffeinated drinks
B. Eat three bland meals
C. Continue drugs till you are symptom free
D. Avoid taking over-the-counter drugs unless prescribed by the physician

Q56. Physician has prescribed omeprazole for a patient for 4 weeks. Nurse understands that this medicine is given to treat:

A. Constipation
B. Abdominal distention
C. Heartburn
D. Burning micturition

Q57. Which of the following medications represents the category of proton pump inhibitors?

A. Ranitidine
B. Pantoprazole
C. Sucralfate
D. Clarithromycin

Q58. Physician prescribes sucralfate to a patient with gastric ulcer. The nurse teaches the patient to take the medicine:

A. With meals
B. Before meals
C. At bedtime
D. 1 hour before meals and at bedtime.

Q59. The nurse taking care of a patient with duodenal ulcer is aware that the patient is at high-risk of injury related to perforation. Which of the following sign and symptoms would indicate the possibility of perforation?

A. Soft, large, distended abdomen
B. Sudden, sharp, severe pain
C. Borborygmi
D. Decreased pulse rate and raised blood pressure

Q60. A patient with recurrent peptic ulcer disease is to undergo a Billroth I procedure. Preoperatively the nurse explains to the patient that Billroth I procedure involves:

A. Cutting the right and left vagus nerves and widening the pyloric end of stomach
B. Removal of entire antrum of the stomach and anastomosis of the remaining portion of the stomach to the duodenum
C. Removal of the distal portion of the stomach and proximal ramnants is anastomosed with duodenum
D. Removal of the distal portion of the stomach and proximal ramnants is anastomosed with jejunum

Q61. A patient who had undergone a subtotal gastrectomy returned to the ward with a nasogastric tube to decompress the remaining portion of the stomach. Which of the following nursing interventions is appropriate to take care of the nasogastric tube and prevent it from clogging?

A. Check tube periodically for its proper placement and reposition whenever needed
B. Apply suction every hourly and clamp the tube in between suction
C. Increase the suction level if the tube is found to be not draining
D. Gently irrigate the tube with normal saline if it is found to be clogged

Q62. A patient who has undergone Billroth I procedure, experiences cramping abdominal pain, weakness, tachycardia, and dizziness after meals. The nurse understands that the patient is experiencing dumping syndrome which is caused by:

A. A slow passage of food through stomach into small intestine
B. A rapid passage of liquid food mixture into the small intestine
C. A rapid passage of hyperosmolar fluid mixture into the small intestine
D. Rapid passage of hypoosmolar fluid into the small intestine

Q63. The nurse is teaching a patient who is complaining of dumping syndrome after gastric resection regarding modification

of diet. Which of the following instructions is most appropriate?

- **A.** Eat three regular meals a day
- **B.** Take a high protein, high fat, and low carbohydrate diet
- **C.** Decrease fat content in the diet
- **D.** Increase carbohydrate content in the diet

Q64. Maintaining which of the following precautions may minimize distressing symptoms of dumping syndrome?

- **A.** Drink fluids only with meals
- **B.** Avoid fluids 2 hours before meals
- **C.** Drink fluids only before meals
- **D.** Lying down for 1 hour after meals

Q65. A patient attends hospital with the complains of epigastric fullness, pain, distention, nausea, vomiting and anorexia. Past medical history reveals repeated ulceration and healing of ulcers distal to the pyloric sphincter. The nurse suspects:

- **A.** Peptic ulcer perforation
- **B.** Acute gastritis
- **C.** Pyloric obstruction
- **D.** Paralytic ileus

Q66. Which of the following statements best describes Crohn's disease?

- **A.** A chronic nonspecific inflammatory bowel disorder
- **B.** An inflammation and ulceration of colon and rectum
- **C.** An inflamed outpouching of the intestine
- **D.** An erosion of the intestinal mucosa

Q67. Which of the following section of the bowel is mostly affected in Crohn's disease?

- **A.** Rectum and sigmoid colon
- **B.** Entire colon
- **C.** Terminal ileum
- **D.** Duodenum

Q68. A patient has been admitted to the hospital with Crohn's disease. During assessment which of the following symptoms the nurse is expected to find?

- **A.** Bloating and flatulence
- **B.** Diarrhea and abdominal pain
- **C.** Jaundice and steatorrhea (fatty stools)
- **D.** Halitosis and sour taste in the mouth

Q69. Which of the following pathophysiological changes found in Crohn's disease?

- **A.** Out pouching of the intestinal wall
- **B.** Atrophy and fattening of the intestinal villi
- **C.** Diffuse ulceration involving mucosa and submucosa of intestinal wall
- **D.** Discontinuous, deep longitudinal ulceration involving all layers of intestinal wall

Q70. The most conclusive diagnostic study for Crohn's disease is:

- **A.** Stool examination
- **B.** Barium study of the upper gastrointestinal tract
- **C.** Serum chemistries
- **D.** Abdominal X-ray

Q71. Which of the following intestinal disorders is responsible for fistula formation as complication?

- **A.** Chronic gastroenteritis
- **B.** Ulcerative colitis
- **C.** Crohn's disease
- **D.** Appendicitis

Q72. All of the following systemic disorders may occur in a patient with Crohn's disease *except*:

- **A.** Arthritis
- **B.** Erythema nodosum
- **C.** Malnutrition
- **D.** Toxic megacolon

Q73. Which of the following interventions should be included in the medical management of Crohn's disease?

- **A.** Restricting fluids and fibers
- **B.** Administering antidiarrheal agents

C. Providing cold food
D. Encouraging activity

Q74. A 25-year-old young woman with Crohn's disease is being treated with corticosteroid. Which of the following findings would indicate that the corticosteroid therapy has been effective?

A. Increase in body weight
B. Increase in the bulk of the stool
C. Moon face
D. Decreased complaints of abdominal pain

Q75. A 30-year-old patient is admitted with a possible diagnosis of ulcerative colitis for investigation. Which of the following statements about ulcerative colitis is true?

A. Bloody diarrhea is the most major symptoms
B. Occurs anywhere along the gastrointestinal tract in characteristic skip lesion
C. Heredity is believed to be a factor for development of the disease
D. Transmural inflammation with fistula formation often occurs in patients with ulcerative colitis

Q76. A patient with ulcerative colitis has undergone total proctocolectomy with continent ileostomy. During teaching to the patient the nurse should emphasize which of the following instructions?

A. Increasing fluid intake to prevent dehydration
B. Wearing an appliance all time over the stoma
C. Consuming a high fiber diet
D. To report if he experiences dumping syndrome

Q77. A patient admitted with exacerbation of ulcerative colitis complains of bloody diarrhea. The patient is very much afraid and apprehensive. Which of the following nursing interventions is appropriate?

A. Send the patient's stools for the presence of occult blood
B. Instruct the patient to keep a record of the number and description of stools
C. Inform the patient's physician immediately
D. Explain to the patient that blood in the stools is expected in this condition

Q78. A 30-year-old patient with ulcerative colitis is advised mesalazine for the maintenance of resistance. The nurse explains to the patient that the principal purpose of this medication is to:

A. Decrease gastrointestinal motility
B. Suppress immune response
C. Suppress inflammation of the bowel wall
D. Increase bowel tone

Q79. Physician has prescribed prednisone to a patient with exacerbation of colitis. The nurse explains to the patient that this drug will:

A. Protect the patient from getting an infection
B. Help the patient to gain body weight
C. Achieve remission but will not cure the disease
D. Cure the disease with long term use

Q80. The nurse is assessing a patient who underwent colostomy 24 hours ago. Which of the following findings should the nurse immediately report to the surgeon?

A. Stoma appears red in color
B. Stoma appears dusky blue in color
C. Stoma is slightly edematous
D. Slight oozing from the stoma when touched

Q81. The nurse taking care of a patient with colostomy instructs the patient to take care of the skin around stoma by:

A. Avoiding the use of soap or irritating agents

B. Clean the stoma and surrounding skin with hydrogen peroxide
C. Clean the stoma and surrounding skin with mild soap and water and apply a skin barrier
D. Clean the stoma and surrounding skin with plain water and dry thoroughly

Q82. Patient having left sided colostomy is expected to have:

A. Liquid stool
B. Semisolid stool
C. Formed stool
D. Dry and hard stool

Q83. The nurse is teaching a patient with sigmoid colostomy the ways to regain control of bowel movement. Which of the following is appropriate?

A. Take a balanced diet with adequate fiber
B. Irrigate the stoma daily at a scheduled time
C. Take a soft low residue diet
D. Take at least 3 liters of fluid daily

Q84. The nurse is preparing a 30-year-old male patient with ulcerative colitis, scheduled for a permanent ileostomy. Which of the following statements is appropriate as preoperartive instruction?

A. 'You will have one normal bowel movement per day'
B. 'Liquid stool will drain constantly in the bag attached to the stoma'
C. 'You will be taught how to drain liquid stool at regular intervals with a catheter'
D. 'You will be taught how to irrigate your bowel through the stoma'

Q85. A patient with ulcerative colitis who is unresponsive to prescribed pharmacologic treatment is admitted for a total colectomy with permanent ileostomy. Which of the following nursing actions should the nurse give priority?

A. Teaching the patient about the ostomy care
B. To refer the patient to ostomy association
C. Correcting the patient's fluid and electrolyte imbalance
D. Teaching deep breathing and coughing exercises to be performed postoperatively

Q86. Which of the following statements regarding cancer of the colon is true?

A. Cancer of the colon is usually detected in early stage.
B. It occurs mostly in women.
C. It tends to remain localize
D. Most of the incidences of intestinal obstructions are due to cancer colon.

Q87. Which of the following persons is at high-risk of developing colorectal cancer?

A. A 30-year-old man suffering from familial polyposis
B. A 30-year-old lady with hemorrhoid
C. A 35-year-old man with chronic peptic ulcer disease
D. A 25-year-old man suffering from diarrheal disease

Q88. Which of the following food items should be avoided by a patient with ileostomy to prevent potential obstruction in ileostomy?

A. Eggs
B. Onions
C. Coffee
D. Nuts

Q89. The nurse is caring for a young patient in the immediate postoperative period following a ileostomy for ulcerative colitis. To which of the following nursing diagnoses would she give priority?

A. Pain at the operated site
B. Risk for fluid volume deficit
C. Risk for impaired skin integrity
D. Disturbed body image

Q90. A patient has been admitted in the hospital with gastroenteritis. During assessment the nurse is expected to find:

A. Hypoactive bowel sounds
B. Hyperactive bowel sounds

C. Rigid and board like abdomen
D. Rebound tenderness

Q91. A patient attends hospital with the complain of diarrhea, abdominal pain and cramping. During abdominal assessment which of the following sequences the nurse should follow?

A. Inspection, palpation, percussion, auscultation
B. Inspection, percussion, auscultation, palpation
C. Inspection, auscultation, palpation, percussion
D. Inspection, auscultation, percussion, palpation

Q92. A patient with gastroenteritis is admitted to hospital with severe dehydration and electrolyte imbalance. Diagnostic test reveals vibrio cholera as the cause of gastroenteritis. The nurse is aware that:

A. Enteric precaution must be maintained
B. The patient is to be vaccinated against cholera
C. The disease transmission takes place from living in a over crowded place
D. The patient is to be treated by an antiviral drug

Q93. A patient is being treated with diphenoxylate hydrochloride with atropine sulfate (lomotil) for acute exacerbation of chronic functional diarrhea. In order to assess the effectiveness of therapy the nurse assesses the patient's:

A. Anxiety
B. Frequency of bowel movements
C. Skin turgor
D. Abdominal pain

Q94. Physician has prescribed lomotil (diphenoxylate with atropine) to a patient. The nurse explains about the medication to the patient. Which of the following is appropriate?

A. Insomnia may occur while on this medicine.
B. It is usually prescribed in infectious diarrhea.
C. It should be taken as prescribed for a limited period of time as it may form habit.
D. Laxative should be taken while on this drug.

Q95. Loperamide (Imodium) is prescribed for the treatment of:

A. Abdominal cramps
B. Amoebic dysentery
C. Diarrhea
D. Abdominal distention

Q96. A patient attends hospital clinic with the complain of diarrhea and abdominal cramps. The physician suspects amoebiasis and orders for stool examination. The nurse anticipates that the stool examination will reveal infection of the bowel by:

A. *Giardia lambia*
B. *Entamoeba hystolytica*
C. Coli
D. Enterobius

Q97. A patient on metronidazole therapy for intestinal amoebiasis complains to the nurse that he is having skin rash and feeling feverish. Nurse's response should be:

A. It is a harmless side effect of the drug.
B. Apply some antiseptic lotion after bath.
C. Report to the physician,
D. Discontinue medication.

Q98. Patient taking metronidazole reports dark colored urine. Nurse's advice should be:

A. You need to increase fluid intake
B. Report to the physician
C. Discontinue medication and report to the physician
D. It is a usual and harmless side effect of the medicine

Q99. Diverticulosis is described as:

A. Multiple noninflamed outpouching of the mucosa through the circular smooth muscle of the intestine

B. An inflamed outpouching of the mucosa through the circular smooth muscle of the intestine

C. Partial impairment of the forward flow of intestinal content due to weakness of the intestinal musculature

D. Complete obstruction in the forward flow of the intestinal content due to twisting of the bowel in the abdominal cavity

Q100. Nursing intervention for a patient with acute diverticulitis will include:

A. Providing bed rest and oral fluids

B. Providing bed rest, oral fluids and stool softeners

C. Administering intravenous fluids and broad spectrum antibiotics as ordered

D. Encouraging high fiber diet, oral fluids and laxatives

Q101. A 18-year-old boy has been admitted in the emergency ward with acute abdominal pain. Physician suspects acute appendicitis and palpates abdomen of the patient for the presence of Rovsing's sign. Rovsing's sign is present when:

A. Patient feels pain and tenderness at McBurney's point

B. Patient feels pain in the left lower quadrant on palpation of the right lower quadrant

C. Patient feels pain in the right lower quadrant on palpation of periumbilical area

D. Patient exhibits rebound tenderness on palpation of lower right quadrant

Q102. The most common cause of acute appendicitis is:

A. A fecalith

B. Kinking of the appendix

C. Tumor in the cecum

D. External occlusion of the bowel by adhesions

Q103. To increase the comfort of a patient admitted with acute appendicitis the nurse would instruct the patient:

A. To lie on his abdomen

B. To sit upright

C. To lie supine with legs stretched

D. To lie with knees flexed

Q104. A patient has undergone an emergency surgery for ruptured appendix. The nurse is assessing the patient in the postoperative ward and detects manifestations of shock. What the nurse should do?

A. Inform physician immediately

B. Prepare for a blood transfusion

C. Increase the flow of oxygen

D. Elevate head of bed at 30° angle.

Q105. All of the following conditions may precipitate hemorrhoids *except*:

A. Pregnancy

B. Diverticulosis

C. Portal hypertension

D. Heavy lifting

Q106. Which of the following symptoms is suggestive of internal hemorrhoids?

A. Itching in rectum

B. Bleeding after defecation

C. Bleeding associated with defecation

D. Intermittent pain

Q107. The nurse is preparing a patient for discharge after hemorrhoidectomy. Which of the following teachings is appropriate?

A. To eat a low residue diet for a month

B. To avoid straining during defecation

C. To take oil retention enema if constipated

D. To report to physician if symptoms reappear

Q108. A patient with irreducible hernia has been admitted for surgery. During the preoperative period nurse's priority should be:

A. Monitoring vital signs frequently.

B. Keeping the patient lying down on bed
C. Applying ice pack over the herniated area
D. Observing patient's bowel movements

Q109. The most common pathogenic mechanism involved in acute pancreatitis is:

A. Hyperplasia of pancreatic cells
B. Autoimmune inflammatory reaction of the pancreas
C. Autodigestion of the pancreas
D. Degenerative changes in the pancreas

Q110. The nurse is assessing the probable risk factors present in a patient with acute pancreatitis. Which of the following data is inappropriate?

A. History of alcohol abuse
B. History of fat intolerance
C. History of diabetes mellitus
D. History of corticosteroid use

Q111. The nurse is assessing a patient with acute pancreatitis. While reviewing the laboratory test results, which of the following laboratory values should the nurse expect to be elevated?

A. Serum cholesterol
B. Serum bilirubin
C. Serum amylase
D. Red blood cell counts

Q112. One of the important objectives of nursing management for the patient with acute pancreatitis is:

A. Controlling fluid volume excess
B. Preventing respiratory infections
C. Preventing hypercalcemia
D. All of the above

Q113. A patient with acute pancreatitis has been allowed oral feeding. The nurse plans diet, which is least stimulating to the exocrine portion of the pancreas. Which of the following diet she should plan?

A. High protein, high carbohydrate, low fat
B. High carbohydrate, low fat with fruits and vegetables
C. High carbohydrate, high protein, low fat and low residue diet
D. Small and frequent bland diet containing adequate amount of protein, fat and carbohydrate

Q114. A patient with cancer of the pancreas is scheduled for Whipple's procedure. Whipple's procedure involves:

A. Resection of proximal portion of the pancreas and duodenum and anastomosis of the pancreatic duct, bile duct and stomach to the duodenum
B. Resection of proximal portion of the pancreas, adjoining duodenum, distal portion of the stomach and common bile duct with anastomosis of the pancreatic duct, common bile duct and stomach to the jejunum
C. Resection of whole of the pancreas and the adjoining duodenum with anastomosis of the stomach, common bile duct with jejunum
D. Creating a bypass around the obstruction resulting from the tumor and joining the common bile duct to the jejunum.

Q115. Which of the following persons is at higher risk of developing cholelithiasis?

A. A 30-year-old young man with family history of cholelithiasis
B. A 20-year-old college girl who is fond of fatty foods
C. A 30-year-old young woman complaining of infertility
D. A 50-year-old woman on estrogen replacement therapy

Q116. The nurse is assessing a patient with cholelithiasis with obstruction of the common bile duct. Which of the following clinical findings she may find?

A. Yellow sclera
B. Black and fatty stools
C. Straw colored urine
D. Superficial venous thrombosis

Q117. A 55-year old lady is scheduled for laparoscopic cholecystectomy. When asked by the patient about the procedure the nurse explains that:

A. 'You will have four small punctures in your abdomen'

B. 'The stones will only be removed leaving the gallbladder as it is'

C. 'You will have a small rubber tube draining bile into a bag for a few days'

D. 'You can resume normal activities within a month after surgery'

Q118. A patient after laparoscopic cholecystectomy is complaining of gas pain. Which of the following instructions by the nurse would relieve the patient from pain and discomfort?

A. To lie down on abdomen

B. To increase fluid intake

C. To ambulate and move around

D. To take deep breaths

Q119. Dietary instructions for a patient with cholecystectomy should include:

A. To avoid poultry products

B. To include fresh fruits and vegetables

C. To eliminate fats from the diets

D. To take nutritious diet and avoid excessive fat intake

Q120. The mode of transmission of hepatitis A virus is by:

A. Sexual contact

B. Use of contaminated needles and syringes

C. Perinatal transmission

D. Contaminated food and water

Q121. The nurse is caring for a patient with hepatitis A in prodromal phase. Which of the following nursing actions is most important?

A. Maintaining skin integrity

B. Providing a high carbohydrate and low protein diet

C. Observing enteric precaution

D. Encouraging patient to increase activity gradually

Q122. A nurse is teaching a patient with hepatitis B before discharge regarding prevention of infection to family members. Which of the following instructions is appropriate?

A. Keep separate personal items like toothbrushes, safety razor and utensils

B. Have the family members vaccinated with hepatitis B vaccine (HBV)

C. Have the family members get an injection of HBIG (hepatitis B immunoglobulin)

D. Both B and C.

Q123. Which of the following conditions causes portal cirrhosis?

A. Alcohol abuse

B. Autoimmune hepatitis

C. Chronic biliary obstruction and infection

D. Chronic severe right sided heart failure

Q124. During assessment of a middle-aged woman with cirrhosis of liver, the nurse finds spider angiomas on her cheeks. The nurse is aware that the spider angiomas appear on the skin of the patients with cirrhosis is due to:

A. Pancytopenia secondary to splenomegaly

B. Increased levels of circulating estrogen

C. Decreased synthesis of blood clotting factors by the liver

D. Capillary vasodilation secondary to increased level of ammonia

Q125. The nurse is assessing a 40-year-old male patient with cirrhosis of liver. During assessment she is expected to find all of the clinical findings *except*:

A. Gynecomastia

B. Loss of axillary and pubic hair
C. Enlargement of testes
D. Loss of libido

Q126. While reviewing laboratory data of a patient with cirrhosis the nurse will anticipate an abnormally elevated value of:

A. Alanine aminotransferase (ALT)
B. Serum cholesterol
C. Serum amylase
D. Serum protein

Q127. A patient with ascites has to undergo abdominal paracentesis. To prepare the patient for the procedure the nurse instructs him to:

A. To take a light diet in the evening before the procedure
B. Evacuate bowel in the morning of the procedure
C. Empty the bladder immediately before the procedure
D. Maintain supine position during the procedure

Q128. Definitive diagnosis of cirrhosis is made from:

A. History of long-term alcohol abuse
B. Liver function test
C. Liver ultrasound
D. Liver biopsy

Q129. While caring for a patient with advanced cirrhosis the nurse finds the patient disoriented. What the nurse should do first?

A. Document her observation in nurse's record
B. Inform the physician
C. Provide a railed cot to the patient
D. Perform mental status examination

Q130. Which of the following assessment findings in a patient with advanced cirrhosis would indicate that the patient is at risk of developing hepatic coma (encephalopathy)?

A. Asterixis
B. Hyperactivity
C. Hyperthermia
D. Elevated blood urea level

Q131. A patient with hepatic encephalopathy is advised bed rest, low protein diet, laxative and enema. The nurse is aware that this treatment aims at:

A. Preventing constipation and thus prevent bleeding from hemorrhoidal varices
B. Promoting fluid loss by causing diarrhea
C. Eliminating excess sodium ions
D. Decrease ammonia production and increase ammonia excretion from the colon

Q132. A patient with advanced cirrhosis has developed esophageal varices. Which of the following nursing interventions is appropriate?

A. Observing for hemorrhage
B. Teaching deep breathing and coughing exercises
C. Encouraging adequate nutritional intake according to his choice
D. Teaching patient about varices

ANSWERS AND RATIONALES OF GASTROINTESTINAL SYSTEM AND NUTRITION

1. **D.** Palpation is not used to determine placement of a feeding tube. Injecting enough air before palpation would cause discomfort. All other methods may be employed for correct placement of the enteral tube.

2. **B.** The most accurate assessment for correct placement of a nasogastric tube is a X-ray visualization of the gastric area. With a X-ray, one actually sees if the tube is correctly positioned. Auscultation is the least reliable method and should not be used to determine the tube tip position. Observing the aspirated fluid and checking its pH is more helpful. However, aspiration should not replace a radiographic evaluation after the initial placement or when tube migration is suspected.

3. **C.** Enteral tube for enteral feeding may be placed in the stomach, duodenum and jejunum of the small intestine. Duodenum and jejunum are the major sites of digestion and absorption. So feed is not delivered beyond this point in the gastrointestinal tract.

4. **C.** A patient with high-risk of aspiration is benefited by postpyloric feeding as it reduces the chance of reflux and aspiration. Esophageal and gastric feeding may cause aspiration if not taken care of.

5. **D.** Gastric acid stimulation test is a part of gastric analysis. Gastric acid stimulation test measures the amount of gastric acid for 1 hour after subcutaneous injection of histalog or pentagastrin. A markedly elevated level of gastric secretion may indicate Zollinger-Ellison syndrome. A decreased level is usually seen in gastric ulcer, gastric cancer and pernicious anemia.

6. **C.** The causes of obesity are related to genetics and environmental factors which include socioeconomics and sedentary lifestyle, etc. It is not influenced by the age and sex of the individual.

7. **D.** Obesity is determined by ideal body weight and by body mass index which is obtained by dividing body weight in kilogram by height in meter. Ideal body weight is calculated by the use of formula based on height, weight and body frame size. So body weight or frame size alone is not enough to determine obesity. Circumference measurement, e.g. waist-to-hip ratio is another way to determine obesity, but not a very common one.

8. **D.** Drugs used for weight loss can be classified into two categories: 1) those that decrease food intake by reducing appetite and increasing satiety (sense of fullness after eating) or appetite suppressing drugs and 2) those that decrease nutrient absorption. Satiety inhibiting drugs will decrease satiety and the individual will consume increased amount of food, so is not used in the treatment of obesity.

9. **C.** Orlistat acts by blocking fat breakdown and absorption in the intestine. It inhibits the action of intestinal lipases. The undigested fat is excreted in the feces facilitating weight loss and maintenance.

10. **D.** The patient on drug therapy for obesity must be taught to continue exercise and maintain a weight

reduction diet as exercise and diet is the cornerstone of permanent weight loss. Modification of the dosages by the patient on her own is harmful. Orlistat may prevent absorption of fat-soluble vitamins and its side effects include flatulence, fecal urgency, fecal incontinence and steatorrhea.

11. A. Patients with anorexia nervosa usually manifests as amenorrhea or irregular menstruation. Dry skin, pallor, bradycardia, hypotension, intolerance to cold, and constipation are other manifestations of anorexia nervosa.

12. A. Clinical manifestations of bulimia nervosa include episodes of binge eating followed by purging (self-induced vomiting). Condition is common among young college students and in middle aged women. Persons with bulimia may have normal body weight for height, or their weight may fluctuate with bingeing and purging. Sensitivity to cold is a typical complain of anorexia nervosa and not of bulimia nervosa.

13. D. For gastric feeding the type of administration can be bolus, intermittent and continuous. In bolus feeding, 300–500 mL of enteral formula are delivered several times a day over 10–15 minutes. In intermittent feeding, the formula is paced in gravity bag and dripped in about 30-60 minutes. Infusion pump may also be used. In continuous feeding, the formula is generally infused over 24 hours at a rate of 50–150 mL hour.

14. C. For intestinal feeding continuous feeding is the desired choice as this method is associated with less distention and less chances of metabolic complications.

15. D. Prevention is the best treatment for dental caries. Regular brushing and flossing and regular visits to the dentist for cleaning, examination and treatment of early evidence of caries prevent caries. Person should take diet low in simple carbohydrate, not high.

16. C. The patient should avoid brushing remaining teeth for about 24 hours after dental extraction as brushing may dislodge any clot formed at the site of tooth extraction and cause bleeding. All other instructions as recollected by the patient are appropriate.

17. C. Stomatitis may develop when a patient's lowered resistance allows an opportunistic infection to develop. Systemic disorders that affect oral mucous membrane include allergies, bone marrow disorders, nutritional disorders, immunodeficiency disorders and chemotherapy, radiation therapy or immunosuppressive therapy. Heart failure is not known to cause stomatitis.

18. B. Candidiasis, an overgrowth of normal flora *Candida* occurs when there is a decreased level of other normal flora. This usually occurs with prolonged use of antibiotics. Other major risk factor is immunosuppression. Candidiasis of oral cavity commonly seen in patients receiving chemotherapy, person with HIV infection or AIDS, those who are critically ill with prolonged tube feeding or intubation. It is not related to poor oral hygiene, malnutrition and smoking.

19. C. Vincent's angina is an acute bacterial infection of the gingiva caused by resident flora in the mouth, fusiform bacteria and spirochetes. Aphthous stomatitis is a recurrent and chronic form of infection secondary to systemic disease, trauma, stress or unknown causes. Herpes simplex stomatitis is caused by herpes simplex virus and not a bacterial infection. Oral candidiasis is also an infection of a yeast-like fungus *candida albicans* and not a bacterial infection.

20. B. Since vincents angina is a bacterial infection, treatment includes application of topical antibiotics. Normal saline and hydrogen peroxide, mouthwashes give relief, not viscous lidocaine. Patient should consume soft nutritious foods, not fibrous foods.

21. D. Leukoplakia, a potentially precancerous lesion appears in the mouth due to chronic irritation of oral mucous membrane by physical and chemical factors. It may also be caused by systemic factors like malnutrition and syphilis. Smoking and chewing tobacco is a chemical factor, broken teeth is a physical factor.

22. A. Teaching regarding prevention of oral cancer should include avoidance of tobacco, alcohol, and very hot beverages. Person should maintain meticulous oral hygiene, eat well balanced diet and avoid exposure to sun. Carbonated beverages, fibrous foods and commercial mouthwashes are not known to cause oral cancer.

23. B. 90–95% of the oral cancers is squamous cell cancer. Next in the list is the basal cell carcinoma. Only a small percentage is adenocarcinoma.

24. A. Teletherapy is a common method of treatment of cancer. In teletherapy, an external beam of radiation from a radioactive source is placed at a distance passes through the skin or mucous membrane to the tumor. Teletherapy does not involve use of light waves or laser. In brachytherapy radioactive material is placed at or near the tumor and the tumor is treated with internal beam of radiation.

25. C. Due to the presence of disfiguring oral lesion, drooling, halitosis, patient experiences an alteration in self-image. So, the nursing diagnosis of social isolation related to disease or change in appearance is appropriate. Lesion in the oral cavity cannot block the airway and fatigue and weakness are not the presenting symptoms of oral cancer. So the diagnoses of ineffective airway clearance and activity intolerance are inappropriate.

26. C. The most important postoperative intervention is to maintain a patent airway. Following an extensive surgical procedure respiratory difficulty may occur due to edema of oral and pharyngeal structures and a prophylactic tracheostomy is usually in place to prevent respiratory difficulty. So maintaining the patent airway is most important than the others.

27. D. Prevention of parotitis involves administering frequent oral hygiene, keeping the patient well hydrated, and asking patient to chew on hard sugarless gum or candy and not hard sugar candy.

28. B. Nausea is a common problem of gastrointestinal diseases in general. It is a result of conditions that increase tension on the walls of the stomach, duodenum or lower end of esophagus. Unpleasant stimuli, distention, gastritis and carcinoma of stomach can cause nausea.

29. D. Topical anesthetic agent is applied at the back of the throat to depress gag reflex and facilitate the passage of the endoscope. The patient may aspirate if food and fluids are given before gag reflex returns. Positioning on the right side is not required after endoscopy. Endoscopy is not associated with pain, so administration of analgesics is not required. Endoscopy of upper gastrointestinal tract does not influence gastrointestinal motility, so auscultating abdomen for bowel sounds is not indicated.

30. C. After the test the patient should take a laxative and fluids to promote elimination and thus to prevent impaction of contrast medium (barium sulphate). Iodine is not added to barium sulphate so history of allergy to sea food is not relevant. Patient should be nothing per oral (NPO) for 8–12 hours before the test. The color of the stool may be white for about 72 hours and not black.

31. B. Water should be administered after feeding to maintain the patency of the tube. Placement of tube in the stomach is ensured by aspirating stomach content before feeding. Instilling water to check proper placement is unsafe. The patient should be sitting or lying with the head of the bed elevated 30° to 40° to prevent aspiration. The temperature of the feeding solution should be at body temperature or at room temperature to decrease the likelihood of diarrhea and other gastrointestinal complaints.

32. B. Achalasia is characterized by the impaired motility of lower two-third of the esophagus accompanied by the failure of the lower esophageal sphincter to relax. Diffuse spasm is a motor disorder of the esophagus, characterized by the difficulty or pain on swallowing and chest pain similar to that of coronary artery spasm. In gastroesophageal reflux disease, there is a backward flow of gastric content into the esophagus and in Barretts esophagus there is a replacement of the normal squamous epithelium of the esophagus with columnar epithelium which is a complication of gastroesophageal reflux disease.

33. D. Complication of pneumatic dilation is perforation. So the nurse should monitor the patient for sign and symptoms of perforation which are persistent pain and dysphagia, fever, infection, abdominal tenderness and severe hypotension.

34. D. The exact cause of gastroesophageal reflux disease is unknown but reflux occurs with relaxed lower oesophageal sphincter, displaced angle of the gastroesophageal junction and altered nerve innervation in the region of the gastroesophageal sphincter resulting in low pressure in the region.

35. B. Metoclopramide enhances response to acetylcholine of tissue in the upper gastrointestinal tract which causes contraction of gastric muscle, relaxes pyloric, duodenal segments; increases peristalsis without stimulating secretions. The medicine to be taken half hour before meals in order to allow the medication time to begin working before food intake and digestion. The medication has a sedative action so hazardous activities to be avoided by the patient until he is stabilized on this medicine.

36. B. Most common surgery for gastroesophageal reflux disease is Nissen fundoplication that involves suturing the fundus around the esophagus. Esophagomyotomy and pneumatic dilation of the oesophagus are done in achalasia.

37. A. Since recurrence rate of gastroesophageal reflux disease is significant the patients after surgery must be taught to follow the anti-reflux medical regimen, e.g. continuing medication, observing dietary modifications and lifestyle changes.

38. B. There are two major types of hiatal hernia: sliding or axial hernia or type I hernia and rolling or paraesophageal hernia or type II. Sliding or axial hernia or type I is the most common type of hiatal hernia which accounts for about 90% occurrence.

39. B. A hiatal hernia is caused by structural changes, e.g. weakening of the muscles in the diaphragm around the esophagogastric opening and increased intra-abdominal pressure not intrathoracic pressure. It is not caused by the weakness and dilation of cardiac end of stomach or the lower esophageal sphincter.

40. C. Hiatal hernia may be prevented or at least delayed by the health promotion activities that would prevent intra-abdominal pressure. These activities include avoiding wearing tight constrictive clothing around the waist and avoiding heavy lifting. Other than these measures hiatal hernia are not preventable. Constipation has no effect on the development of hiatal hernia. Extremely hot or cold foods may complicate a sliding hernia but does not cause it.

41. C. Most common symptom of a sliding hiatal hernia is gastroesophageal reflux. This is due to the exposure of gastroesophageal sphincter to the lower pressure of the thorax making it less effective. Feeling of fullness and difficulty in breathing are the symptoms of paraesophageal hernia.

42. D. Resting in sitting position allows gravity to work that helps in forward passage of foods in the stomach and prevents reflux. Lying down in bed after meals will promote reflux of stored gastric contents into esophagus. Drinking water immediately before and after meals will over distend stomach and cause regurgitation. Water should be taken at least 1 hour before meals and 1 hour after.

43. A. Nissen fundoplication operation is the most common and involves suturing the fundus around the esophagus. Hill operation narrows the esophageal opening and anchors the stomach and distal esophagus to the median arcuate ligament. Belsey operation consists of plication of the anterior and lateral aspects of the stomach onto the distal esophagus. In patients with severe reflux angelchik prosthesis is inserted around the distal esophagus to reinforce sphincter pressure.

44. D. Esophageal diverticulum is a sac like outpouching in one or more layers of the esophagus where ingested food is trapped and later regurgitated. Because of the decomposition of retained food in the diverticulum, halitosis and sour taste in the mouth are common symptoms. In achalasia, there is a difficulty in swallowing both solids and liquids. Gastroesophageal reflux presents as burning in the esophagus, indigestion and dysphagia. Hiatal hernia presents as heartburn, regurgitation and dysphagia.

45. B. Emetic center is situated in the chemoreceptor trigger zone in the fourth ventricle. Medications of the phenothiazine derivative group, e.g. chlorpromazine do not stimulate but depress vomiting by blocking receptors in the chemoreceptor trigger zone.

46. B. Atrophic gastritis is associated with pernicious anemia, gastric ulcer and gastric cancer. Atrophic changes of the stomach lining result in a minimal amount of acid being secreted in the stomach. In absence of gastric acid the source of intrinsic factor is lost which results in inability to absorb vitamin B_{12} and development of pernicious anemia.

47. A. Duodenal ulcers are characterized by the high gastric acid secretion. In gastric ulcer, gastric acid secretion is normal to below normal. Gastric cancer is associated with the chronic atrophic gastritis where there is little or no gastric acid secretion.

48. C. The patients with duodenal ulcer are usually well nourished as these patients experience hunger pain, which is relieved on eating. So patient's food intake increases resulting in weight gain.

49. B. Pain of peptic ulcer disease (gastric and duodenal ulcer) has a definite relationship to eating. Pain of gastric ulcer is caused by eating and may be relieved by vomiting. In duodenal ulcer, pain occurs when the stomach is empty and food intake relieves it. Patient with duodenal ulcer experiences pain at night since at that time stomach remains empty.

50. B. Infection with *Helicobacter pylori* is an important etiological factor for the development of chronic atrophic gastritis. Chronic gastritis is more common in older adults and in men. So a 25-year-old lady teacher is less likely to develop chronic gastritis. Metronidazole along with tetracycline is given to eradicate *Helicobacter pylori*, so it is not a risk factor for chronic gastritis rather a cure. Gallbladder disease is not associated with chronic gastritis.

51. C. Chronic gastritis leads to loss of function of parietal cells resulting into decrease gastric acid secretion which is a source of intrinsic factor. In the absence of intrinsic factor vitamin B_{12} cannot be absorbed, giving rise to pernicious anemia which is evident by macrocytic anemia. Patients with chronic gastritis usually lose weight. Dry scaly skin is due to vitamin A deficiency. Bleeding tendencies are due to deficiency of vitamin K. Deficiencies of vitamin A and vitamin K is not associated with chronic gastritis.

52. B. Bleeding from stomach or upper gastrointestinal tract is evident as black, tarry stool or melena. The black color of the stool is due to the degradation of the hemoglobin and the release of iron during the longer passage of blood through the intestine. The patient who is bleeding from stomach is likely to have coffee ground appearance vomitus. Clay colored stool is seen in obstructive jaundice and frank blood in stool is seen in lower gastrointestinal tract bleeding, e.g. rectum or colon.

53. D. Famotidine is a drug belonging to H_2- receptor blocker. It acts by blocking the action of histamine on the H_2 receptors and thus reduces hydrochloric acid secretion. This drug also reduces the conversion of pepsinogen to pepsin and thus accelerates ulcer healing. The drugs forming protective covering on the ulcer belong to cytoprotective drugs, e.g. sucralfate. Antacids neutralize gastric acid and increase gastric pH. Anticholinergic drugs decrease vagal stimulation and reduce hydrochloric acid secretion.

54. D. Ranitidine is a H2-histamine receptor antagonist which inhibits gastric acid secretion. The single daily dose should be taken at the bedtime. Administration of the drug at bedtime prolongs its effect, provides maximum protection of gastric mucosa both during sleep and at daytime. Other timings are not correct for this purpose.

55. D. Patient with peptic ulcer must avoid taking over-the-counter drugs unless prescribed by the physician as the drugs may have an ulcerogenic effect. Patient should not only limit but also completely stop smoking and carbonated beverages. He should take 6 small meals with bland diet and continue treatment and follow-up visits including modification of lifestyle for at least a year for healing of ulcer and prevention of recurrence.

56. C. Omeprazole is a proton pump inhibitor and an antiulcer agent. It acts by inhibiting hydrogen/ potassium ATPase enzyme system in gastric parietal cells thus blocking final step of gastric acid production. The medicine relieves gastric pain experienced as heart- burn arising due to gastric mucosal irritation by the excess acid production. The medicine does not relieve constipation, abdominal distention and burning micturition.

57. B. Pantoprazole belongs to the category of proton pump inhibitors. Other drugs of this group are omeprazole, lansoprazole and esomeprazole. Ranitidine belongs to H_2-receptor blockers, sucralfate belongs to cytoprotective drugs, and clarithromycin is an antibiotic effective against *Helicobacter pylori.*

58. D. Sucralfate is an antiulcer agent. It protects the gastric mucosa by adhering to ulcer site and thus preventing contact of acid on the mucosa. Adult dose of the medicine 14 times a day and is given 1 hour before meals and at bedtime.

59. B. With perforation patient experiences sudden, sharp, severe pain beginning in the midepigastrium. Gradually the pain spreads over the entire abdomen as peritonitis develops. The abdomen becomes tender, hard and rigid and not soft, large and distended. Patient exhibits signs and symptoms of hypovolemic shock, e.g. tachycardia and hypotension and not decreased pulse rate and elevated blood pressure. With peritonitis paralytic ileus develops. So patient will have hypoactive bowel sounds or absent bowel sounds and not borborygmi (hyperactive bowel sounds).

60. C. Billroth I procedure involves removal of distal portion of the stomach including the antrum and anastomosis of proximal portion of the stomach with duodenum. This is also called gastroduodenostomy. In Billroth II, the proximal ramnants is anastomosed with jejunum. Surgical removal of right and left vagus nerves and widening of the pyloric end of stomach is known as vagotomy with pyloroplasty. In antrectomy entire antrum is removed and the remaining stomach is anastomosed with duodenum.

61. D. If the nasogastric tube is found to be not draining or clogged, the nurse can gently irrigate the tube with normal saline. The nurse should never reposition the nasogastric tube but notify the physician because of danger of perforating the gastric mucosa or disrupting the suture line. Suction should be applied continuously and not intermittently. The nasogastric tube should never be clamped because of danger of accumulation of gastric secretions which may put a strain on the anastomosis. Increasing suction level may injure gastric mucosa.

62. C. During the surgery a large portion of stomach and the pyloric sphincter is removed. Without an adequate stomach reservoir and a sphincter the hypertonic concentrated food mass is rapidly dumped into the small intestine, drawing fluid from surrounding tissue and blood causing hypovolemia and symptoms of shock.

63. B. Management of dumping syndrome involves teaching the patient to maintain a high protein, high fat and low carbohydrate, dry diet; taking small amount of food at 1 time and in frequent intervals. Fat content in the diet to be increased not decreased and carbohydrate content to be decreased not increased.

64. D. Distressing symptoms of dumping syndrome may be minimized by delaying the gastric emptying. This may be done by eating in a semi-recumbent or recumbent position, lying down after meals for 1 hour and drinking fluids in between the meals and not drinking fluids with meals, before meals. Fluids should be avoided 1 hour before meals.

65. C. Patient's complains and past medical history is highly suggestive of pyloric obstruction. Repeated ulcers and healing of ulcer causes scarring which is responsible for the development of obstruction at the pyloric end of stomach. Due to obstruction the contents of the stomach are unable to empty properly which causes gastric fullness, pain, distention, nausea, vomiting and anorexia. Symptoms of peptic ulcer perforation include sudden onset of severe upper abdominal pain that spreads rapidly to the whole abdomen. Abdomen becomes rigid and board like. Patient experiences hypovolemic shock. Some of the symptoms of acute gastritis are similar to those of pyloric obstruction but the patient's history of repeated ulceration is suggestive of pyloric obstruction. In paralytic ileus peristalsis of the bowel stops which causes diminished or absent bowel sounds. It usually occurs as postoperative complication and not as a result of previous ulceration.

66. A. Crohn's disease is a chronic nonspecific inflammatory bowel disorder of unknown origin. An inflammation and ulceration of colon and rectum is ulcerative colitis. An inflamed outpouching of the intestine is diverticulitis. Erosion of the intestinal mucosa leading to ulceration happens in ulcerative colitis.

67. C. Any part of the gastrointestinal tract from mouth to anus may be affected by Crohn's disease, but the most common location is the terminal ileum.

68. B. Principal symptoms of Crohn's disease are diarrhea and abdominal pain. Other manifestations being abdominal cramping and tenderness, abdominal distention, fever, fatigue and weight loss. Bloating and flatulence are the symptoms of lactase deficiency. Jaundice and steatorrhea (fatty stools) are the symptoms of gallbladder disease and halitosis and sour taste in the mouth are the symptoms of esophageal diverticulum.

69. D. Crohn's disease is characterized by the inflammation resulting into ulceration of all segments of the GI tract. Inflammaion involves all layers of the intestinal wall, i.e. transmural and are usually discontinuous, i.e. skip lesions. Outpouching of the intestinal wall occurs in diverticulosis, atrophy and fattening of the intestinal villi occurs in celiac disease and in ulcerative colitis diffuse inflammation and ulceration involving the mucous and submucous layer of the intestine occurs.

70. B. The most conclusive diagnostic study for Crohn's disease is a barium study for upper gastrointestinal tract that shows the classic findings, e.g. stricturing of the ileum (string sign). A barium enema may also show ulcerations, cobble stoning of the mucosa, fistulas, and areas of abnormal and normal mucosa. Stool examination may show occult blood and steatorrhea but it is not conclusive of Crohn's disease. Serum chemistries may determine electrolyte imbalance, presence of anemia, etc. but they are not conclusive of Crohn's disease. Abdominal X-ray cannot provide any information regarding the status of bowel as it is not radiopaque.

71. C. A very common complication of Crohn's disease is fistula formation. Since the inflammation extends through all layers of the bowel wall from the intestinal mucosa, fistulas, fissures and abscesses form as the inflammation extends into the peritoneum. Chronic gastroenteritis is not known to cause fistula. In ulcerative colitis inflammation involves only the mucous and submucous layer of the bowel wall hence, fistula usually does not occur. An appendicitis may complicate into perforation which may lead to peritonitis and abscess formation, not fistula.

72. D. Toxic megacolon as a complication is not associated with Crohn's disease. It is associated with ulcerative colitis. Toxic megacolon is an extreme dilation of a segment of the diseased colon that results in complete obstruction. It usually occurs during an acute exacerbation of ulcerative colitis and it may follow hypokalemia, a barium enema, or the use of anticholinergics, narcotics, corticosteroids or antibiotics.

73. B. Management of Crohn's disease involves reducing inflammation, suppressing inappropriate immune responses and providing rest for a diseased bowel. Sedatives, antidiarrheal and antiperistaltic medications are used to reduce peristalsis to a minimum to rest the inflamed bowel. Fibers are restricted but fluid is encouraged and given orally and parenterally if required. Cold foods are avoided as they stimulate peristalsis. Patient is advised bed rest to decrease peristalsis.

74. D. The principal manifestations of Crohn's disease are diarrhea and abdominal pain due to the inflammatory process. Corticosteroid therapy is effective in reducing inflammation and suppressing disease. Decreased abdominal pain indicates a reduction of symptoms and effectiveness of therapy. Increase in body weight and moon face are the result of long-term use of corticosteroid and do not indicate effectiveness of therapy. Effective therapy will control diarrhea by reducing the number and amount of stool and not increase the bulk of stool.

75. A. The major symptoms of ulcerative colitis are bloody diarrhea and abdominal pain. The disease usually begins in the rectum and sigmoid colon and spreads up the colon in a continuous manner and not as a skip lesion. Skip lesion is seen in Crohn's disease. Heredity may be a causative factor in Crohn's disease, not in ulcerative colitis. Ulcerative colitis affects only mucous and submucous layer of the bowel wall, and the disease is not usually related with fistula formation. Transmural inflammation with fistula formation occurs in Crohn's disease.

76. A. The patient with total proctocolectomy with continent ileostomy has a high-risk of dehydration. Since a more proximal portion of the bowel is used to create the ileostomy, fecal output may be as high as 1500 to 2,000 mL per 24 hours. Patient with continent ileostomy need not wear an external appliance to collect the fecal matter; instead an internal pouch is surgically created to collect the fecal matter. Patient should not consume a high fiber diet as it may irritate the intestine and the stool in ileostomy is already liquid. Patients with ileostomy do not experience dumping syndrome, a complication after gastric surgery.

77. D. The nurse should explain to the patient that blood in the stools is most common manifestation of the disease. Understanding the nature and symptoms of the disease process may help to alleviate fear and apprehension. Sending stools for examination for the presence of occult blood is not necessary as blood in the stools is a typical finding and most of the patients in similar conditions have blood in their stools. The patient should record the number and description of stools but simply recording does not alleviate fear and apprehension. It is not necessary to inform the physician, since blood in the stools is expected in this condition.

78. C. The nurse should explain to the patient that the drug would reduce inflammation of the intestine. The drug does not reduce gastrointestinal motility, suppress immune response and does not increase bowel tone.

79. C. Corticosteroid such as prednisone is used to achieve remission. But the drug is not effective in maintaining remission. So it is used in acute flare-ups. It is given for the shortest possible time because of side effects associated with the long-term use. The drug causes immunosuppression so it cannot prevent infection. Weight gain is due to fluid retention is the side effect of this drug and is not desired.

80. B. The nurse should report to the surgeon immediately if the stoma appears dusky blue in color which indicates ischemia. Pink or red color stoma, slightly edematous stoma and slight oozing from the stoma when touched is normal and need not be reported.

81. C. The nurse should teach the patient to clean the stoma and surrounding area with mild soap and water, rinse and dry thoroughly to prevent irritation from intestinal contents and then to apply skin barrier to protect skin and prevent direct contact with intestinal contents. Cleaning the stoma with irritating agents like spirit or hydrogen peroxide should be avoided. Plain water may not be adequate for cleaning. Soap should be used for cleaning provided it is mild and rinsed thoroughly after cleaning.

82. C. Left sided colostomy is usually made on the descending colon. Since most of the fluid would be absorbed in ascending and transverse colon, the stool is expected to be formed.

83. B. Colostomy irrigation daily at a scheduled time helps in developing the habit of opening the stoma at that particular time. It also helps in keeping colostomy bag clean for rest of the day. Patient with this colostomy need to take well balanced normal diet with adequate fiber and fluids.

84. B. The nurse should explain to the patient before surgery that the fecal drainage from the stoma is liquid in consistency and will drain constantly in an ileostomy bag. Patient should know that he could not have normal bowel movement with formed stool. Permanent ileostomy drains liquid stool which is collected in an open-ended plastic, odor-proof pouch or ileostomy bag attached to the stoma. Drainage of liquid stool by inserting a catheter at regular intervals is done in continent ileostomy or Kock pouch. Ileostomy stoma should not be irrigated.

85. C. The patient with ulcerative colitis, unresponsive to prescribed drug treatment is most likely to develop fluid and electrolyte imbalances secondary to severe diarrhea. Therefore, correction of fluid and electrolyte imbalances is most important and should be given priority by the nurse. Teaching patient ostomy care, referring patient to ostomy association and teaching deep breathing and coughing exercises are all important but priority of care is correction of fluid and electrolyte imbalances.

86. D. Mechanical obstruction of the intestine is most often caused by the growth of malignant cells arising in the lumen of intestine. The disease escapes detection as the symptoms in the early stage are usually vague or absent. Incidence of its occurrence is more in men. Benign tumors remain localized but not malignant tumors.

87. A. A person with familial polyposis is at high-risk of developing colorectal cancer. Familial polyposis accounts for at least 1% of all colorectal cancer. If untreated, patients with familial polyposis almost always develop colon cancer before the age of 40 years. Hemorrhoid is not related to any type of cancer. Patient with chronic peptic ulcer disease is at risk of developing gastric cancer. Diarrheal disease is also not related to colorectal cancer.

88. D. The foods which can cause a potential obstruction in an ileostomy include nuts, raisins, popcorn, seeds, raw vegetables and corn. Patient should initially limit the amount of these foods, chew them thoroughly and accompany them with fluids. Eggs are odor-producing foods, onions are gas- forming foods and coffee may cause diarrhea. Since the effect of food on stoma output is individual, patients are not discouraged from eating these foods and beverage.

89. B. During the immediate postoperative period and after, the patient is at high-risk for fluid volume deficit due to excess fluid loss from ileostomy. So the nurse should accurately monitor intake and output, observe sign of dehydration, and electrolyte disturbances and ensure fluid intake of at least 3,000 mL/day in the initial postoperative period. Pain may occur following an ileostomy but management of pain is not a priority over preventing fluid volume deficit. Risk for impaired skin integrity and disturbed body image are appropriate and important nursing diagnosis for a patient with ileostomy, but these are not priority over risk for fluid volume deficit.

90. B. Gastroenteritis is inflammation of stomach and intestinal tract that primarily affects the small bowel. Irritation and inflammation of bowel mucosa gives rise to increased peristalsis which is heard as borborygmi or hyperactive bowel sounds. Hypoactive bowel sounds are generally observed after general anesthesia. Rigid and board-like abdomen and rebound tenderness are found in peritonitis.

91. D. Abdominal examination should always be done systematically in the following sequence: Inspection, auscultation, percussion, and palpation. Because percussion and palpation can alter intestinal activity, these two procedures should be done after inspection and auscultation.

92. A. Cholera is transmitted by oral route, so the disease transmission is prevented by observing enteric precaution. Vaccination has no role in the recovery of the patient suffering from cholera. Recovery from the disease gives immunity. Vaccination of all household contacts should be carried out. The disease is transmitted by oral route from contaminated water, food, etc. and not by living in over crowded place, i.e. by droplet infection. Vibrio cholera is a bacteria, hence the patient has to be treated with antibiotics and not by antiviral agents.

93. B. The nurse should assess the frequency of bowel movements of the patient as lomotil decreases gastrointestinal motility by acting on the mucosal receptors responsible for peristalsis. It does not relieve anxiety and abdominal pain. When diarrhea is controlled skin turgor will also improve. So improvement of skin turgor is a secondary effect of lomotil.

94. C. Diphenoxylate is an opioid used for a limited period for symptomatic relief in noninfective diarrhea. Being an opioid has the potential for habit formation although atropine is added to diphenoxylate to prevent abuse. So physicians instructions with regard to proper dose and duration is required. The drug causes drowsiness not insomnia. Laxative should not be taken as it is an antidiarrhoic drug.

95. C. Loperamide is an antimotility drug used in acute and chronic noninfective diarrhea. It is not used in other conditions.

96. B. Amebiasis is a protozoan infection of the colon. Offending organism is *Entameba hystolytica*. *Giardia lambia* causes giardiasis. *E.coli* causes gastroenteritis and enterobius (pinworm) causes helminthiasis.

97. D. Fever, rash, itching, chills are allergic reactions of metronidazole. If any of the symptoms appear in patient, drug should be discontinued.

98. D. Darkened urine is a usual side effect of the medicine and needs no action.

99. A. Diverticulosis is described as multiple noninflamed outpouching of the mucosa through the circular smooth muscle of the intestine. When these diverticula are inflamed it is termed as diverticulitis. Diverticulosis is not due to weakness of the intestinal musculature. Complete obstruction in the forward flow of intestinal content due to twisting of the bowel is volvulus.

100. C. Initial treatment in acute diverticulitis consists of rest to the bowel. So the patient is kept in nothing per oral (NPO) status. So the fluids to be administered through intravenous route. To control inflammation broad spectrum antibiotics are administered as prescribed intravenously. A high fiber diet, plenty of oral fluids and laxatives are recommended in diverticular disease but not in acute diverticulitis.

101. B. Rovsing's sign, a possible assessment finding in acute appendicitis is positive when patient feels pain in the left lower quadrant on palpation of right lower quadrant. Pain and tenderness at McBurney's point and rebound tenderness after palpation of abdomen are also the assessment findings in acute appendicitis.

102. A. The most common cause of acute appendicitis is a fecalith (accumulated feces) that occludes the lumen of the appendix.

103. D. Lying with knees flexed helps release tension on the abdominal muscles which helps to reduce the amount of discomfort felt. Lying on abdomen or supine with legs stretched or sitting upright would increase discomfort.

104. A. Peritonitis and shock are potentially life-threatening complications after abdominal surgery. Physician should be informed for initiating rigorous treatment. Patient requires fluid to expand and maintain the circulating volume, not blood. Patient should be placed in flat position. Increased flow of oxygen will not help in maintaining circulating volume.

105. B. Diverticulosis is not known to be related with hemorrhoids. The factors that precipitate hemorrhoids are pregnancy, portal hypertension, heavy lifting, prolonged constipation, straining at stool in an effort to defecate, prolonged standing or sitting.

106. B. Symptoms suggestive of internal hemorrhoids are bleeding after defecation. Bleeding associated with defecation is seen in external hemorrhoids. Other symptom of internal hemorrhoids is dull aching discomfort, not intermittent pain which is a symptom of external hemorrhoids. Itching in rectum is also a symptom of external hemorrhoids.

107. B. The patient should be taught to avoid straining during defecation, as straining may cause recurrence of hemorrhoids. Patient should also avoid constipation by consuming a high fiber diet and to take a stool softener for a few days postoperatively and come for regular checkups and not wait for symptoms to reappear.

108. D. In irreducible hernia the contents of the sac cannot be reduced or replaced by manipulation. Irreducible hernias usually become obstructed and strangulated which is a medical emergency. So nurse's priority should be observation of patient's bowel movement. Lying down on bed has no effect on irreducible hernia. Monitoring of vital signs is done for all patients. Application of ice pack cannot prevent an irreducible hernia to become obstructed.

109. C. The most common pahogenic mechanism involved in acute pancreatitis is autodigestion of the pancreas. The causative factors are believed to cause injury to pancreatic cells or activation of the pancreatic enzymes in the pancreas instead of in the intestine resulting in autodigestion of the pancreas. Acute pancreatitis is not due to hyperplasia of pancreatic cells, autoimmune inflammatory reaction of the pancreas or degenerative changes in the pancreas.

110. C. Diabetes mellitus is not identified as etiological factor in the development of acute pancreatitis. The primary etiological factors of acute pancreatitis include alcoholism and billiary tract disease. So the nurse is right in taking history of alcoholism and fat intolerance. Certain drugs like corticosteroids, thiazide diuretics, oral contraceptives, sulfonamides, NSAIDs may also cause acute pancreatitis.

111. C. A patient with acute pancreatitis will show an elevated serum amylase. Elevated serum amylase is the most important aid in diagnosing acute pancreatitis. Other primary diagnostic tests are serum lipase and urinary amylase which are also elevated in this condition. Serum cholesterol and serum bilirubin are not included in the diagnostic tests of pancreatitis. White blood cell counts are elevated in the acute pancreatitis not the red blood cell counts.

112. B. One of the important objectives of nursing management for a patient with acute pancreatitis is prevention of respiratory infections. Respiratory infections are common in patients with acute pancreatitis because the retroperitoneal fluid raises the diaphragm which causes the patient to take shallow, guarded abdominal breaths. In addition the patient with acute pancreatitis is also susceptible to infection. The other objectives of management are correcting fluid volume deficit related to nausea, vomiting and nasogastric suction not fluid volume excess and maintaining normal electrolyte balance which include prevention of hypocalcemia not hypercalcemia.

113. B. The diet for patient with acute pancreatitis should be high in carbohydrate and low in fat content because that is the least stimulating to the exocrine portion of the pancreas. Diet should be small, frequent and bland with no stimulants, e.g. caffeine and alcohol. Patient should be encouraged to take fruits, vegetables and breads in increased amount. Fat-soluble vitamins may be supplemented.

114. B. Whipple's procedure involves resection of the proximal portion of the pancreas (pancreatectomy), the adjoining duodenum (duodenectomy), the distal portion of the stomach (partial gastrectomy), and the distal segment of the common bile duct. An anastomosis of the pancreatic duct, common bile duct and remaining stomach to the jejunum is done.

115. D. A 50-year-old woman on estrogen replacement therapy is at higher risk of developing cholelithiasis since the incidence of cholelithiasis is highest in women who are multiparous, over the age of 40 years, postmenopausal and on estrogen replacement therapy.

116. A. The nurse would find yellow sclera in a patient with cholelithiasis with obstruction of the common bile duct. Due to obstruction of the common bile duct, bile cannot drain from the liver to the duodenum. The bile backs up into the liver and results in obstructive jaundice, which is manifested as yellow sclera. Other manifestations of obstructive jaundice would be dark foamy urine, clay colored stools, steatorrhea, pruritus, intolerance to fatty foods and bleeding tendencies and not black stools, straw colored urine and superficial venous thrombosis.

117. A. In laparoscopic cholecystectomy, four small punctures are made into the abdomen and gallbladder is removed through one of these punctures. One puncture is made slightly above the umbilicus, two punctures just below the ribs, one in the right anterior axillary line and the other on the right midclavicular line and the fourth puncture is made just right of the midsection. In this operation, gallbladder is removed and not left as it is. No drainage tube is left in place and the patient can resume normal activities usually within a week and not within a month.

118. C. Getting up from the bed and moving around relieves gas pain caused by carbon dioxide that is not released or absorbed by the body. If the patient is experiencing dyspnea due to irritation of the phrenic nerve by carbon dioxide he/she is encouraged to lie in Sim's position in left side with right knees flexed and to take deep breaths. Increased fluid intake does not relieve gas pain and discomfort associated with laparoscopic procedures.

119. D. Patient with cholecystectomy should be advised to take nutritious diet and to avoid excessive fat intake. The amount of fat may be consumed by the patient actually depends on the patient's tolerance of fat. A low fat diet is recommended in the early postoperative period and if the patient is overweight. There is no indication of avoiding poultry products, elimination of fats from diets and to increase vegetables and fruits in the diets.

120. D. Hepatitis A virus is transmitted through the fecal-oral route. It frequently occurs in the small outbreaks caused by fecal contamination of food or drinking water. It does not spread by sexual contact, use of contaminated needles and by perinatal transmission.

121. C. Clinical manifestations of viral hepatitis are classified into 3 phases: 1) preicteric or prodromal phase, 2) icteric phase, 3) posticteric phase or convalescent phase. Preicteric or prodromal phase precedes jaundice and is the period of maximum infectivity for hepatitis A. So the nurse must observe enteric precautions to prevent transmission of infection to others. Since the patient has not yet developed jaundice, maintaining skin integrity is not important. Patient requires high carbohydrate, high protein and low fat diet and not high carbohydrate and low protein diet. Rest reduces metabolic demands on the liver and promotes cell regeneration. So the patient should be on bed rest during this period and not to increase activity. Gradual increase of activity is encouraged in posticteric phase or convalescent phase.

122. B. All family members of a patient with hepatitis B should be vaccinated with hepatitis B vaccine (HBV) immediately. Injection with HBIG or hepatitis B immunoglobulin is indicated in acute exposure of a sexual partner with a HbsAg positive person. The patient should not share personal items like razor and toothbrushes. Since it is not spread by fecal-oral route, there is no need in separating household goods like utensils.

123. A. Portal or nutritional or alcoholic cirrhosis is usually associated with alcohol abuse. This type of cirrhosis was previously known as Laennec's cirrhosis. The incidence of portal cirrhosis is highest than the other types of cirrhosis. Autoimmune hepatitis is the cause of postnecrotic cirrosis. Chronic billiary obstruction and infection is associated with billiary cirrhosis and severe chronic right sided heart failure causes cardiac cirrhosis.

124. B. Spider angiomas are small, dilated blood vessels with a bright red center point and spider like branches appearing on the cheeks, nose, upper trunk, neck and shoulders. These lesions are due to an increase in circulating estrogen level occurring as a result of diseased liver's inability to metabolize steroid hormones. Spider angiomas are not due to pancytopenia, decreased synthesis of blood clotting factors and capillary vasodilation secondary to increased level of ammonia.

125. C. Testicular atrophy is a common finding in a patient with cirrhosis, not testicular enlargement. The other findings, e.g. gynecomastia, loss of axillary and pubic hair, impotence with loss of libido is seen in these patients and occurs due to the inability of the liver to metabolize estrogen.

126. A. In cirrhosis, laboratory value of serum alanine aminotransferase (ALT) will be abnormally elevated because of release of enzymes by the damaged liver cells. Other enzymes found to be elevated are aspartate aminotransferase (AST) and gamma-glutamyltransferase (GGT). Due to impairment of fat metabolism serum cholesterol value will be decreased. Serum amylase value is elevated in pancreatitis, not in cirrhosis. Serum protein value is low in cirrhosis, as damaged liver is unable to synthesize albumin.

127. C. The trocar used in paracentesis may injure a distended bladder. So the patient must empty his bladder immediately before the procedure. Patient should be placed in Fowler's position during the procedure in order to promote flow of fluid due to gravity. Taking light diet in the evening or evacuating bowel is not mandatory.

128. D. Definitive diagnosis of cirrhosis is made by the liver biopsy. Liver biopsy is followed by histopathological examination can identify liver cell changes and alterations in the lobular structures occurring in cirrhosis of liver. History of long-term alcohol abuse gives suspicion of only Laennec's cirrhosis, which is only a type of cirrhosis. Liver function test and liver ultrasound provide sufficient cues of cirrhosis of liver but none is definitive than liver biopsy.

129. D. Disorientation is an early sign of hepatic encephalopathy. So the nurse should perform a thorough examination of mental status, document the findings and then inform the physician. Providing a railed cot prevents injury to a disoriented and confused patient, but mental status examination should be done first.

130. A. Characteristic manifestation found in a patient who is at risk of developing hepatic coma is asterixis or flapping tremors or liver flap. This may take several forms but most common is involvement of arms and hands. When the patient is asked to hold the arms and hands stretched out, he is unable to hold this position and there is a series of rapid flexion and extension movements of the hands. Other signs of impending coma are disorientation, hypothermia, hyperventilation, lethargy, depression, drowsiness, etc. In hepatic encephalopathy serum ammonia level rises not urea, as liver is unable to convert ammonia to urea.

131. D. Patient with hepatic encephalopathy is treated with bed rest, low protein or no protein diet, laxatives and enemas. Rest or limitation of activity and low protein diet reduce production of ammonia which is a byproduct of metabolism. Bacterial action on proteins of feces results in ammonia production. So laxatives and enemas are used to decrease bacterial action in the colon and promote expulsion of ammonia. Any gastrointestinal bleeding increases ammonia production by bacterial action. Constipation and straining can induce bleeding. Enemas and laxatives prevent straining and bleeding, but ultimate aim of all these measures is decrease ammonia production and its excretion. This treatment does not aim in promoting fluid loss and sodium elimination.

132. A. The most important nursing intervention for a patient with esophageal varices is to observe for any signs of hemorrhage from the varices, e.g. hematemesis and melena. Prompt recognition of bleeding from the varices will enable the nurse to assess the patient for hemorrhage, notify physician and be ready to assist with whatever treatment is used to control the bleeding as early as possible. Patient may take deep breath but coughing should be avoided, as it may cause rupture of varices and bleeding. Nurse should encourage adequate nutritional intake but foods according to the patient's choice may not be allowed. Patient with esophageal varices should avoid alcohol and irritating foods such as spicy foods. Teaching regarding esophageal varices is important but more important is observing for hemorrhage.

5
CHAPTER

Urinary System

Q1. The followings are the functions of the kidney *except:*

A. Formation of erythropoietin
B. Formation of urea
C. Maintaining water balance
D. Maintaining acid balance

Q2. The diagnosis of a urinary tract infection is confirmed when the bacterial count in the voided specimen is:

A. 10000/mL **B.** 100000/mL
C. 1000000/mL **D.** 10000000/mL

Q3. Common indication of urethritis is:

A. Pus in urine
B. RBCs in urine
C. Casts in urine
D. All of the above

Q4. A patient with suspected urinary tract infection is advised for urine culture and sensitivity. The nurse instructs the patient to collect the specimen from:

A. First stream of urine from bladder
B. Middle stream of urine from bladder
C. Last stream of urine from bladder
D. Full volume of urine from bladder

Q5. Which of the following methods for collection of urine specimen the nurse should teach a patient who has been advised for urine culture?

A. Teach the patient to collect midstream urine in a clean container
B. Clean the foreskin of the penis of uncircumcised men before collection of urine specimen
C. Teach the patient to void into a clean urinal, and then pour some urine into specimen container
D. Teach the patient to begin the stream of urine in the toilet and then continue voiding midstream in the sterile container provided

Q6. Which of the following diagnostic findings may occur with pyelonephritis?

A. Urinalysis reveals pyuria only
B. Urinalysis shows pyuria, bacteriuria, hematuria and white blood cells casts
C. Urine is acidic
D. Intravenous pyelogram reveals shrinkage of the involved kidney

Q7. The nurse recognizes that the most common pathogen in the bladder and upper urinary tract is:

A. *Escherichia coli*
B. *Klebsiella*
C. *Proteus*
D. *Candida*

Q8. A patient is scheduled for an intravenous pyelogram. Which of the following data the nurse would assess and record?

A. Frequency and burning of urination
B. History of hematuria
C. History of allergies
D. Urine positive for sugar and acetone

Q9. A male patient with an indwelling catheter in place complains to the nurse a desire to void. The nurse will:

A. Flush the catheter with normal saline
B. Palpate the suprapubic area gently for signs of bladder fullness
C. Document the color of the urine
D. Encourage the patient to bear down as if trying to void

Q10. The nurse understands that urine flows through a Foley's catheter by the principle of:

A. Higher pressure to lower pressure
B. Gravity
C. Suction
D. Siphoning

Q11. Which of the following statements is not true regarding phenazopyridine (pyridium)?

A. It is an urinary analgesic and anesthetic
B. It causes bladder spasm
C. Causes bright red-orange urine that stains clothing
D. It causes diarrhea

Q12. The amount of blood flowing to the kidneys per minute is:

A. 20–25% of the cardiac output
B. 30–40% of the cardiac output
C. 35–40% of the cardiac output
D. 40–50% of the cardiac output

Q13. Most of the water and electrolytes of the glomerular filtrate is reabsorbed in the:

A. Proximal tubule
B. Descending limb of loop of Henle
C. Ascending limb of loop of Henle
D. Distal tubule

Q14. A patient attends outpatient department with the complain of dysuria, hematuria, urgency and frequency. The nurse understands that the patient is most probably suffering from:

A. Cystitis
B. Cancer of the bladder
C. Stricture of urethra
D. Pyelitis

Q15. Physician prescribes methanamine (mandelamine) to a patient. The nurse is aware that this drug has been prescribed to:

A. Increase urinary output
B. Relieve burning micturition
C. Treat urinary tract infection
D. Decrease bladder muscle spasms

Q16. A patient has been prescribed trimethoprim for urinary tract infection. The nurse is teaching self care to the patient. Which of the following is not appropriate?

A. To take the medicine with full glass of water
B. To take the medicine at specified time as prescribed
C. To report if severe fatigue
D. To discontinue drug if abnormal taste sensations

Q17. A patient is being treated with gentamicin for a lower respiratory tract infection. Being aware that gentamicin may cause nephrotoxicity the nurse monitors which of the following laboratory values?

A. Blood urea nitrogen
B. Urine pH
C. Serum sodium
D. Alkaline phosphatase

Q18. The nurse is assessing a patient admitted with acute pyelonephritis, which of the following symptoms she is expected to find?

A. Urinary retention
B. Feeling of coldness and hypothermia
C. High blood pressure
D. Flank pain on the affected side

Q19. The nurse is teaching a middle aged woman with a lower urinary tract infection. Which of the following statement by the patient indicates the need for further teachings?

A. "I should drink at least 8 glasses of water every day to eradicate the infectious agent"
B. "I need to clean myself by wiping from front to back after urinating"
C. "I should avoid holding urine in bladder for more than 2–4 hours before voiding"
D. "I can drink tea, coffee and cola in liberal amounts to increase my fluid intake"

Q20. A nurse is preparing a patient with acute pyelonephritis for discharge. Which of the following statements she should include in the teaching?

A. "Discontinue antibiotic when symptoms subside"
B. "Don't worry for recurrence as you have been treated with antibiotic"
C. "Return for follow-up urine culture as prescribed"
D. "Restrict sodium in diet"

Q21. Classic signs of acute glomerulonephritis is:

A. Generalized edema especially of the face and periorbital area
B. Fever and sore throat
C. Hypotension and dizziness
D. All of the above

Q22. Which of the following types of renal calculi is radiolucent?

A. Calcium oxalate
B. Calcium phosphate
C. Uric acid
D. Struvite

Q23. 90% of urinary stones are made up of:

A. Calcium
B. Phosphate
C. Oxalate
D. Uric acid

Q24. The technique of removal of a soft bladder stone by crushing with an instrument, lithotrite, (stone crusher) is called:

A. Ureteroscopy
B. Cystoscopic lithotripsy
C. Cystolitholapaxy
D. Ureterorenoscopy

Q25. The technique of removal of calculi using laser together with an ureteroscope is:

A. Laser lithotripsy
B. Extracorporeal shock wave lithotripsy
C. Percutaneous lithotripsy
D. Laser ureteroscopy

Q26. A patient is admitted in the emergency ward with history of sudden severe pain in right flank radiating towards groin. Physician is suspecting urolithiasis. The nursing diagnosis, which requires immediate intervention, is:

A. Acute pain
B. Impaired urinary elimination
C. Risk for fluid volume deficit
D. Risk for infection

Q27. Physician has prescribed allopurinol to a patient with recurrent renal calculi. The nurse understands that the patient is most probably having:

A. Uric acid stone
B. Calcium phosphate stone
C. Struvite stone
D. None of the above

Q28. Aluminium hydroxide (alludrox) has been prescribed to a patient with recurrent renal calculi of phosphate based stone. The nurse understands that aluminium hydroxide will:

A. Prevent absorption of phosphorus in the stomach

B. Binds with phosphorus in the intestine and prevents its absorption

C. Promote excretion of phosphorus in the urine

D. Decreases urinary pH and thus prevents phosphate stone formation

Q29. Which of the following palliative procedures is usually performed when the ureters are obstructed by a tumor?

A. Transurethral resection

B. Cutaneous ureterostomy

C. Pyelostomy

D. Percutaneous nephrostomy

Q30. Urinary diversion procedure where a segment of ileum is constructed as a conduit and the ureters are attached to it and opened through a stoma on the abdomen is called:

A. Illeal bladder

B. Indiana pouch

C. Neobladder

D. Florida pouch

Q31. The two most common complications of urethral trauma are:

A. Urethral strictures and impotence in men

B. Bladder strictures and impotence in men

C. Impotence among men and ectopic ureters

D. Impotence among men and megaureters

Q32. The most common cause of urinary retention in women is:

A. Urethral stricture

B. Spinal cord injury

C. Cystocele

D. Detrusor failure

Q33. The two major problems caused by bladder diverticula are:

A. Distended bladder and urinary tract infections

B. Urinary tract infections and malignancies

C. Malignancies and obstruction

D. Urinary tract infections and urethral stricture

Q34. Involuntary urine loss associated with overdistention of bladder is:

A. Urge incontinence

B. Stress incontinence

C. Reflex incontinence

D. Overflow incontinence

Q35. A postoperative patient has developed urinary retention. To relieve the patient from retention the nurse carries out all of the following *except:*

A. Place the patient in a sitting position

B. Place a hot water bottle over the perineum

C. Get an order for inserting a catheter into bladder

D. Administer a diuretic

Q36. The physician has ordered bladder catheterization for a postoperative patient with persistent urinary retention. Which of the following catheters she should use?

A. Plain catheter

B. Foley's /indwelling catheter

C. 3-way catheter

D. Any of the above

Q37. The most common intrarenal cause of acute renal failure (ARF) is:

A. Acute glomerulonephritis

B. Renal thrombosis

C. Acute tubular necrosis

D. Septic shock

Q38. A patient with chronic renal failure has developed uremic amaurosis. Uremic amaurosis is the:

A. Diminution of the deep tendon reflexes

B. Progressive hearing loss
C. Sudden onset of bilateral permanent blindness
D. Sudden onset of bilateral temporary blindness

Q39. Which of the following conditions is a common cause of prerenal acute renal failure?

A. Glycosuria
B. Myoglobinuria
C. Enlarged prostate
D. Atherosclerosis

Q40. Most important nursing intervention for a patient with acute renal failure in the diuretic phase involves:

A. Providing high calorie diet
B. Restricting fluid and salt intake
C. Encouraging socialization
D. Encouraging deep breathing

Q41. In oliguric phase of acute renal failure the amount of urine output will be:

A. No urine output
B. Urine output of 50–100 mL/day
C. Urine output is less than 400 mL/day
D. Urine output of 600–700 mL/day

Q42. A patient in acute renal failure has been prescribed 50% glucose solution with 10 units of regular insulin and sodium bicarbonate. The nurse understands that this therapy is intended to treat:

A. Hypokalemia
B. Hyperkalemia
C. Hyponatremia
D. Hypernatremia

Q43. A patient with chronic renal failure is considering to be treated with continuous ambulatory peritoneal dialysis. The nurse explains to the patient that the process:

A. Provides continuous contact of dialyzer and blood to clear toxins by ultrafiltration
B. Cleanses blood by correction of serum electrolytes and excretion of creatinine
C. Allows mobility of the patient as it clears toxins in short intermittent period.
D. Uses the peritoneum as a semipermeable membrane to clear toxins by osmosis and diffusion.

Q44. A patient with chronic renal failure treated with continuous ambulatory peritoneal dialysis develops fever, abdominal tenderness and nausea. Physician suspects peritonitis and sends peritoneal fluid for examination of white blood cells count. The diagnosis of peritonitis will be confirmed when:

A. White blood cells count exceeds 100/ cubic milimeter and neutrophil count is more than 50%
B. White blood cells count exceeds 80/ cubic milimeter and neutrophil count is more than 45%
C. White blood cells count exceeds 60/ cubic milimeter and neutrophil count is more than 40%
D. White blood cells count exceeds 50/ cubic milimeter and neutrophil count is more than 30%

Q45. A patient is being treated by intravesical chemotherapy for bladder cancer. Which of the following nursing interventions is appropriate?

A. Flush all urine down the toilet
B. Place the patient in a private room, after the treatment.
C. Restrict fluid intake for 6 hours after treatment
D. Teach patient the sign and symptoms of cystitis

Q46. The nurse is assessing a patient with ileal conduit on the first postoperative day. Which of the following assessment findings should promptly be reported to the physician?

A. A red moist stoma

B. A cyanotic stoma
C. Continuous flow of urine through the stoma
D. Slight bleeding from stoma during change of dressing and appliance

Q47. Physician is planning a total cystectomy and urinary diversion with an Indiana pouch for a patient with carcinoma of bladder. The nurse is explaining the patient about this procedure. Which of the following statements by the patient indicates the need for further explanations by the nurse?

A. "I should drink at least 8 glasses of water daily."
B. "I should take a balanced diet comprising of food from all groups"
C. "I have to wear an external collection bag for the rest of my life"
D. "I shall have to pass a catheter to the stoma made on my abdomen to drain urine at every 2 hour interval."

Q48. In chronic renal failure there is progressive destruction of:

A. Glomerulus
B. Bowman's capsule
C. Tubular system
D. Nephron

Q49. Which of the following conditions may cause the intrarenal form of acute renal failure (ARF)?

A. Bilateral renal artery occlusion
B. Damage to cells in the adrenal cortex
C. Obstruction of the urinary collecting system
D. Nephrotoxic injury secondary to snake bites

Q50. A patient with acute renal failure, receiving peritoneal dialysis suddenly complains of severe respiratory difficulty. The nurse should:

A. Inform the physician
B. Discontinue the dialysis
C. Administer oxygen
D. Drain fluid from the peritoneal cavity.

Q51. A patient with chronic renal failure treated with continuous ambulatory peritoneal dialysis is ready for discharge. The nurse should reinforce which dietary instructions?

A. Limit fluid intake to three glasses of water per day
B. To increase intake of carbohydrate and fiber
C. To restrict salt and use a salt substitute
D. To consume liberal amounts of fruits including bananas

Q52. A patient with chronic renal failure has been ordered Epoietin Alfa (Epogen) subcutaneously 3 times a week. The nurse is aware that this hormone is given to:

A. Increase white blood cells count
B. To stimulate synthesis of platelets
C. To stimulate synthesis of red blood cells
D. To control bleeding

Q53. Therapeutic effect of Epoietin Alfa is seen:

A. After 24 hours of administration
B. After 3 days
C. After 1 week
D. After 2 weeks

Q54. The nurse is teaching a patient receiving Epoietin Alfa regarding its adverse effect. Which of the following is correct?

A. Jaundice
B. Hypertension
C. Irritability
D. Insomnia

Q55. Which steps should the nurse follow to insert an indwelling catheter?

A. Put on gloves, prepare patient and equipment, create a sterile field, test catheter balloon, clean meatus, insert catheter until urine flows, inflate catheter balloon, and attach catheter with drainage bag
B. Prepare patient and equipment, put on gloves, create a sterile field, test

catheter balloon, clean meatus, insert catheter until urine flows, inflate catheter balloon, and attach catheter with drainage bag.

C. Prepare patient and equipment, create a sterile field, clean meatus, insert catheter until urine flows

D. Put on gloves, create a sterile field, clean urinary meatus, insert catheter until urine flows, inflate balloon of catheter, and attach catheter with drainage bag

Q56. A patient with chronic renal failure (CRF) has developed erythrocytopenia. The nurse should monitor the patient for:

A. Dyspnea and cyanosis
B. Bleeding tendencies
C. Fatigue and weakness
D. Development of infection

Q57. Which of the following anatomical facts about kidneys is not true?

A. The left kidney usually is slightly lower than the right one
B. Kidneys lie between the 12th thoracic and third lumbar vertebrae
C. Average adult kidneys are 11 cm in length and 5–7.5 cm in width
D. Kidneys are covered by fibrous capsule

Q58. A patient with renal stone has undergone lithotripsy. The nurse strains all outflow drainage and sends the stone fragments to the laboratory for:

A. Culture and sensitivity
B. Cytological test
C. Analysis of stone's composition
D. All of the above

Q59. The nurse is teaching a patient regarding self care after lithotripsy. Which statement by the patient indicates the need for further teaching?

A. "I need to drink a lot of fluids to flush the urinary tract"
B. "I need not worry about the passage of sand like particles through the drainage tube"
C. "The colour of urine may be dark red for the first week after the procedure"
D. "I need to report about cloudy or foul smelling urine"

Q60. A patient with renal failure is being treated with continuous ambulatory peritoneal dialysis. Which of the following nursing diagnoses is most appropriate?

A. Risk for infection
B. Self care deficit
C. Acute pain
D. Hyperglycemia

Q61. A patient is admitted in the hospital with chronic renal failure. The nurse understands that CRF is characterized by:

A. Progressive irreversible destruction of nephrons in both kidneys
B. Rapid loss of renal function with an elevated BUN
C. Increased creatinine clearance and reduced urine output
D. Low serum creatinine level, severe azotemia, electrolyte imbalances and impaired urine dilution

Q62. Which one of the following conditions may cause prerenal form of acute renal failure?

A. Benign prostatic hyperplasia
B. Myocardial infarction
C. Hemolytic blood transfusion reaction
D. Septic shock and nephrotoxic injury from radiocontrast agents

Q63. A patient with acute renal failure is admitted in hospital. During the oliguric phase the nurse should monitor the patient for:

A. Kussmaul respiration and hypotension
B. Crackles and ECG changes
C. Urine for high creatinine and low sodium concentration
D. Hypernatremia and fatigue

Q64. In diuretic phase of renal failure, which electrolyte imbalances the nurse should monitor?

A. Hypernatremia, hypokalemia
B. Hyponatremia, hypokalemia
C. Hypocalcemia, hypophosphatemia
D. Hypercalcemia, hypophosphatemia

Q65. Dietary restrictions for a patient with chronic renal failure involve:

A. Low protein, carbohydrate, fluid, sodium and potassium intake
B. High carbohydrate, low protein, fluid, sodium and potassium intake
C. High protein and carbohydrate low fluid, sodium and potassium intake
D. High carbohydrate and fluid, low protein, sodium and potassium intake

Q66. To obtain vascular access for patients with long-term hemodialysis either an arteriovenous fistula (AVF) or an arteriovenous graft (AVG) is surgically prepared. An AVF is preferred over AVG because an AVG:

A. Is more likely to clot
B. May become infected
C. May cause distal ischemia (steal syndrome)
D. All of the above

Q67. The nurse teaches a patient with arteriovenous fistula for long-term hemodialysis to:

A. Palpate thrill over the area of anastomosis daily
B. Squeeze a rubber ball in the affected side
C. Avoid taking injections in the affected side
D. All of the above

Q68. Which of the following drugs should be withheld before hemodialysis?

A. Insulin
B. Calcium preparations
C. Digoxin
D. Antihypertensives

Q69. Which of the following drugs is preferably administered to reduce the serum phosphorus level of a patient with chronic renal failure?

A. Sodium bicarbonate
B. Sorbitol
C. Calcium carbonate
D. Aluminium hydroxide

Q70. A patient admitted with the diagnosis of renal calculi is complaining of severe pain in right flank and nausea. Immediate nursing goal for this patient would be:

A. Relief of pain
B. Prevention of infection due to stasis
C. Prevention of recurrence of stone formation
D. Promoting normal voiding pattern

Q71. The following clinical findings are usually present in a patient with chronic renal failure (CRF) *except:*

A. Uremia
B. Hypertension
C. Metabolic alkalosis
D. Anemia

Q72. During preparation of a patient for routine physical examination the nurse finds the patient unusually anxious. She understands that anxiety can affect the genitourinary system by:

A. Slowing glomerular filtration
B. Increasing glomerular filtration
C. Stimulating or hindering micturition
D. Increases sodium reabsorption and potassium excretion

Q73. The most accurate laboratory test for renal function is:

A. Blood urea nitrogen
B. Urinalysis
C. Creatinine clearance
D. Serum creatinine

Q74. A patient with chronic renal failure is undergoing hemodialysis for the first

time. Which of the following interventions the nurse should carry out in order to prevent disequilibrium syndrome?

A. Monitor patient's mental status at 15 minutes interval

B. Run the dialysate at a faster rate and allow rapid removal of fluid

C. Allow first few dialysis sessions for longer time

D. Dialyze for shorter times at a reduced blood flow rate for the first few sessions

Q75. Which of the following nursing interventions are appropriate for a patient with renal calculi?

A. Provide pain medications, promote complete bed rest

B. Provide low protein, high fluid diets, encourage ambulation

C. Strain all urine, provide pain medications, force fluids and encourage ambulation

D. Insert an indwelling catheter, check intake and output, and provide pain medications

Q76. The nurse is reviewing the findings of the laboratory test just received of a patient with chronic renal failure. Which of the following test results should be immediately reported to the physician?

A. Hb%–8.5 g/dL

B. Serum potassium – 7 mEq/L

C. Serum creatinine 6 mg/dL

D. Blood urea nitrogen 60 mg/dL

Q77. A patient who is receiving hemodialysis for chronic renal failure is especially prone to develop:

A. Peritonitis **B.** Hepatitis C

C. Renal calculi **D.** Bladder tumor

Q78. Which of the following lifestyle factors is most closely related to bladder cancer?

A. Sedentary lifestyle

B. Drinking 2 bottles of cola daily

C. Smoking 2 packs of cigarettes daily

D. Living in an industrial area

Q79. A renal stone located in the pelvis of the kidney will alter the function of the kidney by:

A. Obstructing the arterial supply of the kidney

B. Obstructing the venous return of the kidney

C. Obstructing collection and drainage of urine from the kidney

D. All of the above

Q80. A 22-year-old patient is waiting for a kidney transplant. The nurse is teaching the anxious mother about the transplant. Which of the following statements is appropriate?

A. 'It will take at least 48 hours for the transplanted kidney to form urine.'

B. 'Your son has to take immunosuppressive drugs prescribed by the physician lifelong'

C. 'Your son has to lead a sedentary lifestyle for the rest of his life.'

D. 'Symptoms of rejection include fever, malaise and hypotension.'

Q81. Which of the following symptoms indicate acute rejection of a transplanted kidney?

A. Fever, weight loss, oliguria, high blood pressure, pain at graft site

B. Fever, weight gain, polyuria, low blood pressure

C. Fever, weight gain, oliguria, high blood pressure, pain at graft site

D. Fever, weight loss, polyuria, low blood pressure, pain at graft site

ANSWERS AND RATIONALES OF URINARY SYSTEM

1. **B.** Use of amino acids for gluconeogenesis results in the formation of ammonia as a byproduct. Liver converts this ammonia into urea. Others are the functions of the kidney.

2. **C.** Diagnosis of a urinary tract infection is typically confirmed on the basis of a certain number of microorganisms in the urinary system, usually 10 to the power 5 /mL, although manifestation may begin with many fewer organisms than that.

3. **A.** Presence of pus in the urine is a common indication of urethritis. RBCs and casts are found in upper urinary tract infections, e.g. pyelonephritis, glomerulonephritis.

4. **B.** For urine culture and sensitivity test, clean catch midstream urine specimen is preferred. Normally bladder is sterile, but urethra contains bacteria and a few WBCs. The initial voided (first stream) urine flushes out most of the bacteria in the urethra so the middle stream urine, if properly collected, stored and handled would contain < 10000 organisms/mL and indicates no infection. Full volume of urine is not required for the said test.

5. **D.** Collecting urine midstream reduces the amount of contamination by microorganisms at the meatus. A clean container has to be used for a random specimen, not a clean catch specimen for urine culture. Voiding in the urinal, which is not sterile will contaminate the specimen. The male patient should retract the penis and clean the glans penis before voiding to prevent contamination.

6. **B.** Patient with pyelonephritis will have bloody or cloudy urine. Analysis reveals pyuria, bactriuria, hematuria and white blood cell casts. Urine pH tends to be alkaline. Intravenous pyelogram will look for underlying disease or the cause of reflux not shrinkage.

7. **A.** *Escherichia coli* bacteria are the cause of about 80% of urinary tract infection in persons who do not have urinary tract structural abnormalities or calculi. Other organisms responsible for urinary tract infection are *Klebsiella, Proteus, Candida, Enterococcus, Enterobacter, Pseudomonas, Staphylococcus,* etc.

8. **C.** Intravenous pyelogram involves intravenous injection of a contrast medium containing iodine and obtaining series of X-rays in regular intervals as the contrast medium moves through the tract. Some people develop serious allergic reactions, e.g. urticaria, itching and respiratory distress or failure to this contrast medium. Hence, it is absolutely essential to obtain history of allergies of the patient before the procedure. Other options are not essential for this procedure.

9. **B.** The first action of the nurse should be assessment for bladder fullness by gently palpating suprapubic area. In case the bladder is found to be full, catheter blockage is suspected and attempts to flush the catheter may be taken. Color of the urine is insignificant in this case. The patient should be reassured that it is a normal symptom often found due to the presence of the foreign substance.

10. **B.** Urine flows through the catheter to the drainage bag is by gravity. So the drainage bag is always positioned lower than the level of the bladder

with the catheter. Other options do not operate during urinary drainage.

11. B. Phenazopyridine (pyridium) does not cause bladder spasms contrary it provides a soothing effect on the urinary tract mucosa. It is an urinary analgesic and anesthetic. It causes bright red orange urine that stains clothing. Adverse effect may be diarrhea, rash and blue to purple skin discoloration.

12. A. The kidneys receive 20–25% of the cardiac output under resting conditions, averaging more than 1 liter of arterial blood per minute.

13. A. Most of the water (65%) and electrolytes of the glomerular filtrate is reabsorbed in the proximal tubules, then the descending limb of loop of Henle. Ascending limb of loop of Henle and distal tubule are water impermeable.

14. A. Sign and symptoms of cystitis is frequency, urgency, dysuria and hematuria. Most common manifestation of cancer of the bladder is microscopic or gross, painless hematuria. Pyelitis is the infection of the pelvis of kidney manifested as flank pain, chills, fever and weakness. Patient with stricture urethra will usually complain of diminished flow of urinary stream, straining to void and feelings of incomplete bladder emptying with urinary frequency and nocturia.

15. C. Methanamine (mandelamine) is an urinary antiseptic, given to treat urinary tract infection. Under acidic condition the drug decomposes into ammonia and formaldehyde, which denatures bacterial proteins causing death of the organisms.

16. D. Patient should not discontinue drug as abnormal taste sensation is a harmless side effect of trimethoprim. The medicine should be taken with full glass of water as well as adequate fluid intake must be maintained to decrease bacterial load in the bladder. The drug must be taken in equal interval around clock as prescribed by physician to maintain blood levels. Nausea, vomiting, rash, severe fatigue and sore throat to be reported to the physician.

17. A. Abnormal values of blood urea nitrogen, creatinine clearance and serum creatinine are indicative of renal impairment. Urine pH should be alkaline when gentamicin is used to treat urinary tract infection.

18. D. The patient may complain of pain on the affected side because the kidney is enlarged and might have formed an abscess. Patient will have dysuria, urgency and frequency not retention. Onset of the disease is often with chills and fever, and not hypothermia. High blood pressure is not associated with pyelonephritis.

19. D. Caffeine, alcohol, citrus juices, chocolate, carbonated beverages and highly spiced foods are considered to be bladder irritants and should be avoided. Other statements reflect adequate learning regarding prevention of recurrence of UTI.

20. C. It is vital that the patient returns for follow-up urine cultures, because bacteriuria may be present but may produce no symptoms. Antibiotics need to be taken for the full course of therapy regardless of symptoms. Pyelonephritis often recurs within 2 weeks of completing therapy. There is no need to restrict sodium unless it is otherwise contraindicated. Patient with chronic pyelonephritis has hypertension, so the need to restrict sodium.

21. A. Classic signs of acute glomerulonephritis is generalized

edema especially of the face and periorbital edema. Fever with sore throat or impetigo precedes 2–3 weeks before the onset of disease. Urine is scanty and smoky and contains red blood cells, white blood cells and cast. Pus cells are present in pyelonephritis. Patient has moderate to severe hypertension but not hypotension.

22. C. Uric acid stones and cystine stones are radiolucent, i.e. not visible on plain X-ray. Others are radiopaque, i.e. a plain film can identify larger stones.

23. A. Calcium is the most common substance of urinary stones and is found in up to 90% of stones. Calcium stones exist as calcium oxalate, calcium phosphate, or a mixture of both. Uric acid stones account for about 5–8% of all kidney stones.

24. C. Cystolitholapaxy is performed when a bladder stone is soft enough to crush by a lithotrite (stone crusher). In cystoscopic lithotripsy, an ultrasonic lithotrite is used to crush the stone and then removed by flushing. Ureteroscopy is passing a flexible ureteroscope through a cystoscope to collect stones located in ureter. Ureterorenoscope can be passed to collect stones located in the entire upper urinary tract.

25. A. Laser lithotripsy involves use of lasers together with a ureteroscope to remove or loosen impacted stone. In extracorporeal shock wave lithotripsy sound waves are applied externally to break up stones in the kidney or ureter. Percutaneous lithotripsy involves the insertion of a guide percutaneously under fluoroscopy near the area of the stone and then passing of ultrasonic wave to break the stone in fragments. Small stones lodged in ureter may be removed by passing a flexible ureteroscope through a cystoscope, but no laser is used.

26. A. Urolithiasis causes sudden severe colicky pain that the patient becomes increasingly restless and anxious. So relieving severe pain is the highest priority. Other nursing diagnoses may be appropriate when pain is controlled and therapeutic measures are undertaken to treat urolithiasis.

27. A. Allopurinol is an antigout drug. It inhibits the enzyme xanthine oxidase, reducing uric acid synthesis and thus preventing uric acid stone formation in kidney. The drug also prevents calcium oxalate stone in kidney, not calcium phosphate. Struvite stone is treated with long-term antibiotic therapy.

28. B. Aluminium hydroxide binds phosphorus in the intestine and prevents its absorption. This helps in decreasing serum phosphate level and prevents stone formation in the kidneys. Phosphorus is not absorbed in the stomach, the drug does not promote urinary excretion of phosphorus and phosphate stone is not formed in acidic urine.

29. B. In cutaneous ureterostomy surgeon attaches the ureter to the surface of the abdomen, where urine flows directly in to a drainage appliance. This is done when ureters are obstructed by a tumor. Transurethral resection is conducted in a very early stage of bladder cancer. Pyelostomy or percutaneous nephrostomy is usually performed to prevent obstruction in patient with inoperable bladder cancer.

30. A. Ileal bladder also known as ileal conduit or ureteroileostomy. In Indiana pouch or Florida pouch a reservoir is created in the ileum and then ureters are implanted in to the side of the diversion. In neobladder a bladder is created which empties via a pelvic outlet to the urethra.

31. A. Most commom complications of urethral trauma are urethral strictures and impotence among men due to damage of corpora cavernosa of the penis, blood vessels or nerves supplying this area. Ectopic ureters, mega-ureters (abnormal dilation of ureters) are congenital anomalies and cannot be the effect of trauma.

32. D. Detrusor failure (failure of the bladder to contract) is the most common cause of urinary retention in women. Urethral stricture is a common cause in men. Spinal cord injury if occurs can cause urinary retention in both men and women. Cystocele is another common cause of urinary retention in women.

33. B. Diverticulum is pouch or sack resulting from the herniation of the mucous membrane lining caused by weakness in the muscular wall. Bladder diverticula can give rise to two major problems: 1.Urinary tract infections resulting from stasis, 2. Malignancies, which may develop due to chronic irritation by persistent infection. There is no stricture in the urethra.

34. D. Overflow incontinence is defined as involuntary urine loss with overdistention of the bladder. Urge incontinence occurs randomly when involuntary urination is preceded by the warning of a few seconds to a few minutes. Stress incontinence is an involuntary loss of urine that occurs without detrusor contraction when intravesical pressure exceeds urethral pressure. Reflex incontinence is periodic involuntary urination without any warning or stress.

35. D. In urinary retention bladder is distended with urine, but the patient is unable to pass. Diuretic will further increase the discomfort by producing more urine and distending the bladder. Placing the patient in sitting position often help by increasing intra-abdominal pressure. Warm hot water bottle may promote muscle relaxation. In persistent retention the nurse needs to insert a catheter into the bladder but this requires an order from the physician.

36. A. Postoperative urinary retention is usually a temporary problem. So a plain catheter for single use is adequate to relieve retention. Foley's/ indwelling catheters remain in bladder for longer times for longer-term problems. 3-way catheter is used for bladder irrigation, e.g. after resection of prostate.

37. C. Acute tubular necrosis is the most common intrarenal cause of ARF and accounts for about 75%of cases. Acute glomerulonephritis and renal thrombosis are the less common causes. Septic shock giving rise to decreased peripheral resistance is one of the prerenal causes of ARF.

38. D. Uremic amaurosis is the sudden onset of bilateral blindness, which seems to be reversed in hours to days. Diminution of deep tendon reflexes, progressive hearing loss, or sudden onset of bilateral permanent blindness is not termed as uremic amaurosis.

39. A. Prerenal causes of renal failure are those that interfere with renal perfusion. Severe untreated glycosuria leading to osmotic diuresis may severely deplete circulatory volume resulting in acute renal failure. Myoglobinuria and atherosclerosis are the renal causes of acute renal failure. Enlarged prostate is the example of post-renal cause of renal failure.

40. A. Patient with renal failure must be provided with adequate energy from carbohydrate and fat sources to prevent ketosis from endogenous fat breakdown and gluconeogenesis from muscle protein breakdown. Fluid and electrolytes should be provided adequately to prevent dehydration, hyponatremia and hypokalemia in diuretic phase. Infections must be avoided by protecting the patient from other individuals with infections and restricting visitors. Deep breathing has no special indication in acute renal failure.

41. C. Oliguria, i.e. less than 400 mL of urine in 24 hours is the primary manifestation of acute renal failure. In an elderly patient with oliguric renal failure urine output may be 600–700 mL/day, as the sagging kidney normally loses its concentrating ability. Urine output of less than 100 mL/24 hours is called anuria.

42. B. Emergency pharmacologic management of hyperkalemia is done by administering hypertonic glucose solution along with insulin. IV administration of regular insulin with hypertonic glucose solution causes temporary shift of potassium ion into the cells and reduces its concentration in the extracellular fluid. Sodium bicarbonate alkalinize the plasma and cause temporary shift of potassium into the cells. Hyponatremia and hypokalemia is treated by replacing sodium and potassium. Hypernatremia is treated by infusion of hypotonic saline solution.

43. D. Continuous peritoneal dialysis uses the peritoneum as a semipermeable membrane to clean toxins by osmosis and diffusion. In hemodialysis patient's toxin laden blood comes in contact of the dialyzer for cleaning. In intermittent peritoneal dialysis, dialysis continues for short intermittent period.

44. A. Peritonitis is a common complication of peritoneal dialysis. Symptoms include fever, rebound tenderness, nausea, malaise and cloudy dialysate output. The diagnosis of peritonitis is confirmed when White Blood Cells count is above 100/ cubic millimeter and neutrophil count is more than 50% in the peritoneal effluent.

45. D. Cystitis is a common side effect of intravesical chemotherapy. So patient should be taught the sign and symptoms of cystitis in order to detect early its occurrence. For 6 hours after treatment urine and toilet bowl must be disinfected with bleach before flushing to provide a safe environment for others, as chemotherapeutic agents are toxic. Patient need not be placed in private rooms. Fluids are restricted for 4 hours before the treatment to decrease the need to void for 2 hours after treatment. After two hours of treatment fluids are encouraged to flush the bladder.

46. B. Normal healthy stoma should be red and moist. Stoma becoming pale, dark, dusky, gray or cyanotic means loss of vascular supply, which should be immediately reported to the physician. Continuous flow of urine through the stoma is normal. No urine flow for more than 15 minutes should be reported. Slight bleeding from the stoma during dressing or change of appliance is normal as the intestinal mucosa is very fragile.

47. D. Indiana pouch is an internal pouch, which allows the patient to perform self-catheterization for ileal drainage. As the pouch is made internally the patient does not need to wear an external pouch. The pouch is evacuated every 2 hours in the beginning. The interval between catheterization is increased gradually. Patient should drink a lot of water to prevent infection and calculi formation.

48. D. Pathogenesis of chronic renal failure involves deterioration and destruction of nephrons with progressive loss of renal function. The glomerulus, Bowman's capsule and tubular system are components of the nephron.

49. D. Intrarenal causes of acute renal failure (ARF) involve parenchymal changes caused by disease or nephrotoxic substances. Various agents, e.g. antibiotics, contrast media, heavy metal, poisons, bacterial toxins, etc causes nephrotoxic injury to renal parenchyma. Bilateral renal artery occlusion giving rise to poor perfusion to the kidneys is an example of prerenal cause of ARF. Obstruction of the urinary collecting system is an example of post renal cause of ARF. Damage to adrenal cortex is not related with ARF.

50. D. Respiratory distress experienced by the patient is probably due to the pressure of the dialysate on the diaphragm. So fluid should be removed immediately and patient's respiratory status and vital signs observed. Physician should be notified after immediate action is taken. Oxygen may have to be administered after the removal of fluid and diaphragmatic pressure decreased. Treatment should not be discontinued unless it is ordered.

51. B. A patient with chronic renal failure on continuous peritoneal dialysis should consume high carbohydrate diet to prevent weight loss and protein breakdown. Food should contain high fiber to prevent constipation. Patient should drink at least 2 litres of fluid daily. He should avoid high sodium foods and should avoid salt substitute as they contain potassium. Patient on peritoneal dialysis need not restrict potassium but certain fruits and vegetables contain high potassium (oranges, bananas, tomatoes, etc) so should not be taken in liberal amounts.

52. C. Erythropoietin a hormone produced in the kidney stimulates red blood cells production. Anemia secondary to chronic renal failure is treated with Epogen, a form of erythropoietin produced by recombinant deoxyribonucleic acid (DNA) technology. Epogen is not known to produce any effect on white blood cells, platelets or clotting.

53. D. Epoietin alfa stimulates erythropoiesis. Onset of increased reticulocyte count occurs in 2–6 weeks. So immediate correction of severe anemia is not possible with this drug.

54. B. The most serious adverse effect is hypertension. Hypertension may occur rapidly leading to hypertensive encephalopathy. Other adverse effect is seizures. The medicine is usually well tolerated and patient has a sense of well being while on this drug.

55. B. Option describes all the important steps for inserting an indwelling catheter. Option A is not correct, as gloves to be worn after preparation of patient and equipment. In option C wearing of gloves is omitted. Other steps are for inserting a plain catheter. In option D preparation of patient and equipment has been omitted.

56. C. Erythrocytopenia or decreased number of red blood cells is responsible for diminished cellular oxygenation, leading to fatigue and weakness. Dyspnea and cyanosis in CRF is due to fluid overload resulting in pulmonary edema. Bleeding tendencies develop in advanced CRF due to platelet abnormalities. Accumulation of uremic toxins also hinders platelet adhesiveness. Development of infection is due to the impairment of immune system not due to erythrocytopenia.

57. A. The left kidney is slightly higher than the right one because liver is lying above the right kidney. All other facts are true.

58. C. Stone fragments should be analyzed for composition to determine treatments, e.g. medications and dietary modifications. Culture and sensitivity of the stone fragments and cytological test are not done as stones are not usually due to infection and neither they are made up of abnormal cells. Culture and sensitivity of the urine may be done to detect any associated infection.

59. C. It is expected to have dark red urine for the first 24 hours after the procedure. Persistence of dark red urine beyond 24 hours indicates haemorrhage and must be reported. Patient needs to drink a lot of fluid in order to have more than 3 litres of urine output. Passage of sand like particles through the drainage tube is normal. Cloudy or foul smelling urine indicates infection and must be reported.

60. A. The most important complication of peritoneal dialysis is peritonitis. So risk for infection is the most appropriate nursing diagnosis. The process of ambulatory peritoneal dialysis is relatively simple requiring no machinery. So the patient can carry out any activity even during the procedure. So self care deficit is not an appropriate nursing diagnoses. Some pain, not acute pain may occur during dialysis due to rapid instillation, incorrect dialysate pH or temperature. Hyperglycemia may result in a diabetic patient as the dialysate fluid contains high concentration of glucose. In a non-diabetic, concentrated glucose dialysate gives rise to weight gain.

61. A. Chronic renal failure is characterized by a progressive reduction of functioning renal tissue or nephrons. It usually develops insidiously over many years. Rapid loss of renal function with elevated blood urea nitrogen, creatinine, electrolytes, etc. occurs in acute renal failure. The diseased kidney fails to excrete waste product, e.g. urea and creatinine. So creatinine clearance is low in renal failure, resulting in increased level of serum creatinine, blood urea nitrogen, electrolytes, etc.

62. B. Prerenal ARF is due to factors that reduce renal blood flow and lead to decreased glomerular perfusion and filtration. Myocardial infarction may severely reduce cardiac output resulting in decreased renal blood flow and decreased glomerular perfusion. Benign prostatic hyperplasia is one of the post-renal cause of ARF. Hemolytic blood transfusion reaction causes nephrotoxic injury and is one of the intrarenal cause of ARF. Septic shock also causes prerenal form of ARF but nephrotoxic injury from radiocontrast agents causes intrarenal form of ARF.

63. B. In oliguric phase of acute renal failure patient develops fluid overload due to oliguria. Fluid overload may lead to pulmonary edema. So the nurse needs to auscultate lungs for crackles. Kidney loses ability to excrete potassium, resulting in hyperkalemia. Hyperkalemia may potentiate cardiac arrhythmias and arrest. Warning signs of arrhythmia is ECG changes of tall peaked T waves. So the nurse needs to monitor ECG changes. In oliguric phase the patient develops hypertension due to fluid excess and not hypotension. Urine will have low creatinine and high sodium concentration as damaged kidney will have low creatinine clearance and will conserve low sodium. Low sodium conservation and fluid volume excess will result in hyponatremia not hypernatremia.

64. B. In diuretic phase of renal failure, urine output increases and approximates 1–3 litres /day. Because of high urine output, electrolytes, e.g. sodium and potassium are also lost giving rise to hyponatremia, hypokalemia and dehydration. Damaged kidney cannot activate vitamin D, so calcium is not absorbed from the GI tract resulting in hypocalcemia. Phosphate level increases with decrease in calcium concentration giving rise to hyperphosphatemia.

65. B. The patient with chronic renal failure who is not on dialysis should be provided with restricted diet. Low protein intake of ·6–·75/kg of body weight per day, high carbohydrate with appropriate amount of fat to maintain 30–35 kcal/kg of body weight, low fluid intake of 600 mL plus an amount of previous day's output, sodium and potassium restricted to 2–4 g per day is desirable.

66. D. Because the grafts are made of artificial materials, they can easily become infected and thrombosed. AVGs may cause the development of distal ischemia (steal syndrome) as too much of the arterial blood is being shunted or stolen from the distal extremity.

67. D. Maintaining the vascular access patent and free of infection is important. Patency of the vascular access needs to be assessed regularly by palpating the thrill over the area of anastomosis. Injections and blood pressure measurement should not be carried out in the affected arm to prevent chance of infection and clotting. Patient should exercise by squeezing a rubber ball in order to increase the size of the vessels.

68. C. Digoxin should be withheld before dialysis. Although dialysis does not affect digoxin level, it causes hypokalemia. Hypokalemia can potentiate arrhythmias secondary to digoxin toxicity. Insulin can be administered because they are not removed by dialysis. Calcium preparations are often added in the dialysate to prevent renal osteodystrophy. The dosage of antihypertensives may be modified as dialysis may cause hypotension due to removal of fluid.

69. C. To reduce the serum phosphorus level of a patient with chronic renal failure calcium based phosphate binders like calcium carbonate or calcium acetate is administered. Aluminium hydroxide gel or aluminium antacids were formerly used. But their use nowadays is not recommended since they cause dementia due to excessive absorption of aluminium. Sodium bicarbonate is used to control acidosis. Sorbitol a laxative promotes potassium removal from bowel.

70. A. Since the patient is having severe pain, it has to be controlled with adequate analgesic as prescribed. Nausea and vomiting are usually associated with severe pain and will be relieved as pain subsides. Other nursing goals have to be attained gradually. Relieving pain is the priority.

71. C. In chronic renal failure (CRF) metabolic acidosis occurs due to failure of the kidneys to excrete hydrogen ions. Uremia is the build up of nitrogen wastes in the blood, anemia is due to failure of the kidney to produce erythropoietin and hypertension from fluid overload are consistent manifestations of CRF.

72. C. The most common manifestation of anxiety in urinary system is stimulation of micturition seen as frequent voiding and urinary urgency. If anxiety leads to generalized muscle tension it may hinder micturition because perineal muscle must relax for successful micturition. Anxiety has no effect on glomerular filtration rate and reabsorption and excretion of electrolytes.

73. C. Creatinine clearance is the most accurate test for renal function as it determines the glomerular filtration rate and tubular excretion ability of the kidney. Results from other options may be influenced by different conditions and are not specific. Although serum creatinine is most commonly used for usual purpose.

74. D. Disequilibrium syndrome develops from rapid changes in composition of blood. Solutes are removed more readily from blood than cerebrospinal fluid and brain. This creates high osmotic gradient in brain resulting in cerebral edema. This is prevented by dialyzing for a shorter times at a reduced blood flow rate for the first few sessions. Monitoring mental status will help in early detection of the problem, will not prevent it.

75. C. The appropriate nursing actions are to strain all urine and save any stone for examinations, provide pain medications as kidney stones are painful, force fluids to flush the kidney from small stones if any and encourage ambulation for the easy passage of stone down the ureters by gravity. Indwelling catheter is not needed and should be avoided to prevent infection.

76. B. Normal serum potassium level is 3.5–5.5 mEq/L. Fatal dysrhythmias may occur when the serum potassium level reaches 7–8 mEq/L. So this finding should immediately be reported and precautionary measure taken. Other findings are all consistent with chronic renal failure. Elevated levels of serum creatinine and Blood urea nitrogen may give rise to central nervous system manifestations but none of these findings require emergent care.

77. B. Hepatitis C is transmitted by blood or blood products. Hemodialysis and blood transfusion needed for a patient with renal failure exposes him to the possibility of transmission. Peritonitis is a complication of peritoneal dialysis. Renal calculi and bladder tumor are not known to be the complication of hemodialysis.

78. C. There is a strong correlation between smoking and bladder cancer. Industrial exposure to certain substances, e.g. dyes, asbestos and aromatic amines may also cause bladder cancer but living in an industrial area is not known to be related. Artificial sweeteners have been weakly linked with bladder cancer and cola drinks may be a source of this substance. Sedentary lifestyle is unrelated to bladder cancer.

79. C. Renal pelvis is the funnel shaped sac where the major calices merged. The major calices transport urine to the renal pelvis and then through the ureter to the bladder. Hence a stone in the pelvis will obstruct the collection and drainage of urine from kidney. The entry and exit point of renal artery and vein respectively as well as ureter is the hilus not the renal pelvis.

80. B. In order to prevent the rejection of the transplanted kidney the patient has to take immunosuppressive drug for the rest of his life. The transplanted kidney if taken from a living donor starts functioning immediately, but if taken from a cadaver it may take 24 hours time to start functioning. The patient after transplant is able to lead a normal life. Regular exercises and play are encouraged except contact sports. Symptoms of rejection include, fever, malaise, anemia and hypertension not hypotension.

81. C. Sign of rejection of a transplanted kidney include fever, weight gain, decreased urine output, increased blood pressure and tenderness over the graft area. Serum creatinine and blood urea will also be elevated.

6
CHAPTER

Endocrine System and Diabetes

Q1. Which of the following statements correctly describes the characteristics of hormones?

A. Hormones are chemical substances synthesized and secreted by a specific organ or tissue called glands
B. Circulated through the blood to reach to target tissue
C. Bind to specific cellular receptors either in the cell membrane or within the cell
D. All of the above

Q2. Hormones have their effect on specific body tissue or organ called target. Target tissue for thyroxine (T4) and triiodothyroxine (T3) is:

A. Thyroid gland
B. All body tissues
C. Bone tissue
D. All of the above

Q3. Which of the following groups of hormones is produced by thyroid gland?

A. Thyrotropin, oxytocin and calcitonin
B. Thyrotropin, triiodothyronine and thyroxine
C. Triiodothyronine, thyroxine and calcitonin
D. Triiodothyronine and thyroxine

Q4. Enlargement of the thyroid gland occurs in:

A. Hypothyroidism
B. Hyperthyroidism
C. Tumors of thyroid
D. All of the above

Q5. Endemic goiter:

A. Is more common in men
B. Is more common in middle age
C. Occurs due to excessive consumption of sea foods
D. Occurs in areas where soil and water are deficient in iodine

Q6. The most common type of goiter is:

A. Endemic or simple
B. Sporadic
C. Nodular
D. Toxic

Q7. The most common type of hypothyroidism is:

A. Thyroid hypothyroidism
B. Central hypothyroidism
C. Secondary hypothyroidism
D. Tertiary hypothyroidism

Q8. The most common type of autoimmune hypothyroidism is:

A. Graves' disease
B. Addison's disease
C. Hashimoto's disease
D. Cushing's disease

Q9. A patient attends hospital with complain of intolerance to cold and extreme fatigue. The physician suspects hypothyroidism. Which of the following tests should be ordered?

A. Serum TSH and T4 concentration
B. Thyroid antibodies
C. Thyroid scan
D. All of the above

Q10. The drug that will probably be ordered for the patient with hypothyroidism is:

A. Potassium iodide
B. Lugol's iodine
C. Propylthiouracil
D. Levothyroxine sodium

Q11. Which of the following symptoms are associated with hypothyroidism?

A. Lethargy, constipation, thick brittle nails and weight gain
B. Intolerance to heat, diarrhea, tachycardia and nervousness
C. Polyuria, polyphagia and weight loss
D. Buffalo hump, oily skin, weakness and depression

Q12. While assessing a patient with hypothyroidism the nurse should be alert for:

A. Irritability and restlessness
B. Bounding rapid pulse
C. Puffiness of face
D. Tremors of fingers and tongue

Q13. L-thyroxine sodium has been ordered for a patient with hypothyroidism as replacement therapy. The nurse should teach the patient to take the drug:

A. In the morning at empty stomach
B. In the morning after breakfast
C. At bedtime
D. Whenever convenient

Q14. A 55-year-old female patient is diagnosed with hypothyroidism is on thyroid replacement therapy. The nurse understands that this patient is at the risk of developing:

A. Nephropathy
B. Angina and cardiac dysrhythmias
C. Allergies
D. Thyroid storm

Q15. A 60-year-old woman receiving thyroid replacement therapy has to undergo an emergency internal fixation for fracture neck femur. The nurse is aware that postoperatively the patient is at the risk of developing:

A. Wound infection
B. Hyperthermia
C. Thyroid crisis
D. Myxedema coma

Q16. A 70-year-old female patient suffering from hypothyroidism tells the nurse that she often forgets to take her daily dose of thyroid hormone. The nurse understands that the patient is at risk of developing:

A. Polycythemia
B. Hyperglycemia
C. Myxedema coma
D. Heart failure

Q17. An appropriate nursing intervention for a patient with hypothyroidism is:

A. To encourage the patient to speed up his activities of daily living
B. To provide a low calorie and low roughage diet
C. To provide a comfortable and cool environment
D. To teach patient minimum use of soap for bathing and application of lotion to prevent skin breakdown

Q18. The nurse teaches a patient who is on thyroid replacement therapy for hypothyroidism to report immediately if she experiences:

A. Dyspnea on exertion

B. Fine tremors of hands
C. Chest pain
D. Worsening fatigue

Q19. The nurse is teaching a patient with hypothyroidism for self-care. Which of the following is not appropriate?

A. To take thyroid hormone lifelong
B. To avoid exposure in cold climate for a long time
C. To take a low calorie and low residue diet
D. To avoid sedatives

Q20. The nursing diagnosis for an elderly female patient admitted with hypothyroidism may be all of the following *except*:

A. Imbalanced nutrition: More than body requirements related to hypometabolism
B. Activity intolerance related to hypometabolism and mucin deposits in joints and interstitial spaces
C. Hypothermia related to cold intolerance
D. Fluid and electrolyte disturbances secondary to gastrointestinal hypermotility

Q21. Which of the following conditions is characterized by an excessive secretion of thyroid hormone?

A. Hypothyroidism
B. Hyperthyroidism
C. Exophthalmos
D. Thyrotoxic crisis

Q22. Hyperthyroidism is characterized by:

A. Loss of the normal regulatory controls of thyroid hormones
B. Hypometabolism
C. State of nutritional deficiency and weight loss
D. Both A and C

Q23. Which of the following statements best describes Graves' disease?

A. The most common form of hyperthyroidism
B. Autoimmune disease of unknown etiology
C. Gives rise to exophthalmos, goiter and hyperthyroidism
D. All of the above

Q24. Which of the following conditions is the most common form of hyperthyroidism?

A. Addison's disease
B. Cushing's disease
C. Graves' disease
D. Hashimoto's disease

Q25. A patient attends hospital with the complaint of weight loss instead of increased appetite and frequent defecation. The nurse finds her intensely nervous and a diffuse swelling in the neck. She suspects that the patient may be suffering from:

A. Hypothyroidism
B. Hyperthyroidism
C. Diabetes mellitus
D. AIDS

Q26. The major complications of Graves' disease are:

A. Heart disease and exophthalmos
B. Thyroid storm
C. Only B
D. Both A and B

Q27. Nursing intervention for a patient with hyperthyroidism having exophthalmos involves:

A. Limiting salt intake and elevating the head of the bed at night
B. Lightly tape the eyes shut with non-allergenic tape at night
C. Both A and B
D. Only B

Q28. One of the antithyroid drugs prescribed to control hyperthyroidism in Graves' disease is:

A. Beta blockers
B. Corticosteroids
C. Nonsteroidal anti-inflammatory drugs
D. Propylthiouracil

Q29. Which of the following symptoms are associated with hyperthyroidism?

A. Restlessness, agitation, weight loss and increased appetite

B. Protruding eyeballs, sluggishness and slow pulse

C. Swelling in neck, weight gain and loss of appetite

D. Dry skin, slow pulse and increased appetite

Q30. Nurse is reviewing the laboratory test results of a patient with hyperthyroidism. Which of the following findings she should anticipate?

A. Serum TSH- 12 microunit/mL, FT4 -.5 ng/dL

B. Serum TSH -.28 microunit/ml, FT4 – 2.4 ng/dL

C. Radioactive iodine uptake – 50%

D. Both B and C

Q31. A patient with hyperthyroidism has been ordered a radioactive iodine uptake test. Before administering the dose of radioactive isotope the nurse should ask the patient all of the following *except*:

A. 'Have you eaten sea food within the last 2 weeks?'

B. 'Are you on antihypertensive drugs?'

C. "Are you on estrogen replacement therapy?'

D. 'Have you taken any iodine containing medications within the last 30 days?'

Q32. The action of propylthiouracil in the control of hyperthyroidism is by:

A. Inhibiting synthesis of thyroid hormones

B. Blocking the action of thyroid hormone in the body

C. Blocking peripheral conversion of T4 to more active T3

D. Both A and C

Q33. The purpose of giving Lugol's iodine in Graves' disease is:

A. To reduce vascularity of the thyroid gland

B. To increase vascularity of the thyroid gland

C. To treat thyroid storm

D. Both A and C

Q34. The nurse is teaching a patient with hyperthyroidism regarding antithyroid therapy. Which statement by the patient indicates further teaching?

A. 'I may expect some improvements in my condition after 4-8 weeks'

B. 'I may stop taking the drug after my symptoms improve'

C. 'I may get some allergic rashes or pruritus during the course of my treatment'

D. 'I would stop taking medicine if I get sore throat or fever and report immediately'

Q35. The first line antithyroid drugs used in the treatment of hyperthyroidism are:

A. Propylthiouracil, potassium iodide, and triiodothyronine

B. Methimazole, carbimazole, and Lugol's iodine

C. I-thyroxine sodium, carbimazole, and Lugol's solution

D. Methimazole, potassium iodide, radioactive iodine

Q36. All of the following statements describe radioactive iodine therapy for hyperthyroidism *except*:

A. Radioactive iodine has a delayed action

B. It is a treatment of choice in pregnant and nursing mothers as many of the adverse effect of antithyroid drugs are avoided

C. Lifelong thyroid hormone replacement is necessary in patients treated by this therapy

D. All of the above

Q37. A challenging nursing intervention for a patient with hyperthyroidism is:

A. Providing an adequate diet

B. Restricting visitors

C. Keeping the bed linen neat

D. Providing sufficient rest

Q38. A patient with hyperthyroidism is scheduled for subtotal thyroidectomy. An important preoperative nursing goal for this patient is:

A. To maintain normal body temperature
B. To gain confidence and reduce anxiety
C. To encourage increased independence
D. All of the above

Q39. Which of the following positions is given to a patient after thyroidectomy?

A. Sidelying position with the head elevated by a pillow
B. Recumbent position with the head elevated by a pillow so that the neck is slightly flexed
C. Semi-Fowler's position with the head supported by pillows
D. Any position to make the patient comfortable

Q40. Following a thyroidectomy, the nurse suspects injury to one laryngeal nerve when the patient develops:

A. Laryngeal stridor
B. Hoarseness
C. Respiratory obstruction
D. Both B and C

Q41. The nurse is taking care of a patient with thyroidectomy in the immediate postoperative period. Anticipating bilateral laryngeal nerve damage the nurse should assemble which of the following equipments at the patient's bedside?

A. Blood pressure cuff and stethoscope
B. Oxygen cylinder
C. Tracheostomy set
D. Ampoules of calcium gluconate

Q42. One of the complications of thyroidectomy is injury to parathyroid glands. Which of the following symptoms indicate injury to or removal of parathyroid glands?

A. Hoarseness
B. Dyspnea
C. Muscular weakness
D. Laryngeal stridor

Q43. After thyroidectomy a patient develops tetany. Which of the following drugs the nurse should administer?

A. Calcium gluconate
B. Calcium carbonate
C. Calcium chloride
D. Calcium phosphate

Q44. Postoperative care for a patient with thyroidectomy includes all of the following *except*:

A. Placing the patient in the semi-Fowler's position
B. Instructing patient to bend head in front every 2 hourly
C. Assess patient every 2 hours for signs of hemorrhage
D. Encouraging patient to talk after recovery from anesthesia

Q45. The pituitary gland is located:

A. In the sella turcica at the base of the brain above the sphenoid bone
B. In the mediastinum anterior to the trachea
C. In the central part of the diencephalon area of the brain
D. In the brain above the hypothalamus

Q46. Which of the following groups of hormones is secreted by the anterior pituitary gland?

A. Somatropin, prolactin, oxytocin
B. Somatostatin, luteinizing, prolactin
C. Gonadotropic, prolactin, somatotropin
D. Thyrotropin releasing hormone, prolactin inhibiting hormone, adrenocorticotropic hormone

Q47. The target tissue for somatotropin hormone is:

A. Bone tissue
B. Reproductive system
C. Adrenal cortex
D. All body cells

Q48. Antidiuretic hormone (ADH) or vasopressin is secreted by:

A. Hypothalamus

B. Posterior pituitary
C. Adrenal gland
D. Kidney

Q49. The most important stimulus to antidiuretic hormone secretion is:

A. Decreased plasma osmolality
B. Increased plasma osmolality
C. Decreased blood volume
D. Both B and C

Q50. Acromegaly is due to:

A. Overproduction of growth hormone by the pituitary
B. Deficient production of growth hormone by the pituitary
C. Overproduction of androgens by the adrenal
D. Deficient production of androgens by the adrenal

Q51. Hypersecretion of which of the following hormones is the cause of pituitary gigantism?

A. Adrenocorticotropical hormone
B. Growth hormone
C. Thyroid stimulating hormone
D. Parathyroid hormone

Q52. Which of the following groups of symptoms describes acromegaly?

A. Excessive bone growth, mental sluggishness, hypoglycemia
B. Short attention span, excessive weight gain, excessive thirst
C. Enlargement of bony and soft tissue over the head and face, deep voices, glucose intolerance
D. Irritability, menstrual disturbances, hypertension

Q53. Excess secretion of luteinizing hormone (LH) and follicle stimulating hormone (FSH) from pituitary tumors can produce which of the following conditions in children?

A. Gigantism
B. Dwarfism
C. Sexual precocity
D. Sterility

Q54. The symptoms of hyperprolactinemia are all of the following *except*:

A. Galactorrhea
B. Failure of lactation
C. Amenorrhea
D. Decreased libido in men

Q55. A patient attends hospital clinic with the complaint of galactorrhea (abnormal lactation in nonlactating breast). On examination, no evidence of pituitary tumor was found. The nurse anticipates that the patient will be treated by:

A. Prophylactic surgery
B. Administration of prolactin
C. Administration of bromocriptin
D. Both A and B

Q56. Which of the following disorders that results from hypopituitarism may lead to an absence of lactation in the postpartum woman?

A. Hypothyroidism
B. Secondary adrenocortical insuffiency
C. Short stature
D. Hypoprolactinemia

Q57. Which of the following conditions is a major disorder of the neurohypophysis?

A. Diabetes insipidus
B. Gigantism
C. Secondary hypogonadism
D. None of the above

Q58. Diabetes insipidus results from:

A. Deficiency of epinephrine
B. Excessive secretion of epinephrine
C. Deficiency of vasopressin
D. Excessive secretion of vasopressin

Q59. A patient is recovering from surgery of pituitary gland. The nurse is aware that the patient may develop:

A. Cushing's syndrome
B. Hyperthyroidism

C. Diabetes insipidus
D. Diabetes mellitus

Q60. A patient with acromegaly associated with pituitary tumor has undergone hypophysectomy. Postoperatively the nurse notices sudden increase in urine output and suspects diabetes insipidus as complication. Which laboratory findings are helpful to support nurse's suspicion of diabetes insipidus?

A. Low urine and serum osmolality levels
B. Elevated urine and serum osmolality levels
C. Elevated urine osmolality and low serum osmolality levels
D. Low urine osmolality and elevated serum osmolality levels

Q61. Diagnosis of diabetes insipidus is confirmed by:

A. Water deprivation test
B. Capillary blood glucose test
C. Urine test for specific gravity
D. Urine test for glucose

Q62. While caring for an elderly patient with diabetes insipidus the nurse assesses patient's ability to drink copious amounts of fluids, as she is aware of the fact that the patient is likely to develop:

A. Overhydration and hyponatremia
B. Dehydration and hypernatremia
C. Hypertension and bradycardia
D. Weight gain and hyperglycemia

Q63. Excessive secretion of vasopressin is responsible for which of the following disorders?

A. Diabetes insipidus
B. Syndrome of inappropriate antidiuretic hormone
C. Cushing's syndrome
D. Addisonian crisis

Q64. Which of the following statements characterizes syndrome of inappropriate antidiuretic hormone (SIADH)?

A. Results in concentrated urine inspite of normal intravascular volume and renal function
B. Results in diluted urine, serum hyperosmolality and hypernatremia
C. Results in fluid retention, serum hypoosmolality and hyponatremia
D. Both A and C

Q65. The nurse is assessing a patient with syndrome of inappropriate antidiuretic hormone secretion. Which of the following signs would indicate that the patient might develop complications?

A. Weight loss
B. Sudden increase in urine output
C. Hypotension
D. Neck vein distention

Q66. The nurse is caring for a patient with SIADH. Which of the following symptoms she should include in her assessment?

A. Increased appetite
B. Mental alertness
C. Tetanic contractions
D. Abdominal cramps

Q67. The nurse is taking care of a patient hospitalized with acute onset of SIADH. Which of the following interventions is not appropriate?

A. Restricting total intake of fluids no more than 1000 mL/day
B. Supplementing sodium and potassium in diet
C. Positioning the patient at semi Fowler's position
D. Observing seizures precautions

Q68. A patient is admitted in the hospital ward with a provisional diagnosis of hypoparathyroidism. The nurse caring for the patient should observe closely for the occurrence of:

A. Severe hypertension
B. Excessive thirst
C. Tetany
D. Polyuria

Q69. An elderly patient attends hospital clinic with the complaint of backache and skeletal pain, weakness, increased need for sleep, irritability, anorexia, consti-

pation and polyuria. Based on these subjective data the nurse would suspect which of the following conditions?

A. Hypoparathyroidism
B. Hyperparathyroidism
C. Hypothyroidism
D. Hyperthyroidism

Q70. An elderly woman with hyperparathyroidism is being treated with estrogen supplementation and biphosphonates (alendronate). Which of the following instructions would be most important to include in the patient's teaching plan?

A. To rest as much as possible
B. To maintain a moderate exercise program
C. To adopt a weight reducing diet
D. To perform weight bearing exercises daily

Q71. A 50-year-old woman has been diagnosed with hypoparathyroidism. The nurse anticipates that the patient will be prescribed a daily supplements of calcium 2 g/day and:

A. Phosphorus
B. Folic acid
C. Vitamin D
D. Vitamin C

Q72. The nurse encourages patient with hyperparathyroidism to force fluids, as she is aware that the patient may develop kidney stones. Which of the following electrolytes are responsible for stone formation in these patients?

A. Calcium and magnesium
B. Calcium and phosphorus
C. Calcium and chlorides
D. Calcium and potassium

Q73. Which of the following nursing interventions is not appropriate for a patient who has just been diagnosed with hyperparathyroidism and is on medical treatment?

A. Providing a low bed with side rails
B. Providing high calorie low residue diet
C. Encouraging plenty of fluids including fruit juice
D. Encouraging regular exercise under supervision

Q74. The nurse was checking the blood pressure of a patient with hypoparathyroidism. During inflation of the blood pressure cuff patient experienced spasms of the wrist and hand of the side examined. The nurse identified the phenomenon as:

A. Positive Chvostek sign
B. Positive Trousseau sign
C. Hyperactive deep tendon reflex
D. None of the above

Q75. Which of the following groups of hormones is produced by the adrenal cortex?

A. Adrenocorticotropic hormone (ACTH), aldosterone, androgens
B. Cortisol, aldosterone, androgens
C. Cortisol, aldosterone, catecholamines
D. Catecholamines, aldosterone, cortisol

Q76. Which of the following disorders causes secondary adrenal insufficiency?

A. Hyposecretion of somatotropin by pituitary
B. Hyposecretion of corticotropin by pituitary
C. Hyposecretion of cortisol by adrenal
D. Hypersecretion of corticotropin by pituitary

Q77. The most common cause of primary adrenal insufficiency (Addison's disease) is destruction of the adrenal gland by:

A. Infection
B. Ischemia
C. Autoimmune process
D. Metastatic invasion by tumor

Q78. A patient attends the hospital with the complain of progressive weakness, anorexia, dark pigmentation of skin and

laboratory findings of low serum sodium and high serum potassium. The nurse anticipates that the patient may be presenting with:

A. Addison's disease
B. Cushing's syndrome
C. Diabetes mellitus
D. SIADH

Q79. What may occur if a patient with adrenocortical insufficiency has been under stress?

A. Addison's crisis
B. Osteoporosis
C. Adrenocortical hyperfunction
D. All of the above

Q80. A patient with Addison's disease has been prescribed corticosteroids for replacement. The nurse instructs the patient to take the medicine preferably:

A. Daily at bedtime
B. After each principal meal
C. On awakening and in the late afternoon
D. Every 6 hourly after food

Q81. A patient has been admitted with addisonian crisis. Which of the following assessment the nurse should perform frequently?

A. Body weight
B. Vital signs
C. Urine for sugar
D. Neckvein distention

Q82. During discharge a patient with Addison's disease should be instructed to do which of the following before undergoing dental extraction or minor surgery?

A. Continue to take his usual dose of hydrocortisone
B. Administer hydrocortisone IM
C. Contact physician to obtain a dosage increase
D. Take hydrocortisone at 50% reduced dosage for a period of 1 week after the surgery

Q83. Which of the following nursing goal is appropriate for a patient with Addison's disease?

A. Teaching patient self-care
B. Managing fluid volume excess
C. Promoting early ambulation
D. Improving nutritional status

Q84. The nurse is assessing a patient with Addison's disease during follow-up visit. Which of the following indicates that the patient has a desirable outcome with prescribed treatment?

A. Patient maintains same body weight for the last 3 months
B. Vital signs within normal limits
C. Patient states that the fatigue has decreased
D. All of the above

Q85. A patient in Addisonian crisis has been admitted in the hospital. Which of the following nursing interventions would be most appropriate?

A. Placing the patient in a separate room
B. Assessing vital signs every 4 hourly
C. Encouraging a high carbohydrate diet every 2 hourly
D. Allowing ambulation as tolerated

Q86. A 30-year-old female patient attends hospital with the complaints of weight gain, facial hair, acne, absent menstruation and frequent bruising. The nurse suspects that the patient may be suffering from:

A. Myxedema
B. Addison's disease
C. Cushing's syndrome
D. Graves' disease

Q87. The most common cause of Cushing's syndrome is:

A. Tumor of adrenal gland
B. Pituitary adenoma that produces ACTH
C. Hyperplasia of adrenal gland
D. Ectopic corticotropin secreting tumor

Q88. The clinical manifestations of Cushing's syndrome include all of the following *except*:

A. Hyperglycemia
B. Hypoglycemia
C. Hypokalemia
D. Immunosuppressive responses

Q89. The nurse is assessing a patient with Cushing's syndrome. Which of the following signs she is expected to find?

A. Hypotension
B. Truncal obesity and supraclavicular fat pad
C. Hyperkalemia
D. Thick coarse skin

Q90. A patient with unilateral adrenalectomy has been prescribed spironolactone (aldactone). Which of the following adverse effects the patient may experience during the therapy?

A. Breast tenderness
B. Menstrual irregularities
C. Increased facial hair
D. Hair loss

Q91. The nurse is giving dietary advice to a patient with Cushing's syndrome. Which of the following diet she should advise?

A. Diet high in calorie, protein, potassium and calcium; low in fat and sodium
B. Diet high in protein, calcium and potassium; low in fat, sodium and simple sugars
C. Diet high in protein and calorie; low in potassium and calcium
D. Diet high in carbohydrate, potassium and calcium; low in protein and fat

Q92. Which of the following nursing diagnoses is appropriate for a patient with Cushing's syndrome?

A. Fluid volume deficit
B. Disturbed self esteem
C. Ineffective thermoregulation
D. Improper nutrition less than body requirements

Q93. The nurse is taking care of a patient with Cushing's syndrome. Which of the following nursing actions she should perform?

A. Teach handwashing to patient engaged in self-care
B. Explain rational for increasing salt and fluid intake in times of illness, increased stress or hot weather
C. Teach patient to consume diet high in calorie and protein
D. Encourage patient to take rest as much as possible

Q94. An important nursing intervention when caring for a patient with Cushing's syndrome is to:

A. Provide a low protein diet
B. Observe for signs of hypotension
C. Provide extra blankets to prevent hypothermia
D. Encourage good grooming and use of attractive clothing

Q95. The most common cause of primary hyperaldosteronism is:

A. Excessive sodium intake
B. Adrenal adenoma
C. Pituitary adenoma
D. Chronic renal disease

Q96. Hyperaldosteronism exhibits which of the following symptoms?

A. Hypertension
B. Hypernatremia
C. Hypokalemia
D. All of the above

Q97. A patient with hypertension has been admitted for the diagnostic tests and diagnosed with primary hyperaldosteronism. Diagnosis indicates that patient's hypertension is caused by excessive secretion of aldosterone by:

A. Adrenal cortex
B. Adrenal medulla
C. Pituitary
D. Testis

Q98. Which of the following statements about pheochromocytoma is true?

A. Characterized by a tumor of the adrenal medulla that produces excessive catecholamines
B. Characterized by atrophy of adrenal medulla resulting in deficient catecholamines
C. Severe hypotension and collapse are the common features of this disease
D. This condition commonly occurs in old age

Q99. A patient is admitted in hospital with the diagnosis of pheochromocytoma. Which of the following sign and symptoms the nurse is expected to find?

A. Pounding headache, hypertension, hypoglycemia, confusion
B. Pounding headache, tachycardia, diaphoresis, hypertension
C. Bradycardia, hypotension, agitation, weight gain
D. Hypometabolism, weight gain, nausea, vomiting

Q100. Diabetes mellitus is a chronic disease characterized by:

A. Deficiency of insulin
B. Oversecretion of insulin
C. Decreased ability of the body to use insulin
D. Both A and C

Q101. The following statements about type 1 diabetes mellitus are all true *except*:

A. Type 1 diabetes mellitus usually occurs in older adults
B. Patients with type 1 diabetes mellitus are insulin dependent
C. Endogenous insulin production is little or none in these patients
D. Islet cell antibodies are found in these patients

Q102. The most common form of diabetes mellitus is:

A. Type1 diabetes mellitus
B. Type 2 diabetes mellitus
C. Gestational diabetes mellitus
D. Secondary diabetes mellitus

Q103. Which of the following events does not occur in the pathogenesis of type 1 diabetes mellitus?

A. Genetic predisposition
B. Environmental triggers
C. Inactive autoimmunity
D. Progressive beta cell destruction

Q104. Which of the following phenomenon precisely describes the pathogenesis of type 2 diabetes mellitus?

A. Sensitization and insulin resistance
B. Desensitization and insulin resistance
C. Sensitization and insulin tolerance
D. Desensitization and insulin tolerance

Q105. Which of the following metabolic problems occurs when pancreas fails to produce insulin?

A. Decreased glucose utilization
B. Increased protein utilization
C. Increased fat metabolism
D. All of the above

Q106. Which of the following signs and symptoms are associated with type 1 diabetes mellitus?

A. Polyuria, polydipsia and weight loss
B. Polyphagia, weight gain and tiredness
C. Diaphoresis, excessive hunger, irritability and tachycardia
D. Bradycardia and hypertension

Q107. The clinical characteristics associated with type 2 diabetes mellitus is:

A. Loss of body weight
B. Presence of islet cell antibodies
C. May develop ketosis suddenly after remaining asymptomatic initially
D. Only exercise and diet therapy may be enough to control hyperglycemia

Q108. Polyuria and polydipsia in diabetes mellitus are primarily caused by:

A. The release of ketones from cells during fat metabolism
B. Fluid shifts resulting from the osmotic diuresis caused by high blood glucose level
C. Damage to kidney tubules from constant exposure to high blood glucose level
D. High blood glucose level inhibits secretion of antidiuretic hormone

Q109. Which of the following blood test values confirms the diagnosis of diabetes mellitus?

A. Fasting blood glucose level of 120 mg/dL
B. Random plasma glucose measurement of 175 mg/dL
C. Two hour oral glucose tolerance test level of 220 mg/dL
D. None of the above test results indicative of diabetes mellitus

Q110. Physician has ordered a repeat fasting blood sugar test to an individual whose previous test result was 124 mg/dL. The nurse instructs the individual not to consume any nutrient other than water for:

A. 2-4 hours
B. 4-6 hours
C. 6-8 hours
D. 8-12 hours

Q111. A middle aged woman who has recently been diagnosed with type 2 diabetes and was advised diet therapy and exercise program has come for follow-up after 3 months. Which of the following tests will be most conclusive in evaluating the response of the prescribed regimen?

A. Fasting blood glucose
B. Postprandial blood glucose
C. Random blood glucose
D. Glycosylated hemoglobin

Q112. Effective collaborative management of diabetes includes:

A. Administering insulin to all patients to achieve glycemic control
B. Instituting nutritional therapy mainly as initial therapy for all patients with diabetes
C. Depending on the physician as central figure in the program for diabetic control
D. Aiming for a balance of diet, activity and medications together with appropriate monitoring and patient and family teaching

Q113. Oral hypoglycemic agents are indicated in patients with type 2 diabetes mellitus when:

A. Loosing body weight is a problem
B. Endogenous insulin is totally absent
C. Random blood glucose level is more than 400 mg/dL
D. Inadequate control of blood glucose level after exercise and diet therapies

Q114. Regular consistent exercise is considered an essential part of diabetes management because exercise:

1. Lowers blood glucose level by increasing carbohydrate metabolism and insulin sensitivity
2. Contributes to weight loss that decreases insulin resistance
3. Lowers blood pressure, improves circulation and reduces stress and tension
4. Increases high density lipoprotein level and decreases triglyceride level
5. Decreases need for diabetes medicines to reach target blood glucose goals

A. All of the above
B. 1,2 and 5
C. All except 3
D. All except 4

Q115. The nurse is teaching a 45-year-old lady recently diagnosed with type 2 diabetes

regarding exercise. Which of the following aspects she should include in the teaching?

A. The blood glucose lowering effects of exercise can only be attained with vigorous exercise

B. Exercise is best done after meals

C. Exercise should always be done before meals

D. A and C only

Q116. The nurse who is teaching a diabetic patient regarding nutritional therapy provides with the knowledge that diabetic diet is designed:

A. To be used only for type 2 diabetes

B. To control excessive blood glucose by elimination of sugar

C. To be used only when patient is unable to exercise

D. To help normalize blood glucose through a balanced diet

Q117. Diabetic meal plan focuses on the percentage of calories to come from carbohydrate, fats and proteins. Which of the following caloric distribution is desirable for a patient with diabetes to achieve total caloric requirements?

A. 30-35% of daily calories from carbohydrate, 30-35% from fat and 30-35% from protein

B. 35-40% of daily calories from carbohydrate, 30-35% from fat and 25-30% from protein

C. 45-50% of daily calories from carbohydrate, 35% from fat, 15-20% from protein

D. 50-60% of daily calories from carbohydrate, 30% from fat, 10-15% from protein

Q118. The nurse is teaching a group of newly diagnosed diabetic patients regarding oral antidiabetic agents. Which of the following statements regarding oral antidiabetic agents is appropriate?

A. Oral antidiabetic agents are effective in type 1 diabetes

B. Oral antidiabetic agents are effective in type 2 diabetes

C. Oral antidiabetic agents are especially indicated in pregnant women with type 2 diabetes

D. Oral antidiabetic agents are oral preparation of insulin

Q119. The physician has prescribed tolbutamide (orinase) 100 mg BD for a patient with type 2 diabetes. The nurse understands that this drug will lower blood glucose level by:

A. Increasing metabolism of carbohydrate

B. Stimulating the pancreas to secrete more insulin

C. Delaying digestion of complex carbohydrates

D. Decreasing insulin resistance

Q120. The nurse is teaching a patient with type 2 diabetes who has been prescribed glipizide (glynase) 5 mg BD. Which of the following teaching is not appropriate?

A. Avoid using over-the-counter medication unless prescribed by the physician

B. Avoid alcohol to prevent hypoglycemia

C. Always wear medic alert bracelet

D. Delay or skip lunch unless hungry to lower hyperglycemia

Q121. Acarbose (glucobay) has been ordered in conjunction with metformin to an elderly patient with type 2 diabetes mellitus. Which of the following the nurse should emphasize?

A. To take high fiber diet to prevent constipation

B. To take glucose tablets if symptoms of hypoglycemia

C. It is natural to experience abdominal distention and flatulence

D. B and C only

Q122. A patient with type 1 diabetes mellitus has been prescribed 15 units of humin-

sulin 30/70. The nurse understands that this insulin contains:

A. 30 units of regular insulin and 70 units of NPH insulin
B. 30% of regular insulin and 70% of NPH insulin
C. 70 units of regular insulin and 30 units of NPH insulin
D. 70% of regular insulin and 30% of NPH insulin

Q123. Which of the following type of insulin is the treatment of choice in diabetic ketoacidosis?

A. Regular insulin
B. NPH insulin
C. Ultralente insulin
D. NPH/regular 70/30

Q124. The nurse is teaching a patient who is on continuous subcutaneous insulin infusion regarding self-management of blood glucose and insulin doses. Which of the following statements by the nurse is appropriate?

A. Continuous subcutaneous insulin infusion involves the use of short acting insulin only
B. Teflon catheter inserted in the subcutaneous tissue may be left in place for months
C. Required doses of insulin are automatically delivered and patient need not worry about dosing
D. All of the above

Q125. Which of the following types of insulin is least allergic?

A. Beef insulin
B. Monkey insulin
C. Pork insulin
D. Human insulin

Q126. While teaching a patient about the sites of insulin injection the nurse states that insulin is most rapidly absorbed in the:

A. Arm
B. Abdomen
C. Buttocks
D. Thigh

Q127. The nurse is teaching a patient about self-administration of insulin. Which of the following instructions is not appropriate?

A. Wash hands thoroughly
B. Inspect insulin bottle before using it
C. Inject insulin at a 90° angle into the abdomen
D. Withdraw needle by applying some pressure with a dry cotton ball at the site and then massage the site with it

Q128. A patient with type 1 diabetes has to receive 10 units regular insulin and 30 units NPH insulin before breakfast and dinner. Which instruction about the administration of the insulin prescribed should the nurse give to the patient?

A. Shake the bottle of NPH insulin vigorously before withdrawing insulin
B. Draw up regular insulin first then draw NPH insulin
C. Clean the site with alcohol
D. Aspirate syringe before pushing insulin

Q129. The nurse who is teaching a diabetic patient about insulin injection provides with the knowledge that discomfort associated with subcutaneous injection of insulin may be minimized by administering it at a temperature of:

A. Room temperature
B. Just above room temperature
C. Just below room temperature
D. Temperature of insulin does not make any difference in pain sensation

Q130. Symptoms of hypoglycemia usually does not occur until the blood glucose level is less than:

A. 60–70 mg/dL
B. 50–60 mg/dL
C. 40–50 mg/dL
D. 30–40 mg/dL

Q131. A patient with type 2 diabetes mellitus who is being treated with chlorpropamide (diabenes) wakes up in the morning with headache, palpitation, tachycardia, diaphoresis and hunger. Which of the following actions the family members should take?

A. Call for the physician

B. Administer sublingual nitroglycerin tablets

C. Administer 20–30 g of carbohydrate, e.g. orange juice 1 cup

D. Administer glucagon 1 mg subcutaneously

Q132. Which of the clinical manifestations will be seen in a patient with hypoglycemia?

A. Dry skin, hypotension, bradycardia, deep rapid respiration

B. Polyuria, polydipsia, hypernatremia, hypotension

C. Polyuria, polydipsia, hunger, and weight loss

D. Anxiety, palpitation, tachycardia, cool moist skin, headache

Q133. A patient has type 1 diabetes. In the early morning his wife finds him unconscious at bed and administer glucagon 1 mg SC after 5 minutes the patient wakes up and is offered a snack of toast and milk. What is the rational behind this action?

A. To prevent nausea and vomiting associated with glucagon

B. To prevent recurrence of hypoglycemia

C. To stimulate his appetite

D. It was time for his breakfast

Q134. A newly diabetic patient on oral hypoglycemic drug experiences recurrent hypoglycemic episodes. The nurse providing dietary instructions to the patient should emphasize:

A. Increasing saturated fat intake

B. Eating glucose tablets or simple sugar whenever light headedness occur

C. Consuming a meal or a snack every 4-5 hours while awake

D. Increasing the amount of saturated fat and protein foods in the meal

Q135. A patient with type 1 diabetes is advised to avoid over-the-counter drugs. Which of the following over-the- counter drugs the patient should avoid?

A. Valium

B. Ibuprofen

C. Antacids

D. Aspirin

Q136. Which of the followings is not a common cause of diabetic ketoacidosis?

A. Taking too much insulin

B. Skipping doses of insulin

C. Inability to meet an increased need for insulin

D. Developing insulin resistance

Q137. An insulin dependent patient (type 1) who fails to take insulin regularly is at risk of developing which of the following complications?

A. Diabetic ketoacidosis

B. Hypoglycemia

C. Hyperosmolar hyperglycemic nonketotic syndrome (HHNS)

D. Diabetic nephropathy

Q138. A patient with history of type 1 diabetes is admitted to the hospital with abdominal pain, nausea and vomiting. On admission his blood glucose level is 430 mg/dl. What are the other assessment findings the nurse would possibly find?

A. Cool moist skin, palpitation, faintness, dizziness

B. Warm dry skin, hypotension, tachycardia, hyperpnea, breath odor of ketones

C. Profound dehydration, increased serum osmolality, polyuria, confusion

D. Inability to concentrate, irrational behavior, lethargy, loss of consciousness

Q139. A patient with type 1 diabetes mellitus has been admitted in the intensive care unit with the diagnosis of diabetic ketoacidosis. To correct this acute diabetic

emergency which of the following actions should the health team members take first?

A. Monitoring vital signs, oxygen saturation
B. Initiate fluid replacement therapy
C. Administer insulin
D. Determine the cause of DKA

Q140. Which of the following is the most common cause of hyperosmolar hyperglycemic nonketotic syndrome (HHNS)?

A. Insulin overdose
B. Undiagnosed untreated hyperpituitarism
C. Undiagnosed untreated hypercortisolism
D. Undiagnosed untreated diabetes mellitus

Q141. Which of the following conditions can differentiate hyperosmolar hyperglycemic nonketotic syndrome from diabetic ketoacidosis?

A. Hyperglycemia
B. Hyperosmolality
C. Absence of ketonuria
D. Electrolyte imbalance

Q142. A patient is admitted in the intensive care unit with excessive thirst, altered level of consciousness, and manifestations of dehydration. Patient gives the history of fever for 4 days and type 2 diabetes mellitus, which was controlled with oral antidiabetic agents. Physician suspects hyperosmolar hyperglycemic nonketotic syndrome (HHNS) and orders for which of the following test to confirm?

A. Blood glucose
B. Serum electrolytes and BUN
C. Arterial blood gas
D. Serum osmolarity

Q143. Treatment of hyperosmolar hyperglycemic nonketotic syndrome (HHNS) focuses on replacement of fluid and electrolytes. Which of the following statements about fluid replacement is appropriate for a patient with HHNS?

A. Administer normal saline 2-3 liter rapidly over a period of 2 hour
B. Administer ringer lactate for the first 2 hour
C. Administer 5% glucose saline 1L/hour for the first 4 hours
D. Administer IV fluid cautiously to prevent circulatory overload

Q144. A type 1 diabetic patient is scheduled for bilateral herniorrhaphy. Which of the following nursing consideration must be taken into account on the morning of surgery?

A. Eliminate the morning dose of insulin
B. Eliminate regular insulin and administer half the dose of intermediate acting NPH or lente insulin
C. Administer the full daily dose of insulin
D. Start an IV insulin infusion

Q145. A diabetic patient has upper respiratory tract infection accompanied by fever 101°F. Which action regarding his daily insulin administration is appropriate?

A. Administer insulin in reduced dose, as he is not eating much due to anorexia
B. Administer daily dose of insulin
C. Administer increased dose of insulin
D. Gets him admitted in the hospital for a continuous IV infusion of insulin

Q146. In teaching a newly diagnosed type 1 diabetic 'survival skills' the nurse includes information about:

A. Weight loss measures
B. Eliminating sugar from diet
C. Need to increase rest
D. Prevention of hypoglycemia

Q147. The nurse is teaching a group of diabetic patients regarding prevention of foot ulcer. Which of the following she should emphasize in her teaching?

A. Wash and inspect all surfaces of the feet daily

B. Cut the toenail by rounding edges

C. Treat small cuts promptly by disinfecting with iodine

D. Use hot water bottles to warm feet in winter to improve circulation

Q148. A patient has been admitted in an unconscious state. Blood sugar of the patient on admission is 790 mg/dL. Which of the following assessment findings provides cue to the diagnosis of diabetic ketoacidosis (DKA) rather than hyperosmolar hyperglycemic nonketotic syndrome

A. Dehydration

B. Rapid thready pulse

C. Kussmaul's respirations

D. Hypokalemia

ANSWERS AND RATIONALS OF ENDOCRINE SYSTEM AND DIABETES

1. **D.** A hormone is a chemical substance synthesized and secreted by a specific organ or tissue called glands. There are two types of glands–endocrine and exocrine. Hormones of endocrine glands are secreted into blood and carried by it to different target tissue or organ where they bind to specific cellular receptors either in the cell membrane or within the cell.

2. **B.** The primary function of the thyroid hormone (T3 and T4) is to control the cellular metabolic activity. These hormones accelerate metabolic processes by increasing the level of specific enzymes that contribute to oxygen consumption and altering the responsiveness to tissues to other hormones. They influence the cell replication and necessary for normal growth. Through their widespread effects on cellular metabolism influence every major organ system.

3. **C.** Triiodothyronine, thyroxine and calcitonin are secreted by the thyroid gland. Thyrotropin or thyroid stimulating hormone and oxytocin are secreted by the pituitary gland.

4. **D.** Enlargement of the thyroid gland known as goiter occurs in hypothyroidism, hyperthyroidism and tumors of thyroid.

5. **D.** Endemic goiter is caused principally by nutritional iodine deficiency. It tends to occur in geographical areas where soil and water are deficient in iodine. Goiter is less common in coastal areas since iodine is readily available in salt water and sea foods. Incidence of goiter is twice in women as that in men and it commonly occurs in adolescents, pregnant and lactating women because during these periods there is increased need for thyroid hormone.

6. **A.** Endemic or simple goiter is the most common type of goiter, encountered chiefly in certain geographical areas where natural supply of iodine is deficient. Second most common type is sporadic goiter which is not restricted to any geographical area. When goiter is associated with hyperthyroidism, it is called toxic goiter. In some persons thyroid glands contain areas of hyperplasia which appears as nodular. Frequency of both nodular and toxic goiter is less.

7. **A.** 95 percent of patients with hypothyroidism have primary or thyroidal hypothyroidism, which refers to dysfunction of the thyroid gland itself. When thyroid dysfunction is caused the by failure of the hypothalamus or pituitary or both, it is central hypothyroidism. When it is entirely due to disorder of pituitary gland it is secondary hypothyroidism and when it is entirely due to disorder of hypothalamus it is tertiary hypothyroidism.

8. **C.** Chronic inflammatory or autoimmune diseases like Hashimoto's disease, amyloidosis and sarcoidosis can give rise to hypothyroidism. Among them Hashimoto's disease is the most common. Graves' disease is also an autoimmune disease of thyroid is characterized by hyperthyroidism and goiter. Addison's disease is due to hypofunction of adrenal cortex and Cushing's disease is due to increased production of adrenocorticotropic hormone (ACTH) by the pituitary.

9. A. Diagnosis of hypothyroidism is confirmed by measuring serum concentration of thyroid stimulating hormone (TSH) and thyroxin (T4). Thyroid antibodies are tested when thyroiditis is suspected. Thyroid scan is ordered when a nodule is present in the thyroid gland.

10. D. Levothyroxine, a synthetic form of the thyroid hormone T4 is the medication of choice for treating hypothyroidism. Potassium iodide is given in thyroid storm. Lugol's iodine is given to reduce vascularity of thyroid gland before thyroidectomy and propylthiouracil is given in hyperthyroidism.

11. A. Lethargy, constipation, thick brittle nails and weight gain are the symptoms of hypothyroidism secondary to a decrease in cellular metabolism. Polyuria, polyphagia and weight loss are the symptoms of type 1 diabetes mellitus. Intolerance to heat, diarrhea, tachycardia and nervousness are symptoms of hyperthyroidism. In Cushing's syndrome patient develops buffalo-hump, oily skin and acne, weakness and depression.

12. C. Patient with hypothyroidism develops mucinous edema, characterized by dry, waxy type non-pitting swelling in skin and other tissues especially in the periorbital or facial areas. This mucinous edema causes the characteristic facies of hypothyroidism, i.e. puffiness, periorbital edema and mask-like effect. Other signs listed are manifestations of hyperthyroidism.

13. A. The thyroid hormone should preferably be taken in the morning at empty stomach for maximum absorption. The timing also mimics normal hormone release and prevents insomnia.

14. B. Anginal pain or cardiac dysrhythmia are often a serious complication of hypothyroid treatment particularly in the elderly or in patient with compromised cardiac status due to increased myocardial oxygen demand. Nephropathy is usually a complication of diabetes mellitus. Allergies are not related to hypothyroid or its treatment. Thyroid storm is a complication of hyperthyroidism.

15. D. Myxedema coma is a life-threatening complication may be precipitated by stress, e.g. surgery, infection or trauma. Drugs, e.g. narcotics, tranquilizers and tricyclic antidepressants may precipitate myxedema coma. Wound infection, hyperthermia and thyroid crisis are not related to hypothyroidism.

16. A. Myxedema, the major complication of hypothyroidism is brought on by stress, e.g. surgery, injury or infection or by noncompliance with thyroid treatment. In hypothyroidism, there is anemia which is due to low level of erythropoietin. In severe hypothyroidism the patient has hypoglycemia due to decreased absorption of glucose. Heart failure is associated with hyperthyroidism.

17. D. Patient with hypothyroidism usually has dry coarse skin. So sparing use of soap and application of lotion keeps skin soft and supple. These patients are lethargic due to hypometabolic state which would improve with hormone replacement therapy. So these patients should be encouraged to carry out activities with frequent rest periods in between instead of speeding up of activities. These patients have sensitivity to cold, so they should be kept comfortable in a warmer climate.

18. C. The patient who is on thyroid replacement therapy for

hypothyroidism may complain of anginal pain or chest pain which should be immediately reported. Dyspnea on exertion is a symptom of heart failure and may be present in hyperthyroidism. Fine tremors of hands are also associated with hyperthyroidism. Fatigue which is associated with hypothyroidism disappears with thyroid replacement therapy and is not a complication of thyroid replacement therapy.

19. C. The patients with hypothyroidism should be taught measures to minimize constipation. The teaching should include an increase intake of fibers and not a low residue diet. Other measures to minimize constipation are—gradual increase in activity and exercise, use of stool softeners and maintenance of a regular bowel elimination time.

20. D. In hypothyroidism, gastrointestinal motility is decreased. So constipation is a common complain instead of diarrhea. All other nursing diagnoses are appropriate to hypothyroidism.

21. B. Excessive secretion of thyroid hormone is known as hyperthyroidism. Hypothyroidism results from suboptimal levels of thyroid hormones. Exophthalmos is the bulging of eyes, usually seen as a manifestation of hyperthyroidism. Thyrotoxic crisis is a complication of hyperthyroidism.

22. D. In hyperthyroidism, there is a sustained increase in synthesis and release of thyroid hormone due to loss of normal regulatory mechanism (negative feedback by T4 on thyroid stimulating hormone). The action of thyroid hormone on the body is stimulatory resulting in hypermetabolism. Hypermetabolism leads to a negative nitrogen balance, lipid depletion and a state of nutritional deficiency and weight loss.

23. D. Graves' disease is an autoimmune disease of unknown etiology marked by diffuse thyroid enlargement (goiter), hyperthyroidism and exophthalmos. It accounts for 75% of the cases of hyperthyroidism.

24. C. Grave's disease is the most common form of hyperthyroidism accounts for about 75% of the cases. Addison's disease is insufficiency of adrenocortical hormone. Cushing's disease is an excess production of adrenocorticotropic hormone by the pituitary. Hashimoto's disease is the most common type of autoimmune hypothyroidism.

25. B. The early sign and symptoms of hyperthyroidism may be only weight loss, increased nervousness, frequent defecation. On examination, diffuse swelling in the neck and fine tremors of hands may also be present. Hypothyroidism usually presents with weight gain, constipation, mental sluggishness and lethargy. In diabetes mellitus, patient complains of polydipsia and polyuria with polyphagia. Patient with AIDS may have weight loss, diarrhea, fever, night sweat and exhibits signs of one or more of opportunistic infections.

26. D. The three major complications of Graves' disease are exophthalmos, heart disease and thyroid storm. Exophthalmos develops as a result of proptosis, lid retraction, muscle swelling and tissue edema from a prolonged hyperthyroid condition. Heart disease includes tachycardia, atrial fibrillation and heart failure among the elderly which poses a serious threat. Thyroid storm is a potentially fatal, acute episode of thyroid overactivity characterized by high fever, severe tachycardia, delirium, dehydration and extreme irritability.

27. C. Elevating head of the bed at night and limiting salt intake relieves periorbital edema and reduces discomfort. Taping the eyes shut during sleep is helpful to avoid getting dirt and dust in eyes and also prevent drying which is the cause of corneal ulceration.

28. D. To control hyperthyroidism antithyroid drugs are given. One of the antithyroid drugs is propylthiouracil. It controls hyperthyroidism by impairing thyroid hormone synthesis. Beta-blockers are given in Graves' disease as adjunctive therapy to treat tachycardia and palpitations. Corticosteroids may be given to treat exophthalmos and thyroid storm. It does not control hyperthyroidism. NSAIDs have no role in the management of Graves' disease.

29. A. Restlessness, agitation, weight loss and increased appetite are the all symptoms of hyperthyroidism. Protruding eyeball or exophthalmos is a sign of hyperthyroidism but mental sluggishness and slow pulse are manifestations of hypothyroidism. Swelling in neck may be in hypo- or hyperthyroidism but weight gain, dry skin, loss of appetite and slow pulse are seen in hypothyroidism.

30. D. In hyperthyroidism, serum TSH levels are decreased (normal .38-6.15 microunit/mL) and elevated free thyroxine levels (normal- .9-1.7 ng/dL). Patients with hyperthyroidism will show a high uptake of radioactive iodine (35 to 95%).

31. B. Iodine uptake test provides direct measure of thyroid activity. Patient should not have supplemental iodine or iodine rich food before the test as it distorts test results. Estrogen containing medication can falsely elevate test results. Antihypertensive drugs have no known relation with test results.

32. D. Propylthiouracil acts by blocking the utilization of iodine in the synthesis of thyroid hormone. It also blocks extrathyroidal conversion of T4 to T3. It does not interfere with release or block the activity of previously formed thyroid hormones. So several weeks of treatment with this drug is necessary for relief of symptoms.

33. D. Although iodine is a constituent of thyroid hormones, it is the fastest acting thyroid inhibitor. The gland if enlarged, shrinks, becomes firm and less vascular. The thyroid status starts returning to normal. With daily administration peak effects are seen in 10-15 days. So it is given in the treatment of thyroid storm and as a preoperative preparation for surgery.

34. B. Antithyroid drug has to be taken life-long. After initial therapy when the patient is euthyroid a maintenance dose is given. The major problem of this therapy is noncompliance by the patient. Improvement usually begins after 1-2 weeks of therapy and good results are seen after 4-8 weeks. Less serious side effects of this drug are skin rash, joint pain and gastrointestinal intolerance. Less common but serious side effect is agranulocytosis. So patient should be instructed to stop medicine and report sore throat, fever or rash so that white blood cells count is done.

35. B. Drugs that inhibit synthesis of thyroid hormones are called antithyroid drugs, e.g. propylthiouracil, methimazole and carbimazole. Potassium iodide and Lugol's solution inhibit hormone release and are termed as thyroid inhibitors. Radioactive iodine damages thyroid tissue thus limiting thyroid hormone secretion. Triiodothyronine and L-thyroxine sodium are thyroid hormone given in hypothyroidism as a replacement therapy.

36. B. Radioactive iodine therapy is contraindicated in pregnancy and in nursing mothers as radioiodine crosses the placenta and is secreted in breast milk. It is a method of choice in most adults beyond the childbearing years. Response from this therapy may be seen after 2–3 months. So patient is usually treated with antithyroid drugs before and during the first 3 months of therapy. One of the biggest disadvantages of this therapy is high incidence of posttreatment hypothyroidism, requiring lifelong thyroid replacement therapy.

37. D. Providing sufficient rest is a challenge because of the patient's irritability and restlessness. Patient may be placed in a cool room, away from ill patients and away from noisy areas. A high carbohydrate and high protein diet to be provided. Visitors who upset the patient may only be restricted. Frequent changing of bed linens is necessary if the patient is diaphoretic.

38. B. Patients with hyperthyroidism are restless, irritable and nervous. Impending surgery may cause additional tension and stress which may precipitate thyroid storm. Hence, it is absolutely necessary to gain confidence and reduce anxiety. The patients are treated with appropriate medication so that they are euthyroid. When euthyroid, patients will maintain normal body temperature. Encouraging independence may not be an appropriate goal for these patients as they are already restless and hyperactive.

39. C. After thyroidectomy, the most comfortable position is semi- Fowler's position with the head supported by pillows so that the head is neither hyperextended nor hyperflexed. This position reduces stress on the suture line and avoids flexion of the neck.

40. B. Injury to one of the laryngeal nerves gives rise to weakness or hoarseness of the voice. Injury to bilateral laryngeal nerve gives rise to vocal cord paralysis resulting into spastic airway obstruction. Laryngeal stridor (harsh, vibratory sound) may occur as a result of tetany.

41. C. Bilateral laryngeal nerve damage will cause vocal cord paralysis resulting into spastic airway obstruction which will require immediate tracheostomy. Blood pressure cuff and stethoscope are required to monitor blood pressure, oxygen cylinder to facilitate breathing in postoperative period and calcium gluconate to treat tetany which may develop due to injury to one or more of parathyroid glands.

42. D. Laryngeal stridor or harsh, vibratory sound during inspiration or expiration occurs as a result of tetany which is a consequence of injury to or removal of parathyroid glands. Hoarseness occurs due to injury of one laryngeal nerve. Dyspnea is the result of bilateral laryngeal nerve injury. In tetany there is a painful tonic spasm of skeletal muscle instead of muscle weakness.

43. A. To treat hypocalcemia and tetany in patient, calcium gluconate IV is administered. Calcium gluconate ampoules should always be available at bedside and the patient should have a patent IV line. Others are not indicated.

44. B. After thyroidectomy the patient should not hyperextend his head neither hyperflex or bend forward. Semi-Fowler's position is most comfortable. Checking for hemorrhage is very important as postoperative hemorrhage after thyroidectomy is very common. Patient should be encouraged to talk to check hoarseness of voice which is a sign of laryngeal nerve injury.

45. A. Pituitary gland is located in the sella turcica at the base of the brain above the sphenoid bone. Thymus gland is situated in the mediastinum anterior to the trachea. In the central part of the diencephalon area of the brain hypothalamus is located. Pituitary gland is located below the hypothalamus not above.

46. C. Gonadotropic hormones, prolactin, somatotropin or growth hormone secreted by anterior pituitary. Other hormones secreted by this gland are thyroid stimulating hormone or thyrotropin, adrenocorticotropic hormone and melanocyte stimulating hormone. The posterior pituitary secretes oxytocin. Somatostatin is produced and secreted by the delta cells of pancreas and thyrotropin releasing hormone is the hormone secreted by the hypothalamus.

47. D. Somatotropin or growth hormone has effects on all body tissue. It affects the growth and development of skeletal muscles and long bones. It has numerous biologic functions including protein, fat and carbohydrate metabolism. The target organs for gonadotropic hormone is reproductive system. Adrenocorticotropic hormone acts on the adrenal cortex. Calcitonin and parathyroid hormone act on bone tissue.

48. A. Antidiuretic hormone and oxytocin are actually produced in the hypothalamus. These hormones travel down the nerve tracts (the communication between hypothalamus and pituitary) from the hypothalamus to the posterior pituitary and are stored until their release is triggered by appropriate stimulus. Adrenal gland and kidney have no role in the production or in release of ADH

49. D. Increased plasma osmolality (decrease in the extracellular fluid and increase in the solute concentration) and decreased in blood volume both stimulate ADH release. When the ADH is released, the renal tubules reabsorbs water creating more concentrated urine. Decreased plasma osmolality will inhibit ADH release, and when ADH release is inhibited, the renal tubules do not reabsorb water, thus creating more dilute urine.

50. A. Overproduction of growth hormone by the pituitary in adults causes acromegaly. Deficient production of growth hormone in adults causes nonspecific clinical findings, e.g. truncal obesity, decreased muscle mass, decreased energy and reduced exercise capability. Overproduction of androgens by adrenal will cause pronounced acne, virilization in women and feminization in men. Deficient production will cause in females oligomenorrhea or amenorrhea and in males no symptoms as testis produces enough sex hormones.

51. B. Hypersecretion of growth hormone causes pituitary gigantism. Adrenocortical hyperfunctions will cause hypercortisolism and primary aldosteronism. Hypersecretion of thyroid stimulating hormone will result in hyperthyroidism and hypersecretion of parathyroid hormone will result in hyperparathyroidism.

52. C. Enlargement of bony and soft tissue over the head and face, deep voices, glucose intolerance are manifestations of acromegaly. Mental sluggishness, excessive weight gain are the seen in hypothyroidism. Hypoglycemia is seen in Addison's disease. Short attention span, irritability are seen in hyperthyroidism.

Menstrual disturbances and hypertension occur in Cushing's syndrome. Excessive thirst is seen in diabetes insipidus.

53. C. Excess secretion of LH and FSH in children causes sexual precocity. Gigantism is the result of excessive growth hormone in children (before closure of the epiphysis). Dwarfism is caused by the deficiency of growth hormone in children. Sterility is the result of deficiency of LH and FSH.

54. B. Clinical manifestations due to hyperprolactinemia are galactorrhea (abnormal lactation in nonlactating breast), amenorrhea, decreased vaginal lubrication, decreased libido in men, impotence, depression, anxiety, etc. Failure of lactation in postpartum women is due to deficiency of prolactin hormone.

55. C. Bromocriptin, a dopamine agonist, inhibits prolactin secretion. So patients with prolactinomas (hyperprolactinemia) can be successfully treated with bromocriptin. Surgery is not the treatment of choice in most cases.

56. D. Prolactin deficiency (hypoprolactinemia) due to hypopituitarism is indicated by the absence of lactation in the postpartum woman. All other conditions are due to hypopituitarism but does not cause failure of lactation.

57. A. The posterior lobe of pituitary or the neurohypophysis produces antidiuretic hormone and oxytocin. Diabetes insipidus is a major disorder of the posterior lobe of the pituitary is due to the antidiuretic hormone deficiency. Gigantism is caused by excess growth hormone by the adenophysis or anterior lobe of the pituitary. Secondary hypogonadism is due to hyposecretion of gonadotropic hormones by the anterior pituitary.

58. C. Diabetes insipidus results from deficiency of vasopressin or antidiuretic hormone by the posterior pituitary. Excessive secretion of vasopressin causes syndrome of inappropriate antidiuretic hormone (SIADH). Hypo- or hypersecretion of epinephrine by the adrenal gland are not related to diabetes insipidus.

59. C. Diabetes insipidus may result after surgery of the pituitary gland. Other risk factors for diabetes insipidus include head injury, brain infections, pituitary or hypothalamic tumors, etc. Removal of pituitary may give rise to the absence of tropic hormones resulting in adrenal insufficiency and hypothyroidism not Cushing's syndrome and hyperthyroidism. Diabetes mellitus is due to the deficiency of insulin by pancreas.

60. D. Diabetes insipidus results in excretion of large amounts of urine with low specific gravity and an elevated serum osmolality due to dehydration and hypernatremia, if water is not adequately replaced. Elevated urine osmolality and low serum osmolality will be found in syndrome of inappropriate antidiuretic hormone. Others are not appropriate to diabetes insipidus.

61. A. Water deprivation test is usually done to confirm the diagnosis of diabetes insipidus. Capillary blood glucose test and urine test for glucose is done in diabetes mellitus. Urine specific gravity of less than 1.005 is suspicious of diabetes insipidus but does not confirm the disease and its type.

62. B. The patient with diabetes insipidus is at risk of developing severe dehydration and hypernatremia if the fluid intake cannot keep up with urinary losses. So, the nurse needs to assess patient's ability to drink copious amounts of fluids otherwise fluids to be replaced intravenously. Overhydration and hyponatremia are not the manifestations of diabetes insipidus. A patient with diabetes insipidus resulting in fluid deficit may experience hypotension and tachycardia not bradycardia. Patient with diabetes insipidus usually looses weight. The disease has no effect on blood glucose.

63. B. Syndrome of inappropriate antidiuretic hormone occurs due to excessive secretion of vasopressin or antidiuretic hormone. Diabetes insipidus occurs due to the deficiency of vasopressin. Cushing's syndrome is caused by excessive secretion of corticosteroids. Addisonian crisis is an acute condition of adrenocortical insufficiency.

64. D. Sustained secretion of antidiuretic hormone in SIADH increases distal tubule and collecting duct permeability and reabsorption of water into the circulation resulting in retention of fluid, serum hypo-osmolality and dilutional hyponatremia. Patient will experience concentrated urine inspite of normal extracellular volume and renal function. Dilute urine, serum hyperosmolality and hypernatremia occurs in diabetes insipidus.

65. D. SIADH causes fluid retention. Severe SIADH may cause fluid overload. Sustained increase in fluid volume may potentiate heart failure and pulmonary edema. Fluid overload is signalled by neck vein distention. Weight loss, increase in urinary output and hypotension are the signs of fluid excretion and are desired.

66. D. Patient with SIADH develops fluid retention and hyponatremia. Symptoms of hyponatremia include vomiting, abdominal cramps, muscle twitching and seizures. If the situation continues, patient will develop cerebral edema which will manifest as confusion, lethargy, anorexia, headache, seizures and coma.

67. C. The patient with SIADH should be positioned so that the head is placed flat on the bed or no more than 10° of elevation to enhance venous return to heart and increase left atrial filling pressure, reducing antidiuretic hormone release. Other nursing interventions are appropriate for the patient with SIADH.

68. C. Hypoparathyroidism slows bone resorption, reduces serum calcium level and causes profound neuromuscular irritability manifested by tetany. Hypoparathyroidism does not alter blood pressure or affect thirst mechanism. Polyuria is due to hypercalciuria is a symptom of hyperparathyroidism.

69. B. Hyperparathyroidism is most common in older women and is characterized by the bone pain and weakness from excess parathyroid hormone (PTH). Increased need for sleeping, anorexia, irritability, constipation and polyuria from hypercalciuria are other manifestations of the disease. Hypoparathyroidism is characterized by tetany, and urinary frequency rather than polyuria. Hypo- and hyperthyroidism do not cause bone pain.

70. B. A moderate exercise program will promote bone calcification and prevent bone loss from excess parathyroid hormones. Too much of rest is harmful as immobility aggravates the bone loss. Patient may benefit from a reducing diet, but regular exercise program is more beneficial. Weight bearing exercises should be discouraged due to weakened bones. Walking and swimming are most beneficial.

71. C. Patients with hypoparathyroidism are prescribed daily supplements of calcium along with vitamin D, because vitamin D helps in calcium absorption from the intestine. Patient does not require phosphorus, as increased phosphorus level will reduce calcium absorption. Hypoparathyroidism does not cause deficiency of folic acid and vitamin C. So daily supplements of folic acid and vitamin C are not needed to maintain adequate calcium level in blood.

72. B. Calcium and phosphorus are responsible for calcium phosphate stones in the kidney. The other type of calcium stones frequently found in kidney is calcium oxalate stone. Magnesium and potassium are not known to form stones. Chlorides in the form of ammonium chlorides are thought to prevent stone formation in the kidney.

73. B. Due to adverse effects of hypercalcemia on gastrointestinal tract patient develops constipation. So these patients require high calorie and high fiber diet and not low residue diet. All other nursing interventions are appropriate and aim at preventing injury, e.g. fractures, renal stones and bone demineralization.

74. B. Spasms of the wrist and hand after compression of the upper arm as by a blood pressure cuff indicates presence of Trousseau sign. Positive Chvostek sign means spasms of facial muscles after a tap over the facial nerve. Deep tendon reflex examined by percussion hammer. All these signs are related to hypocalcemia produced in hypoparathyroidism.

75. B. The hormones of the adrenal cortex are the aldosterone (mineralocorticoid), cortisol (glucocorticoid) and androgens. ACTH is secreted by anterior pituitary. Catecholamines (epinephrine and norephinephrine) are the hormones of the adrenal medulla.

76. B. Secondary adrenal insufficiency results from hypofunction of the pituitary-hypothalamic unit resulting in deficient corticotropin hormone. Hyposecretion of somatotropin leads to dwarfism. Hyposecretion of cortisol by adrenal gland results in primary adrenal insufficiency and hypersecretion of corticotropin by pituitary causes Cushing's syndrome.

77. C. Autoimmunity is the most common cause (75%) of adrenal insufficiency. Infection especially tuberculosis is the cause in about 20% of cases. Adrenal metastasis and hemorrhagic infarction may also cause adrenal insufficiency in rare cases.

78. A. The clinical picture of Addison's disease include progressive muscle weakness, fatigue, anorexia, weight loss, hyperpigmentation of the skin, hyponatremia, hyperkalemia, nausea, vomiting and diarrhea. Clinical picture of Cushing's syndrome is buffalo hump, moon faces and thin extremities. In diabetes mellitus patient may experience weakness and fatigue but skin pigmentation, hyponatremia, etc. are not present. Patient with SIADH experiences low urinary output, hyponatremia, muscle weakness and weight gain but no skin pigmentation.

79. A. Patients with adrenocortical insufficiency are at risk for an acute adrenal insufficiency or Addisonian crisis if under stress. Stressors being infection, surgery, trauma, hemorrhage or psychological distress. Osteoporosis develops with excessive secretion or use of glucocorticoids. Patient with adrenocortical insufficiency under stress exhibits severe manifestations of glucocorticoid and mineralcorticoid deficiency, not adrenocortical hyperfunction.

80. C. Corticosteroids especially glucocorticoids are given in divided doses, two-third in the morning and one-third in the afternoon. Mineralocorticoids are given once daily in the morning. This dosage schedule reflects normal circadian rhythm in endogenous hormone secretion and decreases side effects associated with corticosteroid replacement therapy.

81. B. Patient in Addisonian crisis develops circulatory collapse and shock. So vital signs including blood pressure should be assessed every 30 minutes to 4 hours interval depending on the patient's condition for the first 24 hours. Assessment of daily body weight is adequate. Urine testing for sugar is not required as these patients develop hypoglycemia. Neck vein distention is also not expected, as there is circulatory collapse and shock.

82. C. During a stressful situation, e.g. dental extraction, minor surgery, upper respiratory infections or mental disturbances, the dosage of hydrocortisone should be increased (usually double) by physician's order. Hydrocortisone by self-injection is required when the patient experiences acute stress, e.g. automobile accident, trauma or cannot tolerate the medication orally, e.g. nausea or vomiting.

83. A. Management of patients with Addison's disease in the community takes place with regular medical follow-up. Hence, the focus of management is on self-care. Patient must learn how to take steroids lifelong. Patients with Addison's disease exhibit fluid volume deficits not excess. Early ambulation is not a desired goal for these patients. Due to fatigue activity may be limited. Patient with Addison's disease has loss of weight and water and sodium deficit, but correction of these problems will automatically occur when patient learns self-care.

84. D. Patient with Addison's disease after proper exogenous steroid balance will live a normal active life, which will be manifested by decreased fatigue, maintenance of stable body weight, vital signs including blood pressure within normal limits and a normal level of cortisol.

85. A. Patient with Addison's disease cannot tolerate stress. Stress might have been the cause for Addisonian crisis. So the patient must be protected from further physical or emotional stress. A separate room free from environmental noises will be helpful to minimize extra stress on the patient. Patient's vital signs should be checked every 30 minutes till stable. This patient is critically ill so no oral feeds should be given until condition stabilizes which usually takes about 24 hours. Ambulation is not important for this patient.

86. C. The typical picture of a patient with Cushing's syndrome is truncal obesity, thin limbs, moon-shaped face, thinning of scalp hair, but excessive bodily and facial hair, virilization, etc. In myxedema patient gains weight but no symptoms of virilization. Patients with Addison's disease lose weight and complain of weakness, anorexia, and dark pigmentation of skin. Patients with Graves' disease have symptoms of heat intolerance, irritability, bulging eyes, etc.

87. B. The most common (about 85%) cause of Cushing's syndrome is tumor of the pituitary gland that produces adrenocorticotropic hormone which stimulates the adrenal cortex to increase its hormone secretion despite adequate amounts being produced. Other causes listed are less common.

88. B. In Cushing's syndrome, excess of glucocorticoids result in persistent hyperglycemia (steroid diabetes) and not hypoglycemia. Excess mineralocorticoids promote sodium retention and potassium excretion giving rise to hypokalemia. These patients also manifest immunosuppressive responses and demonstrate poor wound healing.

89. B. Patients with Cushing's syndrome exhibit abnormal fat distribution, which results in moon face, truncal obesity with thin limbs and supraclavicular fat pad (buffalo hump). These patients have hypertension, hypokalemia and thin brittle easily bruised skin.

90. B. Spironolactone causes menstrual irregularities and decreased libido. Men may also experience gynecomastia and impotence. Others do not occur with spironolactone.

91. B. Patient with Cushing's syndrome require low calorie but nutritious diet containing high protein, calcium and potassium because excess corticosteroids produce weight gain and loss of protein, calcium and potassium.

92. B. Patients with Cushing's syndrome usually have disturbed self-esteem related to altered body image, emotional lability and diminished physical capabilities. Fluid volume deficit related to inadequate adrenal hormones is common in patients with Addison's disease. Ineffective thermoregulation is a problem in patients with hyperthyroidism. Patients with Cushing's syndrome usually have imbalanced nutrition, more than body requirements as manifested by increased appetite and body weight more than optimum for height.

93. A. Patients with Cushing's syndrome have increased susceptibility to infection. So patient engaged in self care should be taught to prevent infection. One of the important ways of preventing infection is hand washing. Patients with Addison's disease, not Cushing's syndrome should increase salt and water intake in time of stress to prevent hypotension. Patient with Cushing's syndrome should consume a high protein but low calorie diet. Patient must maintain a balance between rest and activity as too much rest may promote abnormal thromboembolic phenomena.

94. D. The nurse should encourage good grooming and use of attractive clothing to improve patient's appearance and self-esteem which is usually disturbed by altered physical appearance. These patients need high protein diet. They are usually hypertensive and do not exhibit hypothermia.

95. B. Primary hyperaldosteronism occurs most commonly from a small aldosterone-producing adenoma of the adrenal glands. Hyperplasia of the adrenal glands is the second most common cause. It is not caused by excessive intake of sodium. Pituitary adenoma gives rise to Cushing's syndrome. Chronic renal disease may give rise to secondary hyperaldosteronism.

96. D. Elevated levels of aldosterone in hyperaldosteronism are associated with sodium retention and elimination of potassium. Sodium retention leads to hypertension and hypernatremia. Potassium wasting leads to hypokalemia.

97. A. Aldosterone is secreted by adrenal cortex. Adrenal medulla secretes catecholamines. Pituitary secretes adrenocorticotropic and other hormones. Testis produces testosterone.

98. A. Pheochromocytoma is a condition characterized by a tumor of the adrenal medulla that produces excessive catecholamines (epinephrine and norepinephrine). The secretion of excessive catecholamines results in severe hypertension not hypotension. This is a rare condition occurring in young to middle aged adults.

99. B. Patient with pheochromocytoma may present with manifestations of diabetes mellitus, hypertension, hyperthyroidism and psychoneurosis (emotional instability). But hypertension is the principal manifestation and can be persistent, fluctuating, intermittent or paroxysmal. The classic triad of symptoms of pheochromocytoma is pounding headache, tachycardia, and profuse sweating. Manifestations of diabetes mellitus include hyperglycemia and glycosuria not hypoglycemia. Manifestations of hyperthyroidism include hypermetabolism, weight loss, diaphoresis, agitation, emotional outburst and not hypometabolism, confusion, weight gain, etc.

100. D. Diabetes mellitus is a chronic systemic disease characterized by either a deficiency of insulin or a decreased ability of the body to use insulin. It is not due to oversecretion of insulin.

101. A. Type 1 diabetes can develop at any age usually it is diagnosed before the age of 30 years. Type 1 diabetes is characterized by destruction of pancreatic beta cells, usually leading to absolute insulin deficiency. With the destruction of beta cells by an autoimmune process islet cell antibodies appear. Patient requires exogenous insulin to survive.

102. B. Type 2 diabetes mellitus accounts for about 90 to 95% of all known cases of diabetes mellitus. Type 1 diabetes affects 10% of people who have diabetes. Gestational diabetes mellitus develops in 2 to 5% of all pregnant women but disappears when the pregnancy is over. Secondary diabetes mellitus accounts for 1 to 2% of all diagnosed cases of diabetes.

103. C. Type 1 diabetes results from destruction of pancreatic beta cells due to an autoimmune process in susceptible individuals. Auto-antibodies to the islet cells can cause a reduction of 80 to 90% of normal beta cell function before hyperglycemia and other manifestations occur. A genetic predisposition and exposure to an environmental factors, e.g. virus may appear to trigger the autoimmune process.

104. B. Two pathologic processes, e.g. desensitization and insulin resistance play a role in the development of type 2 diabetes mellitus. Desensitization is the phenomenon of progressive loss of efficiency of beta cells. Beta cells chronically exposed to high blood levels of glucose become less efficient when responding to further glucose elevation. The second pathologic process is insulin resistance. This is a condition in which body tissues do not respond to the action of insulin. This is due to insulin receptors that are either unresponsive to the action of insulin and/or insufficient in number. When insulin is not properly used, the entry of glucose into the cells is impeded resulting in hyperglycemia.

105. D. Skeletal and cardiac muscles and adipose tissue require insulin for glucose transport. Without adequate insulin much of the ingested glucose cannot be used, decreasing glucose utilization. Without insulin amino acids are converted to glucose in the liver. Lack of insulin leads to increased catabolism thus protein wasting. When body tissue cannot utilize glucose due to lack of insulin it turns to fat stores for energy production. Fat metabolism causes breakdown products, e.g. ketones.

106. A. The classic clinical manifestations of diabetes mellitus are polyuria, polydipsia and weight loss despite increased food intake or polyphagia. Weight gain and tiredness may be noticed in type 2 diabetes mellitus. Diaphoresis, excessive hunger, irritability and tachycardia are seen in hyperthyroidism. Bradycardia and hypertension are not due to diabetes.

107. D. In type 2 diabetes, the pancreas usually continues to produce some endogenous insulin which may not be enough for the need of the body or is poorly utilized by the tissues. Hence for some individuals with type 2 diabetes, a regimen of proper nutrition, regular exercise and maintenance of a desirable body weight is sufficient to attain an optimal level of blood glucose control. Patients with type 2 diabetes are usually obese at the time of diagnosis. They do not contain islet cell antibodies and do not develop ketosis.

108. B. When blood sugar level exceeds renal threshold excess glucose is excreted in the urine, accompanied by the large amounts of water and electrolytes called osmotic diuresis. With diuresis extracellular fluid volume is depleted, serum osmolality increases, thirst center is stimulated resulting in polydipsia. Ketones do not cause diuresis. Polyuria is not due to damage to kidney, although long standing untreated diabetes may cause damage to kidney after 10 to 15 years. Secretion of antidiuretic hormone is not related to blood glucose level.

109. C. Two hour oral glucose tolerance test result of more than 200 mg/dL is indicative of diabetes. Fasting blood glucose level of more than 126 mg/dL and random plasma glucose level of more than 200 mg/dL are indicative of diabetes.

110. D. The fasting blood sugar sample is drawn when the individual has not ingested any nutrients other than water for 8-12 hours.

111. D. Glycosylated hemoglobin is the most reliable indicator of glucose utilization because the result of this test shows the average blood glucose level over the previous 3 months.

112. D. Effective collaborative management of diabetes includes a combination of nutritional therapy, drug therapy, exercise and self-monitoring of blood glucose level. Patient and family teaching is an essential component in the management of diabetes. Teaching enables the patient to become an active participant in his/her own care. All patients with diabetes do not require insulin neither only nutritional therapy is adequate as initial management.

Patient has to learn to control his own blood sugar as an active participant not relying solely on the physician.

113. D. Oral hypoglycemic agents are indicated in patients with type 2 diabetes mellitus who cannot attain normal or near normal blood glucose levels with exercise and diet therapies. Other indications for oral agents are: 1) random blood glucose level is less than 300 mg/dL and 2) fasting blood glucose level is less than 250 mg/dL. Body weight is not a criterion for prescribing oral agents. Oral agents are not effective in the absence of endogenous insulin.

114. A. A program of planned exercise is a crucial part of the treatment plan for a diabetic patient. Because exercise lowers blood glucose by increasing carbohydrate metabolism, increases insulin sensitivity, reduces weight, so decreases insulin resistance, increases high density lipoprotein level, decreases triglyceride level, lowers blood pressure and reduces stress and tension. All these therapeutic effects of exercise thus help in decreased need for diabetes medicines in order to reach target blood glucose level.

115. B. The diabetic patients who are on insulin or oral medication should exercise 1 hour after meals to prevent hyperglycemia or they should consume a carbohydrate snack before exercise. Exercise need not be vigorous. Exercise like brisk walking is equally effective for desired outcome typically for a woman of 45 years of age.

116. D. The nurse should provide patient with the knowledge that nutritional therapy for the management of diabetes is based on a plan of healthy eating that is appropriate and beneficial to most people. The same principles of good nutrition that apply to the general population also apply to the person with diabetes which means adhering to a balanced diet comprising of all essential nutrients according to his need. Diabetic diet is designed for both type1 and type 2 diabetes. Only controlling sugar in the diet is not enough for control of hyperglycemia. Diet therapy and exercise program should be used concurrently.

117. D. The dietary management for diabetes includes identification of the person's daily caloric requirements and choosing foods from different food groups in amounts sufficient to meet the total daily calories. Recommended dietary composition include 50-60% of total calories from carbohydrate source, 10-15% from protein and 30% from fat which includes 7% of saturated fat.

118. B. Oral antidiabetic agents are effective for patients with type 2 diabetes who have some amounts of endogenous insulin. They are not effective in patients with type 1 diabetes in whom endogenous insulin is totally absent. These agents are contraindicated in pregnancy and lactation since their effects on the fetus are unknown. These agents are not oral preparation of insulin.

119. B. Tolbutamide (orinase) and sulfonylureas primarily act on the beta cells of the pancreas to secrete more insulin. They also increase tissue response to insulin (insulin sensitizer). They do not increase the metabolism of carbohydrates. The drug that delays the digestion of complex carbohydrates is acarbose, a alpha glucosidase inhibitors. The drug belonging to thiazolidinediones decreases insulin resistance.

120. D. Delaying or skipping lunch is harmful for a patient who is on sulfonylurea, oral antidiabetic agent because of risk of developing hypoglycemia.

Some medications may interact with the drug either potentiating hypoglycemic or hyperglycemic effect. Alcohol may cause hypoglycemia and should be avoided. Because of risk of hypoglycemic attack, patient should carry medic alert bracelet/ card.

121. D. Acarbose (glucobay) is a member of alpha glucosidase inhibitors category. It works by delaying digestion of complex carbohydrates and some sugars, so blunts peak of blood glucose levels after meals. If given with sulfonylurea or metformin may produce hypoglycemia. So patient should be advised to take glucose when hypoglycemia, instead of sucrose since sucrose absorption will be blocked. Flatulence abdominal distention and diarrhea are adverse effects which are usually minimized by starting with low dose and increasing gradually.

122. B. Huminsulin 30/70 is mixed insulin. It is a combination of 30% of regular insulin and 70% NPH (neutral protamin hagedorn) insulin.

123. A. Short acting insulin or regular insulin is the treatment of choice in diabetic ketoacidosis, since it has rapid onset of action (30 minutes-1 hour). Onset of action for NPH is 3-4 hours and ultralente is 6-8 hours and cannot be used in diabetic ketoacidosis which requires immediate management of hyperglycemia.

124. A. In continuous subcutaneous insulin infusion short acting or regular insulin is used. The teflon catheter inserted in the subcutaneous tissue (usually on abdomen) is changed at least every 3 days and not left for months. The system involves a continuous infusion of insulin at a rate (basal) of .5-2 units/hour and bolus doses of insulin before every meal which the patient receives by pushing buttons of the pump. The amount of insulin for each bolus dose is calculated by the patient is based on blood glucose level, activity level and amount of food intake.

125. D. Human insulin prepared from common bacteria using recombinant DNA technology is least allergic than the insulin prepared from beef and pork pancreas. Monkey is not the source of insulin.

126. B. The insulin is most rapidly absorbed in the abdomen followed by arm, thigh and buttocks.

127. D. After injecting insulin the needle to be withdrawn by applying some pressure with a dry cotton ball at the site and the cotton ball should be held in the place for a few seconds. Massaging of the site should not be done. All other instructions are appropriate.

128. B. When mixing two insulin together, the clear insulin or the regular insulin should be drawn first and then the intermediate acting (NPH) insulin. Intermediate (NPH) or long acting insulin bottle should gently be rolled between palms of hands to mix insulin and not shaken. The site need not be cleaned with alcohol. Standard cleaning with soap and water is adequate. Aspiration does not need to be done before injection.

129. A. Vials of insulin in use should be kept at the room temperature and not refrigerated. The insulin administered at room temperature is less painful.

130. B. Hypoglycemia—abnormally low blood glucose level (also known as insulin reaction or hypoglycemic reaction) is a common feature of type 1 diabetes mellitus and can also be seen in type 2 diabetes treated with insulin or oral agents. The precise blood glucose level at which patients have manifestations varies but it usually does not occur until the blood glucose level is less than 50-60 mg/dL.

131. C. The patient is exhibiting moderate sign and symptoms of hypoglycemia. Since the patient is awake the family members should administer 20–30 g of simple carbohydrate, e.g. orange juice or 4–6 tsf of simple sugar. Calling the physician is unnecessary and is a waste of time. Sublingual nitroglycerin is not indicated. Administration of glucagon would have been appropriate if the patient was unconscious or semiconscious.

132. D. Clinical manifestations of hypoglycemia include anxiety, nervousness, shakiness, palpitation, tachycardia, diaphoresis, cool moist skin, headache, tremors, paresthesia, irritability, inability to concentrate, drowsiness, slurred speech, visual disturbances, etc.other manifestations listed above are that of diabetic ketoacidosis, diabetes insipidus and diabetes mellitus respectively.

133. B. Patient with hypoglycemia who required glucagon should be given a complex carbohydrate snack as soon as possible. Since the action of glucagon is transient a complex carbohydrate snack would restore the liver glycogen and prevent recurrence of hypoglycemia

134. C. The patient who experiences recurrent hypoglycemia should take regular meal or a snack at 4-5 hours interval. Eating inadequate amount, delaying meal or skipping meal are the most important cause of hypoglycemia. Patient should not increase saturated fat and protein foods excessively for the danger of atherosclerosis and nephropathy. Consuming sugar or glucose tablets will contribute to hyperglycemia.

135. D. Aspirin may interact with insulin and result in hypoglycemia. Other drugs listed do not have such interactions.

136. A. Taking too much insulin is not a common cause of diabetic ketoacidosis, rather it is a cause of hypoglycemia or insulin reaction. Other factors may lead to diabetic ketoacidosis.

137. A. A patient who does not take his insulin regularly is at risk of developing hyperglycemia, which will ultimately cause diabetic ketoacidosis. Hypoglycemia occurs due to excessive insulin. HHNS typically occurs with type 2 diabetes. Diabetic nephropathy is a complication of long standing diabetes of either type.

138. B. The patient with high blood sugar level, complaining of abdominal pain, nausea and vomiting is probably presenting with diabetic ketoacidosis. So the nurse is likely to find other manifestations of diabetic ketoacidosis, e.g. dehydration, hyperpnea, breath odor of ketones, hypotension, tachycardia, warm dry skin, visual disturbances, impaired level of consciousness, etc. Cool moist skin, palpitation, faintness, dizziness, inability to concentrate, irrational behavior, etc. are manifestations of hypoglycemia. Profound dehydration, increased serum osmolality, polyuria, confusion are the manifestations of HHNS.

139. B. DKA is a serious condition that proceeds rapidly and must be treated promptly. Because fluid imbalance is potentially life-threatening, the initial goal of therapy is to establish intravenous access and begin fluid and electrolyte replacement. Hyperglycemia is corrected by IV insulin administration but insulin administration is withheld until fluid resuscitation is underway because insulin allows water to enter the cells along with glucose resulting in depletion of vascular volume. Monitoring of vital sign and oxygen saturation is important but more important is IV fluid replacement. The cause of DKA does not have any effect on treatment modalities.

140. D. Undiagnosed, untreated or poorly controlled diabetes mellitus type 2 is the cause of HHNS. Other conditions do not give rise to this condition.

141. C. The most distinguishing feature of HHNS to DKA is the lack of ketonuria with HHNS. Both conditions share hyperglycemia, hyperosmolality and electrolyte imbalance.

142. D. Serum osmolarity is the most important test for confirming HHNS, which will be more than 350 mOsm/L. Other tests are also important but are not as important as serum osmolarity for the confirmation of diagnosis.

143. A. The patient with HHNS is severely dehydrated. Regardless of patient's medical history, rapid fluid resuscitation is critical for cardiovascular integrity. Aggressive fluid replacement with normal saline followed by hypotonic saline is common intervention. Glucose is the added later when blood glucose level reaches 250 mg/dL. Requirement of Ringer lactate will be judged later in the course of treatment after careful studies of electrolyte levels.

144. B. Since the patient remains NPO before surgery he requires reduced amount of insulin. Even when no food is taken, glucose level may rise as a result of hepatic glucose production. Eliminating total dose of insulin may predispose to hyperglycemia and administering the full dose will also result in hypoglycemia. IV insulin infusions are not needed for routine surgery. They are reserved for more stressful situation like transplants or coronary artery bypass surgery.

145. C. Physiologic stress, e.g. infection and surgery as well as emotional stress contributes to hyperglycemia and may precipitate DKA or HHNS. Hence patient with fever and infection require increased dose of insulin. Continuing with usual dose or reducing the dose may result in hyperglycemia. Continuous IV infusion of insulin is also not required as this management is reserved for more stressful situations.

146. D. A diabetic dependent on insulin must have some basic information which will help him to survive that is to avoid severe hypoglycemic or hyperglycemic complications after discharge. Categories of survival information include – normal blood glucose ranges, diabetes, effect of insulin, diet, exercise and stress, treatment modalities, e.g. insulin administration, monitoring of blood glucose and urine ketones, and recognition, treatment and prevention of hypoglycemia and acute hyperglycemia.

147. A. Patients with diabetes should wash their feet with mild soap and water. Examine feet daily for cuts, blisters, etc. They should cut toenails even with rounded contour of toes, not to cut the corners. Applying iodine, alcohol, etc. on cuts or using hot water bottles should be avoided as the tissue injury caused by these substances or thermal injury will not be felt by patient with insensitive foot.

148. C. The main difference between DKA and HHNS is that in DKA there is ketosis. Ketones are acidic byproducts so there is a metabolic acidosis in DKA. Patients with metabolic acidosis have Kussmaul's respiration (rapid deep breathing). It is an attempt to reverse metabolic acidosis through the exhalation of excess carbon dioxide.

7
CHAPTER

Reproductive System

Q1. The most important function of estrogen is:

A. Development and maintenance of secondary sex characteristics
B. Stimulation of growth and maturity of the ovarian follicles
C. Ovulation of matured follicles
D. Maintenance of the implanted ovum

Q2. During assessment of a woman with disorder of reproductive system the nurse is obtaining history regarding the patient's past medical history. Which of the following information is relevant?

A. Age of initiation of sexual activity
B. Role-related problems with family members
C. Previous sexually transmitted infections
D. History of mumps in childhood

Q3. During physical examination of an elderly woman of 70 years age, which of the following age related changes the nurse is expected to find?

A. Enlargement of breast
B. Increased vaginal discharge
C. Narrower and shorter vagina
D. Enlargement of labia

Q4. The examination technique used to evaluate testicular cancer is:

A. Inspection of scrotum for unilateral swelling
B. Percussion of scrotum to detect dull sound
C. Auscultation of scrotum for presence of bruit
D. Transillumination of scrotum to detect shadow

Q5. Which of the following blood tests should be included in the yearly physical examination of men over 50 years of age?

A. AST
B. CEA
C. PSA
D. ELISA

Q6. Which of the following prostate specific antigen (PSA) levels if detected in a 55-year-old male warrants further and prompt investigation?

A. PSA level undetectable
B. 2 ng/mL
C. 4 ng/mL
D. 10 ng/mL

Q7. Which of the following childhood infections may be a cause of infertility in the male?

A. Mumps
B. Measles
C. Pertusis
D. Diphtheria

Q8. A man attends hospital clinic with a suspected diagnosis of benign prostatic hypertrophy. Which of the following symptoms is suggestive of benign hypertrophy of prostate?

A. Frequency and burning of micturition
B. Stress incontinence
C. Residual urine of more than 50 mL
D. Pain during micturition

Q9. Definitive diagnosis of benign hypertrophy of prostate is made by:

A. Digital rectal examination
B. Elevated level of prostate specific antigen
C. Biopsy of prostatic tissue
D. Transrectal ultrasound

Q10. Which of the following conditions may arise as a complication of benign hypertrophy of prostate?

A. Stone in kidney
B. Stone in bladder
C. Bladder cancer
D. Both B and C

Q11. A patient with BPH complains of incomplete bladder emptying and need to strain during urination. In order to detect the development of complications associated with this condition the nurse should particularly obtain information regarding:

A. Decrease in size and force of urine stream
B. Difficulty in initiating voiding
C. Urgency and dysuria
D. Dribbling at the end of urination

Q12. Which of the following factors may precipitate acute retention of urine in a patient with benign hypertrophy of prostate (BPH)?

A. Exposure to hot humid climate
B. Excessive consumption of alcoholic beverages
C. Excessive exercise
D. Antihypertensive drugs

Q13. A patient with BPH is being treated with prazosin (minipress). Prazosin is effective in reducing the symptoms of BPH as it results in:

A. Regression of hyperplastic tissue of the gland
B. Regression of prostate gland through suppression of androgens
C. Relaxation of the smooth muscles of prostate that facilitates urinary flow through the urethra
D. Improvement of renal function through renal vasodilation

Q14. Physician has prescribed finasteride for a patient with benign hypertrophy of prostate. The nurse is teaching the patient about the medicine. Which of the following is appropriate?

A. To take the drug immediately after food.
B. The drug will reduce the size of the prostate within 3 months of therapy
C. To report to physician if decreased libido or impotence
D. To avoid coitus or to use condom during sexual activity

Q15. A triple lumen Foley's catheter is being used for a patient after transurethral resection of prostate. The nurse is aware that one of the 3 lumen is to be used for balloon inflation and the other 2 lumens to be used for:

A. Continuous inflow of irrigating solution and continuous outflow of urine and irrigating solution

B. Intermittent inflow of irrigating solution and intermittent outflow of urine and irrigating solution
C. Prevention of hemorrhage and continuous flow of urine
D. Intermittent inflow of irrigating solution and prevention of hemorrhage

Q16. A patient who has undergone TURP a few hours ago is on continuous bladder irrigation. He is complaining of increasing pain. Which of the following nursing actions is most appropriate?

A. Reassure the patient that this pain is expected during postoperative period
B. Administer pain medication as prescribed
C. Check the patency of the catheter and drainage
D. Instruct the patient to void around the catheter

Q17. While caring for a patient after TURP the nurse notices clots to pass through the drainage tube. Which of the following actions is appropriate?

A. Increase the flow of irrigating fluid to flush out the clots
B. Decrease the flow of irrigating fluid
C. Prepare to remove the urinary catheter
D. Stop continuous bladder irrigation and inform the physician

Q18. A nurse is preparing a patient for discharge after a transurethral resection of prostate. Which of the following instructions is appropriate for this patient?

A. Limiting intake of fluid
B. Avoiding frequent urination
C. Resuming normal activities as early as possible
D. Continuing to have a yearly digital rectal examination

Q19. The most important dietary risk factor for prostate cancer is the consumption of diet that is high in:

A. Fat
B. Vitamin D
C. Purine
D. Alcohol and caffeine

Q20. While teaching a group of middle aged men regarding early detection of prostate cancer, the nurse advises that they should have an annual:

A. Histopathological test of urethral smear
B. Prostatic ultrasound
C. Digital rectal examination
D. Serum alkaline phosphatase

Q21. Bilateral orchiectomy has been performed for a patient with stage D prostate cancer. The purpose of orchiectomy in this patient includes:

A. Reduction of circulating testosterone and thus arresting tumor growth
B. Prevention of metastasis to the testicles
C. Relief of bone pain associated with advanced cancer
D. Both A and C

Q22. Perineal pain in the absence of an infectious process is suggestive of:

A. Bladder calculi
B. Internal hemorrhoids
C. Acute prostatitis
D. Chronic prostatitis

Q23. The nurse advises the patient with chronic prostatitis that management include:

A. A short course of antibiotic therapy
B. Bladder drainage with suprapubic catheterization
C. Prostatic massage
D. Avoiding sexual activity

Q24. Which of the following measures help prevent develpoment of phimosis in a 25-year-old uncircumcised man?

A. Careful cleaning of the prepuce
B. Regular ejaculation
C. Avoiding multiple sex partner
D. All of the above

Q25. Which of the following discharge instructions should be given to a man who has had a vasectomy?

- **A.** To continue his usual activities
- **B.** Apply hot compress if scrotal edema
- **C.** Do not worry for erectile dysfunction, which is temporary
- **D.** Use an alternative form of contraception for 6 weeks postoperatively

Q26. Which of the following conditions if reported by a young adult is considered to be a risk for development of testicular cancer?

- **A.** Hydrocele
- **B.** German measles
- **C.** Cryptoorchidism
- **D.** Maternal exposure to synthetic progesterone

Q27. A woman complaining of infertility is being advised to record her basal body temperature. Which of the following instructions the nurse should include regarding monitoring of basal body temperature?

- **A.** Take temperature at the same site and at the same time everyday
- **B.** Take temperature in the morning before getting out of bed
- **C.** Take temperature with any standard glass thermometer
- **D.** A slight rise in temperature indicates ovulation

Q28. The cause of primary dysmenorrhea is most commonly due to:

- **A.** Elevated levels of estrogen
- **B.** Elevated levels of uterine prostaglandins
- **C.** Endometriosis
- **D.** Uterine myoma

Q29. The nurse is assessing a 32-year-old woman complaining of dysmenorrhea. In order to differentiate between primary and secondary dysmenorrhea the nurse should ask which of the following questions?

- **A.** "When in your menstrual history did the dysmenorrhea begin?"
- **B.** "Do you get relief from dysmenorrhea by taking nonsteroidal anti-inflammatory drug?"
- **C.** "Is your dysmenorrhea associated with irregular menstrual bleeding?"
- **D.** "How long the pain lasts?"

Q30. Long interval between menses is termed as:

- **A.** Amenorrhea
- **B.** Oligomenorrhea
- **C.** Menorrhagia
- **D.** Metrorrhagia

Q31. Primary amenorrhea refers to the failure of menstrual cycles to begin by age:

- **A.** 10 years
- **B.** 13 years
- **C.** 16 years
- **D.** 19 years

Q32. A 15-year-old girl is brought to the hospital clinic with the complain of primary amenorrhea. The nurse attending the girl should assess:

- **A.** Height and weight
- **B.** Breast tenderness
- **C.** Nausea
- **D.** Secondary sex characteristics

Q33. The most common condition associated with secondary amenorrhea is:

- **A.** Anorexia nervosa
- **B.** Polycystic ovary disease
- **C.** Pregnancy
- **D.** Pseudocyesis

Q34. A 18-year-old girl is complaining of secondary amenorrhea. The cause of her amenorrhea has been identified as anovulation. The girl most probably will

be treated by which of the following hormones?

A. Danazol (antiandrogen)
B. Estrogen
C. Clomiphene citrate
D. Progesterone

Q35. Which of the following is a cause of menorrhagia?

A. Anovulatory menstrual cycles
B. Uterine fibroids
C. Hypothyroidism
D. All of the above

Q36. A patient with menorrhagia has undergone endometrial biopsy to determine the cause of menorrhagia. Which of the following instructions the nurse should include in the discharge teaching plan for the patient?

A. Resume normal activity as early as possible
B. Inform physician if next menses do not occur in time
C. Inform physician if excessive pain occurs
D. Irrigate vaginal canal with sterile normal saline twice a day

Q37. The patient who had a dilatation and curettage procedure is being instructed about some activity limitations. Which of the following instructions by the nurse is appropriate?

A. Stay on bed rest for 1 week then gradually resume normal activities
B. Avoid sexual intercourse for 1 week
C. Avoid strenuous work for 6 weeks
D. Avoid tub bath or pond bath for at least 2 weeks

Q38. A 48-year-old postmenopausal woman reports to the nurse that she has recently experienced some spotting. Which of the following instructions by the nurse is appropriate?

A. "Do not worry. This is not a serious problem"
B. "Keep a menstrual calendar for the next 6 months"
C. "Watch for the next episode of spotting. If it happens come back to the clinic immediately"
D. "You need an endometrial biopsy to determine the cause of spotting"

Q39. Women who have had panhysterectomies are usually prescribed:

A. Estrogen and progesterone
B. Estrogen
C. Progesterone
D. Calcium

Q40. For menopausal women with no surgical histories a combination of estrogen and progesterone is recommended. The reason for this combination is:

A. Reproductive fertility is enhanced with combination
B. Respiratory capacity is increased with combination
C. Regular menstrual cycles resume for a few more years with combination therapy
D. Progesterone in combination therapy prevents hyperproliferation of uterine endometrium

Q41. The most common site of ectopic pregnancy is:

A. Ovary
B. Cervix
C. Fallopian tube
D. Abdomen

Q42. The most significant assessment finding in a patient with ruptured tubal pregnancy is:

A. Severe vaginal bleeding and shock
B. Vague abdominal pain
C. Irregular vaginal bleeding and syncope
D. Hypovolemic shock which does not necessarily correlate with the extent of vaginal bleeding

Q43. The nurse is teaching a postmenopausal woman who is not on hormone replacement therapy about options to minimize unwanted symptoms of menopause. Which of the following instructions is most important and must be included in the teaching?

A. To perform regular aerobic and weight bearing exercises
B. To maintain daily calcium intake of at least 1500 mg
C. To maintain usual sexual activity
D. To avoid obesity

Q44. A patient attending hospital clinic complains of thick, white curdy vaginal discharge and intense itching of the vulva. The patient is most probably suffering from:

A. Gonorrhea
B. Monilial vaginitis
C. Trichomoniasis
D. Gardnerella vaginalis vaginitis

Q45. Which of the following factors increases the risk for candidiasis in a susceptible woman?

A. Anemia
B. Nulliparity
C. Use of broad-spectrum antibiotics
D. Use of spermicidal jelly

Q46. A patient visits hospital with the complain of frothy greenish vaginal discharge and hemorrhagic spots (strawberry spots) on the vaginal wall. The physician suspects trichomoniasis and prescribes which of the following medications?

A. Fluconazole
B. Metronidazole
C. Azithromycin
D. Ciprofloxacin

Q47. A pregnant woman has developed chlamydial infection. The nurse will teach the patient that:

A. Chlamydia is not a sexually transmitted disease
B. Chlamydial infection in pregnancy may lead to stillborn or premature birth
C. If untreated, chlamydial infection may lead to renal failure
D. The treatment of choice for chlamydia in pregnancy is tetracycline 250 mg orally every 6 hours

Q48. Which of the following methods of contraception provides protection against sexually transmitted diseases (STDs)?

A. Oral contraceptive
B. Intrauterine contraceptive devices (IUD)
C. Condom
D. Norplant implant

Q49. While assessing a female sexual partner of a man with gonorrhea, the nurse is most likely to find which of the following symptoms?

A. May not find any symptom
B. Chancres in the vaginal wall
C. Vesicular lesions on the vulva
D. Macular palmer rash

Q50. Which of the following conditions is not a complication of gonorrhea in women?

A. Pelvic inflammatory disease
B. Bartholin's abscess
C. Ectopic pregnancy
D. Urethral strictures

Q51. Which of the following symptoms in men with gonorrhea prompts an individual to seek medical attention?

A. Dysuria and purulent discharge from urethra
B. Sterility
C. Genital ulcer
D. Multiple warts on penis

Q52. The typical sign of untreated primary syphilis is:

A. Foul-smelling urethral discharge
B. Flu-like symptoms and maculopapular rash on palms and soles

C. Painless chancre on the genitalia
D. Unilateral painful swelling of the scrotum

Q53. The recommended drug therapy for a patient with uncomplicated gonorrhea is a single dose of:

A. Ceftriaxone 125 mg IM
B. Ciprofloxacin 500 mg orally
C. Cefixime 400 mg orally
D. Any of the above

Q54. For a patient with gonorrhea, physician has prescribed ceftriaxone 125 mg IM followed by doxycycline 100 mg orally, twice a day for 7 days. Which of the following statements justifies administration of both antibiotics?

A. Combined antibiotic therapy prevents reinfection
B. Resistant strains of *N. gonorrhea* is best treated with combined antibiotic therapy
C. The high rate of coexisting chlamydial and gonococcal infections requires combined antibiotic therapy
D. Coexisting syphilis indicates dual antibiotic coverage

Q55. Which of the following statements about genital herpes is not appropriate?

A. Majority of genital herpes is caused by herpes simplex virus type 2
B. It is a sexually transmitted disease
C. The disease is cured by antiviral medication
D. The condition may result into corneal ulcer

Q56. Which of the following symptoms if found in a patient with the history of genital herpes would indicate that a recurrence is imminent?

A. Headache and fever
B. Fever and regional lymphadenopathy
C. Urinary retention and dysuria
D. Tingling, burning and itching at genitalia

Q57. A woman who had an attack of genital herpes should be advised to:

A. Adopt stress reduction technique
B. Ask her partner to use condom when lesions are present
C. Expose her to sunlight daily
D. Get pelvic examination and Pap smear done every 2 years

Q58. A patient attending gynae outpatient department is diagnosed with genital warts (condylomata acuminate). The nurse is providing information about this condition to the patient. Which of the following information is appropriate?

A. "It is a harmless bacterial infection"
B. "You may have acquired this infection from public washrooms"
C. "The lesion will disappear after 7 to 10 days of treatment with the antibiotic prescribed by the physician"
D. "You need to visit this clinic every year for Pap test as you are at increased risk for genital cancer"

Q59. Pelvic inflammatory disease involves infection of the:

A. Fallopian tubes
B. Ovaries
C. Pelvic peritoneum
D. All of the above

Q60. Pelvic inflammatory disease may result from all of the following *except:*

A. Sexual intercourse
B. Recent abdominal surgery
C. Child birth
D. Termination of pregnancy

Q61. A woman is admitted in hospital with the diagnosis of pelvic inflammatory disease (PID). During assessment the nurse is most likely to find a history of:

A. Recent blood transfusion
B. Multiparity
C. Multiple sex partner
D. Pulmonary tuberculosis

Q62. The nurse taking care of a patient with pelvic inflammatory disease (PID) encourages her to be in semi Fowler's position. The most important rational for this position is to:

A. Relieve pain by relaxing abdominal muscles
B. Prevent abscess formation by promoting drainage
C. Prevent thromboembolism by improving circulation
D. Prevent respiratory complications by easing breathing

Q63. The term endometriosis refers to:

A. Inflammation of the endometrium
B. Hypertrophy of the endometrium
C. Endometrial tissue is located outside the uterus
D. Metaplasia of endometrial tissue within the uterine cavity

Q64. The most common manifestations of endometriosis are:

A. Menorrhagia, dysmenorrhea, dysuria, hematuria
B. Dysmenorrhea, infertility, pelvic pain, dyspareunia
C. Menorrhagia, dysuria, painful bowel movements, dysmenorrhea
D. Amenorrhea, pelvic pain, dyspareunia, dysuria

Q65. Which of the following modalities of treatment is appropriate in a patient with endometriosis to relieve distressing manifestations?

A. To inhibit ovarian estrogen production and shrink the endometrial implants
B. Use of contraceptives to avoid pregnancy
C. Use of analgesics to relieve pain and dysmenorrhea
D. To provide information, support and teach coping strategies for pain management

Q66. While planning care for a patient on hormonal therapy for endometriosis the nurse includes teaching regarding the side effect of:

A. Long-term use of NSAID
B. Synthetic estrogen supplementation
C. Hormonal suppression of ovulation
D. Hormonal stimulation of anterior pituitary

Q67. Which of the following woman is at high-risk of developing leiomyomas?

A. 40-year-old African woman
B. 45-year-old white woman
C. 50-year-old Asian woman
D. 60-year-old Indian woman

Q68. The most common manifestation of leiomyomas is:

A. Profuse vaginal discharge
B. Abnormal uterine bleeding
C. Constipation
D. Hydroureter

Q69. A 30-year-old woman complaining of infertility is diagnosed with leiomyomas. The nurse anticipates that the management of this patient will include:

A. A hysterectomy to treat abnormal uterine bleeding
B. Administration of NSAIDs to relieve dysmenorrhea
C. A myomectomy to remove the tumor and preserve fertility
D. Hormonal therapy to shrink tumor and induce pregnancy

Q70. The findings of Pap test of a woman aged 42 years indicate dysplasia. The nurse is aware that dysplasia indicates:

A. An increase in the number of cells in a tissue
B. A change in the size, shape or arrangement of the cells
C. A reversible transformation of one cell type into another
D. An increase in the size of cells

Q71. A patient has been admitted in hospital with the diagnosis of incomplete abortion. She has abdominal pain and moderate amount of vaginal bleeding. Which of the following nursing actions is most important to include in the care plan of this patient?

A. Observation of the amount and type of vaginal bleeding
B. Restricting food and fluid per mouth
C. Reassuring the patient that one abortion does not prevent future pregnancies
D. Instructing the patient to lie flat on the bed until pain and bleeding stops

Q72. Which of the following women is at greatest risk of developing cervical cancer?

A. Women with history of recurrent candidiasis
B. Women with a pregnancy before age 20 years
C. Women infected with human papilloma virus
D. Women with long history of oral contraceptives

Q73. The nurse is assessing a woman attending gynae outpatient department with the complaint of vaginal discharge. Which of the following subjective data would indicate a risk factor of cancer of the uterine cervix?

A. Diet high in fat
B. Menarche at age 12 years
C. Occupational exposure to aromatic dye
D. Multiple sex partners

Q74. According to American Cancer Society's guidelines all sexually active women should undergo Pap test how frequently?

A. Every 5 years
B. Every 3 years
C. Every 2 years
D. Every year till 3 consecutive negative results

Q75. Which of the following symptoms is an early manifestation of cervical cancer?

A. Malodorous thick vaginal discharge
B. Thin, watery vaginal discharge
C. Vaginal bleeding
D. Aching abdominal pain

Q76. All of the following surgical management for cervical cancer preserve fertility *except:*

A. Conization
B. Loop electrocautery excision procedure (LEEP)
C. Laser therapy
D. Pelvic exenteration

Q77. A patient with cancer of the cervix is scheduled for intracavitary radiation therapy. In preparation of the patient the nurse administers a cleansing enema as prescribed. The rational for administering a cleansing enema is:

A. To prevent bowel movement during the procedure which may result in infection of the uterine cavity through contamination of vagina
B. Feces present in the bowel during radiation may lead to fecal impaction
C. To place the applicator in position accurately when the bladder and bowel is empty
D. To prevent straining at stool, which may cause displacement of the applicator and radiation source

Q78. A patient with cervical cancer is scheduled for internal radiation. As a part of preparing the woman for this procedure the nurse would be most accurate in teaching the patient that:

A. She will be on bed rest with bathroom privileges only
B. Visitors are allowed provided they maintain a distance of 6 feet from the patient
C. She will be placed in high Fowler's position
D. She will be given a low residue diet and antidiarrheal medications to prevent

bowel movement and diarrhea during treatment

Q79. The nurse is taking care of a patient following vaginal hysterectomy. To prevent deep vein thrombosis in the postoperative period, the nurse should plan all of the following *except:*

A. Frequent changes of position
B. High Fowler's position
C. Leg exercises
D. Avoiding pillow under the knees

Q80. The nurse is teaching a 40-year-old woman after hysterectomy regarding restriction of activities after discharge. Which of the following statements by the patient indicates the need for further teaching?

A. "I know that I should not lift heavy objects for at least 2 months"
B. "I should avoid sexual activity for 4–6 weeks"
C. "Swimming would be a good exercise for me"
D. "I should walk swiftly for at least 30 minutes daily to control my body weight"

Q81. Which of the following symptoms is suggestive of breast cancer?

A. Breast enlargement
B. Breast tenderness
C. Darkening of nipple
D. Unilateral discharge from nipple

Q82. A patient with breast tumor is scheduled for breast conservation surgery. Which of the following statements about breast conservation surgery is correct?

A. A portion of the tumor is excised and examined
B. The tumor is removed
C. The tumor and some normal surrounding tissue will be removed
D. The underarm lymph nodes are surgically resected and examined

Q83. A nurse is caring for a patient with modified radical mastectomy. Which of the following potential complications she should assess for?

A. Pneumonitis
B. Rib fracture
C. Lymphedema
D. Compartment syndrome

Q84. Following a left modified radical mastectomy, which of the following nursing measures should not be implemented to prevent postoperative lymphedema in the affected arm?

A. Immobilizing the affected arm with a splint
B. Positioning the affected arm on a pillow
C. Instructing the patient to squeeze a rubber ball with left hand
D. Applying the blood pressure cuff on the patient's right hand while measuring blood pressure

Q85. Breast self-examination involves both:

A. Inspection of breasts and palpation of breast tissue
B. Palpation of breast tissue and cervical lymph nodes
C. Palpation of breast tissue and squeezing nipple for discharge
D. Palpation of breast tissue and axillary lymph nodes

Q86. The nurse is teaching a group of premenopausal women regarding breast self-examination. She tells the women that best time to do the self-examination of breasts is:

A. 7 days before the start of menstruation
B. 7 days after the start of menstruation
C. The first day of opening a new package of oral contraceptive
D. On the birthdate of each month

Q87. The nurse who is planning to teach breast self-examination (BSE) to a

group of young women should include which of the following teaching –learning methods?

A. Lecture emphasizing the value of early detection of breast cancer

B. A film showing the technique of breast self-examination

C. Demonstration of breast self-examination (BSE) on a woman

D. An opportunity to perform a return demonstration by all women of the group

Q88. The nurse is teaching a 20-year-old young woman with fibrocystic breast changes regarding self-care. Which of the following teaching is inappropriate?

A. "You may expect discomfort or pain just before menstruation"

B. "Any lump in breast must be biopsied to rule out malignancy"

C. "You may experience the symptoms off and on throughout your reproductive life"

D. "Restriction of coffee and chocolate, supplementation of vitamin E and use of good support bra may relieve your discomfort"

Q89. Which of the following women is at greatest risk of developing breast cancer?

A. Woman above age 60 years

B. Woman having a maternal grand mother with postmenopausal breast cancer

C. Woman using oral contraceptives for the past 10 years

D. Woman who consumes a high fat diet

Q90. A patient diagnosed with breast cancer has undergone lumpectomy with axillary clearance followed by detailed diagnostic studies of the operated mass. Test result that indicates most favorable prognosis is:

A. Tumor measuring above 5 cm

B. Absence of lymph node involvement

C. Over expression of c-erb-B2 genetic marker

D. Estrogen and progesterone receptor negative tumor

Q91. A patient with breast cancer is considering the treatment choice of breast conservation surgery with radiation or a modified radical mastectomy. When asked by the patient about these options, the nurse informs that breast conservation surgery with radiation involves:

A. A short treatment course with minimum cost

B. Preserves normal texture and sensitivity of breast

C. Results in fewer complications than that of modified radical mastectomy

D. Has about the same survival rate as that with modified radical mastectomy

Q92. A woman who has undergone a modified radical mastectomy is being taught self-care measures to prevent lymphedema of the affected arm. Which of the following teachings is appropriate?

A. To use an elastic bandage during the early postoperative period

B. To avoid trauma to the arm on the affected side

C. To perform weight bearing exercises by the arm on the affected side

D. All of the above

Q93. After a modified radical mastectomy for breast cancer a patient is on adjuvant chemotherapy. In caring for this woman which of the following nursing diagnoses should a nurse give priority?

A. Disturbed body image

B. Altered sexuality pattern

C. Fatigue

D. Impaired physical mobility

ANSWERS AND RATIONALES OF REPRODUCTIVE SYSTEM

1. **A.** The most important function of estrogen is development and maintenance of secondary sex characteristics. The hormone responsible for stimulation of growth and maturity of the ovarian follicles is FSH (follicle stimulating hormone). LH (luteinizing hormone) causes follicles to complete maturation and undergo ovulation and progesterone is mainly responsible for the maintenance of the implanted fertilized ovum.

2. **C.** While taking history of a woman with reproductive disorder regarding past medical history, the relevant information to be obtained is past history of sexually transmitted infections and other infections of the respiratory tract. Age of initiation of sexual activity is relevant while taking history of sexual and reproductive life. History of role-related problems is also not relevant. Obtaining history of mumps from a woman patient is not relevant but it is relevant for a male patient.

3. **C.** The nurse is expected to find narrower and shorter vagina in an older woman due to atrophy of tissue in the vagina. The woman is likely to exhibit decreased size of breast, not enlargement, decreased not increased vaginal discharge and decreased not increased size of labia and clitoris.

4. **D.** Examination technique to detect testicular cancer is transillumination of the scrotum. The examiner should first palpate the scrotum for any mass then transilluminate the scrotum by darkening the room and shining a flashlight through the scrotum behind the mass. A scrotum filled with serous fluid transilluminates as a red glow. A more solid lesion, e.g. hematoma or mass do not transilluminate and may be seen as a dark shadow. Although inspection is carried out at first but inspection alone cannot suspect the presence of mass. Percussion and auscultation are not carried out to detect testicular mass.

5. **D.** The PSA level of 10 ng/mL if detected in a 55-year-old man would warrant prompt investigation. Serum PSA level of 10 ng/mL is abnormally elevated (normal being < 4 ng/mL). Elevated PSA level may be due to condition, e.g. benign prostatic hypertrophy or may be due to a tumor in the prostate gland.

6. **C.** Cancers of the prostate occur in elderly men. Regular physical examination by digital rectal examination and blood test for prostate specific antigen (PSA) should be done yearly for men over 50 years for the early detection of prostate cancer. AST is done during all physical examination. Carcinoembryonic antigen (CEA) is done for diagnosis and monitoring of gastrointestinal cancers. ELISA to detect HIV positive status need not be done for the elderlies as a routine since the largest percentage of HIV positive individuals are young adults.

7. **A.** The cause of infertility in male may be due to mumps. Mumps in young men is associated with sterility. Measles, pertusis and diphtheria are not associated with male sterility.

8. **C.** A residual urine of more than 50 mL after voiding is suggestive of benign hypertrophy of prostate. Hypertrophy of prostate causes urinary outflow problems. The patient experiences

voiding symptoms, e.g. a decrease in the caliber and force of the urinary stream, difficulty in initiating voiding, intermittency, dribbling at the end of urination and incomplete bladder emptying, determined either by catheterization or by ultrasonography after voiding.

9. C. Definitive diagnosis of benign hypertrophy of prostate is made by biopsy followed by histopathological examination of prostatic tissue. Digital rectal examination reveals only size and configuration of prostate gland. PSA level and transrectal ultrasound are helpful in differentiating BPH from prostate cancer but definitive diagnosis is only made by biopsy followed by histopathology.

10. B. Stone in bladder may arise as a complication of BPH. Bladder stones are 8 times more common in men with BPH. Incomplete evacuation of the bladder results in residual urine. Calculi may develop in the bladder because of alkalinization of residual urine. Risk of stone formation in kidney is not increased due to BPH. The possible causes of bladder cancer are cigarette smoking, industrial exposure to certain substances, e.g. asbestos and aromatic amines, artificial sweeteners; chronic cystitis; pelvic radiation, etc.

11. C. Common complication that develops in BPH is urinary tract infection (UTI). Incomplete emptying of the bladder resulting in residual urine provides a favorable environment for bacterial growth. Symptoms associated with urinary tract infection are urgency, dysuria, bladder pain, nocturia and incontinence. So the nurse should obtain information regarding this complication during assessment of the patient. A decrease in size of the urine stream, difficulty in initiating voiding and dribbling at the end of urination are the usual voiding symptoms of partial obstruction due to BPH and not the symptoms of complication associated with BPH.

12. B. Excessive consumption of alcoholic beverages may precipitate acute retention of urine in a patient with BPH. Other factors which may precipitate acute retention are exposure to cold climate not hot, humid climate; bed rest not excessive exercise; use of decongestants, anticholinergics and antidepressants not antihypertensives.

13. C. Prazosin (minipress) belongs to the group alpha-adrenergic blocker. Prazosin and other drugs of this group promote smooth muscle relaxation in the prostate by blocking alpha adrenergic receptors in the gland. Relaxation of smooth muscle ultimately facilitates urinary flow through the urethra. The drug does not reduce the size of the prostate either by regression of hyperplastic tissue of the prostate or by suppression of androgens. These actions are exhibited by finasteride (proscar) and not by minipress. This drug does not also effect renal function through renal vasodilation.

14. D. Pregnant women or women who may become pregnant should not touch the drug or come into contact with semen of a patient taking the drug to prevent adverse effect to the developing male fetus. The drug may be taken any time without regard to meals. The desired therapeutic effect of the drug is not obtained before 6 to 12 months of treatment. So patient must take the medicine on a continuous basis. Decreased libido, impotence and decreased volume of ejaculate is a side effect and not an adverse effect

15. A. After TURP a 3 way indwelling Foley's catheter is inserted. One lumen is used for inflation of the balloon of the self-retaining catheter. The other 2 lumens are used for continuous inflow of the irrigating solution and the other lumen is used for continuous drainage of urine and outflow of irrigating solution. The inflated balloon of the self-retaining catheter provides pressure to prevent hemorrhage. No other lumen is used for extra balloon inflation.

16. C. Pain after prostate surgery is mostly due to obstruction in the urinary catheter and drainage system. Obstruction causes bladder spasm and pain. So the nurse should check the patency of the catheter and drainage system. Some postoperative pain is expected but increasing amount of pain is not expected unless the patient is experiencing bladder spasm. The nurse will administer pain medication as prescribed, but before administering the drug she should check the patency of the catheter and drainage tube. The patient should not void around the catheter. Voiding around the catheter will increase bladder spasm.

17. A. The appropriate action by the nurse is to increase the flow of irrigating fluid to flush out the clots to keep the catheter patent and for easy drainage of urine. The nurse should not decrease the flow of irrigating fluid in such situation, remove catheter or stop continuous bladder irrigation. There is no need to inform the physician.

18. D. After transurethral resection of prostate the patient should be advised to continue to have annual digital rectal examination (DRE) as hyperplasia or cancer may occur in the remaining prostate tissue. The patient should be advised to take 2–3 liters of fluid per day and not limit fluid. He should be encouraged to void every 2–3 hours to flush the urinary tract. Some of the activities are limited after prostatectomy, e.g. sitting for prolonged time, driving or taking prolonged automobile rides for 2 weeks and heavy lifting and strenuous exercise for 4–6 weeks.

19. A. The dietary factor, which may play a role in the development of prostate cancer, is consumption of a high fat diet. High fat consumption can alter cholesterol and steroid metabolism, which may increase the risk of cancer. Diet high in Vitamin D is believed to decrease the risk of prostate cancer. People who receive more sunlight exposure have a lower incidence of and lower death rate from prostate cancer. Diet high in purine causes gout not prostate cancer. No associations have been found with alcohol and caffeine intake and prostate cancer.

20. C. For early detection of prostate cancer middle aged men should undergo annual digital rectal examination and blood test for prostate specific antigen. Histopathological test of urethral smear does not reveal prostate cancer. Prostatic ultrasound helps the surgeon to visualize the abnormality and collect specimen for histopathological examination. Measurement of serum alkaline phosphatase does not help in early detection but it is done to detect bony metastasis in advanced cancer.

21. D. For advanced stages of prostate cancer (stage D), a bilateral orchiectomy is one treatment option for cancer control. Testosterone produced by the testes stimulates growth of the prostate cancer. An orchiectomy reduces the circulating testosterone level by 90%. Another benefit of orchiectomy is rapid relief of bone pain associated with advanced cancer. The purpose of preventing metastasis does not arise as the patient is already in stage D.

22. D. Chronic prostatitis also known as chronic pelvic pain syndrome is characterized by prostate and urinary pain in the absence of an obvious infectious process. In bladder calculi patient usually complains of frequency, dysuria, hematuria due to cystitis. In acute prostatitis patient exhibits fever, chills, back pain, perineal pain along with dysuria, urinary urgency, frequency and cloudy urine, which suggest acute bacterial infection. Internal hemorrhoids cause rectal pain usually during defecation.

23. C. Repetitive prostatic massage is therapeutic for most type of prostatitis except acute bacterial prostatitis. Prostatic massage relieves congestion within the prostate by squeezing out excess prostatic secretions, thus providing pain relief. Other therapeutic measures of chronic prostatitis include long-term administration of antibiotics and anti-inflammatory agents, frequent ejaculations by masturbation and intercourse and increased fluid intake. Suprapubic catheterization may be required in acute urinary retention developed from acute prostatitis, not chronic prostatitis.

24. A. Phimosis is a constriction of the uncircumcised foreskin around the head of the penis, making retraction difficult. It is caused by edema or inflammation of the foreskin due to poor hygienic practices that allow bacterial and yeast organisms to become trapped under the foreskin. Careful cleaning of the preputial area to remove secretions is critical for prevention of phimosis. Regular ejaculation decreases symptoms of chronic prostatitis, but it has no effect on the development of or prevention of phimosis. Avoiding multiple sex partners prevents STDs, not phimosis.

25. D. The man should use an alternative form of contraception for 6 weeks or until semen analysis confirms absence of sperms. Because sperms remain in the semen beyond the point of occlusion of the vas deferense and only gradually disappear from the ejaculate. The person should rest for a few days and continue normal activities including heavy lifting and coitus after a week. He should apply ice pack if scrotal edema, not hot compress. Erectile dysfunction should not result from vasectomy. It may occur in some men due to psychological maladjustment. Careful discussion of the procedure and its outcome before surgery may prevent this problem.

26. C. Cryptoorchidism or undescended testes is considered to be a risk for development of testicular cancer. Other risk factors are family history of testicular cancer, orchitis, mumps, HIV infection, maternal exposure to diethyl stilbesterol, inguinal hernia in childhood and testicular cancer in the contralateral side. Hydrocele, german measles and maternal exposure to synthetic progesterone are not considered as risk factors in the development of testicular cancer.

27. B. The nurse should instruct the woman to take her temperature every morning before getting out of bed and any activity. The temperature should be taken everyday at the same site (e.g. oral or rectal) on awakening but need not be at the same time. For best results basal body temperature should be taken with a

BBT thermometer, which measures temperature between 36° F and 100°F. A slight drop in the temperature graph indicates ovulation.

28. B. The most common cause of primary dysmenorrhea is due to elevated levels of uterine prostaglandins or due to an increased sensitivity to prostaglandins. Prostaglandins are hormone like secretions, which cause smooth muscle contraction. An elevated level of estrogen is not associated with primary dysmenorrhea. An imbalance between estrogen and progesterone may be a causative factor. In primary dysmenorrhea no underlying pathological disorders are present, e.g. endometriosis or uterine myoma. These are the cause of secondary dysmenorrhea.

29. A. The most important distinguishing feature of primary dysmenorrhea to that of secondary dysmenorrhea is its onset. Primary dysmenorrhea begins in the few years after menarche, typically with the onset of regular ovulatory cycles. Secondary dysmenorrhea begins after adolescence, occurring most commonly at 30–40 years of age. Both type of dysmenorrhea may get relief from nonsteroidal anti-inflammatory drug. Dysmenorrhea associated with irregular menstrual bleeding is seen in secondary dysmenorrhea. Duration of pain in primary dysmenorrhea rarely lasts more than 2 days and in secondary dysmenorrhea the pain continues longer than in primary dysmenorrhea.

30. B. Long intervals between menses are termed as oligomenorrhea. Absence of menstruation is termed as amenorrhea, which may be primary or secondary. Menorrhagia is excessive menstrual bleeding and metrorrhagia is irregular bleeding or bleeding between menses.

31. C. Primary amenorrhea refers to the failure of menstrual cycles to begin by age 16 years.

32. D. The nurse should assess secondary sex characteristics in a girl of age 15 years, which include axillary and pubic hair, development of breast and widening of pelvis. Height and weight abnormality is usually not associated with primary amenorrhea unless severe dyscrepancy, e.g. dwarfism or obesity. Breast tenderness and nausea are associated with pregnancy, which must be ruled out to diagnose pathological condition causing secondary amenorrhea.

33. C. The most common condition associated with secondary amenorrhea is pregnancy. Anorexia nervosa, polycystic ovary disease and pseudocyesis (false pregnancy) are associated with secondary amenorrhea but not so common as pregnancy.

34. D. Secondary dysmenorrhea due to anovulation is treated by progesterone or birth control pills. In anovulation the corpus luteum that produces progesterone does not form, giving rise to persistent and excessive build up of the endometrium by the unopposed estrogen. To shed the endometrial lining progesterone is prescribed. Danazol-an antiandrogen, estrogen and clomiphene citrate-an antiestrogen do not cause secretory phase of menstrual cycle.

35. D. Menorrhagia or excessive vaginal bleeding at normal intervals can occur due to various causes. Anovulatory menstrual cycle, uterine fibroids, hypothyroidism can cause menorrhagia. Other causes of menorrhagia include spontaneous abortion, inflammatory process, e.g. endometritis or salpingitis, blood dyscrasias, use of an IUD (intrauterine devices), endometrial carcinoma and medications, e.g. anticoagulants.

36. C. After endometrial biopsy, the patient usually experiences minimal uterine cramping. Excessive pain signals complication and should be promptly reported. The patient should avoid strenuous activity for about 1 week. Following endometrial biopsy the subsequent menstrual periods may or may not be affected. So, physician need not be informed if next menses do not occur in time. Douching / irrigation of vaginal canal is prohibited for the risk of ascending infection.

37. D. After a dilatation and curettage procedure, the patient should be instructed to avoid tub bath or pond bath for 2 weeks to prevent infection. Sexual intercourse should also be avoided to prevent infection for at least 2 weeks. The patient should resume usual activities gradually, reaching preoperative levels within 2 weeks and not 6 weeks, but bed rest is not necessary.

38. D. Whenever spotting is experienced by menopausal women, endometrial cancer must be considered. So the nurse should advise the woman for endometrial biopsy to rule out endometrial cancer. Keeping a menstrual calendar for 6 months and watching for the next episode of spotting will unnecessary delay the diagnosis of endometrial cancer if any, and is harmful for the patient.

39. B. Women who have had panhysterectomies should be prescribed estrogen. Estrogen replacement in perimenopausal, menopausal and postmenopausal women alleviates vasomotor instability, vaginal and urinary tract atrophy and dyspareunia. It also prevents osteoporosis and possibly cardiovascular disease. Progesterone prevents hyperproliferation of uterus with onset of menses, but in the absence of uterus, this function of progesterone is not applicable. Calcium level does not affect hormonal function but it is given for the treatment of osteoporosis, which is common in menopausal women.

40. D. Progesterone prevents hyperproliferation of uterine endometrium and risk of endometrial cancer. So unopposed ERT (estrogen alone) without progesterone is no longer recommended for women with intact uterus. The purposes of postmenopausal replacement therapy are not to enhance reproductive fertility, resuming menstrual cycles for a few more years and to increase respiratory capacity but to relieve distressing symptoms of menopause, prevent osteoporosis and cardiovascular disease.

41. C. The most common site of ectopic pregnancy is fallopian tube. About 97 to 98% of ectopic pregnancies occur at the fallopian tube. The remaining 2 to 3 percent may be abdominal, ovarian or cervical.

42. D. The most significant assessment finding in a patient with ruptured tubal pregnancy is hypovolemic shock due to internal bleeding from the ruptured fallopian tube. External vaginal bleeding is not that obvious, so the manifestation of hypovolemic shock does not correlate with the amount of vaginal bleeding. Severe vaginal bleeding with hypovolemic shock is present with incomplete abortion not in ruptured tubal pregnancy. With tubal rupture the patient will have intense not vague abdominal pain, which may be referred to the shoulder as a result of irritation of the diaphragm by blood released into the abdominal cavity. Irregular vaginal bleeding and syncope are the symptoms of ectopic pregnancy and not ruptured tubal pregnancy.

43. A. Postmenopausal women should follow a regular program of activity and exercise. Regular aerobic exercise and weight bearing exercise improves circulation, maintain muscle tone, delays atherosclerosis and osteoporosis. Calcium intake of at least 1500 mg. daily, maintaining usual sexual activity and avoiding obesity are all important but most important is regular aerobic and weight bearing exercises.

44. B. The symptoms of curdy white, thick vaginal discharge, intense itching of vulva and dysuria is usually associated with monilial vaginitis or vulvovaginal candidiasis. In gonorrhea patient experiences mucopurulent vaginal discharge. Frothy greenish or gray discharge is seen in trichomoniasis and watery discharge with fishy odor is found in gardnerella vaginalis vaginitis.

45. C. Candida is a normal inhabitant of the vagina. When patient receives broad-spectrum antibiotics, protective organisms usually present in the vagina are destroyed and clinical candidiasis may occur. The condition is not associated with anemia but it is associated with diabetes mellitus. Pregnancy, not nulliparity, increases the risk for candidiasis. Oral contraceptives, not spermicidal jelly, increase the risk for candidiasis.

46. B. Trichomonas vaginalis responsible for causing trichomoniasis is a flagellated protozoan. Treatment for this condition includes metronidazole, given in a single loading dose or a smaller dose three times a day for 1 week to both the partners. Fluconazole, an antifungal drug is given in *Candida moniliasis.* Azithromycin and ciprofloxacin are both broad- spectrum antibiotics and is given in bacterial vaginitis, e.g. *Chlamydia, gonorrhea* and *Staphylococcus aureus.*

47. B. The nurse will teach the woman that chlamydial infection in pregnancy may give rise to stillbirth, neonatal death and premature labor. Chlamydia is a sexually transmitted disease and is found in young sexually active people with more than one partner. Untreated chlamydial infection may cause pelvic inflammatory disease but not renal failure. The treatment of choice in pregnant women is erythromycin not tetracycline.

48. C. The condom is considered to be the only contraceptive device that is prophylactic in regard to STDs. Oral contraceptives cause the secretions of the cervix and the vagina to become more alkaline which produces a more favorable environment for the growth of organisms that cause STDs at these sites. Intrauterine devices and norplant implant, a long acting contraceptive confer no protection against STDs.

49. A. Women with gonorrhea are frequently asymptomatic or may have minor symptoms, which are usually overlooked by them. A few women may complain of vaginal discharge, dysuria, frequency of urination, changes in menstruation and redness and swelling at the site of contact, e.g. cervix or urethra. Chancres in the vaginal wall, vesicular lesions on the vulva and macular palmer rash are not associated with gonorrhea.

50. D. Urethral stricture is not a complication of gonorrhea in women, but it is a common complication in men.

The complications associated with gonorrhea in women are pelvic inflammatory disease, Bartholin's abscess, ectopic pregnancy and infertility. Complications associated with gonorrhea in men are prostatitis,urethral stricture, sterility from orchitis or epididymitis.

51. A. In men the symptoms of gonorrhea are obvious and distressing. The early symptoms of gonorrhea are dysuria and purulent, foul-smelling urethral discharge. These symptoms are obvious and distressing and prompt an individual to seek medical care. Sterility is a late complication of gonorrhea. Genital ulcers and multiple warts on penis are not the symptoms of gonorrhea for which an individual seeks medical attention early.

52. C. The typical sign of untreated primary syphilis is painless chancre on the genitalia. The chancres may also appear on vulva, lips, mouth, vagina and rectum. Foul-smelling urethral discharge is seen in gonorrhea. Flu-like symptoms and maculopapular rash on palms of the hands and soles of the feet are seen in secondary stage of syphilis. Unilateral painful swelling of the scrotum is due to chlamydial epididymitis.

53. D. Any of the drug regimen may be used to treat uncomplicated urogenital and anorectal gonococcal infections. Traditionally penicillin was the drug of choice but due to penicillin resistant strains, ceftriaxone, a penicillinase resistant cephalosporin or cefixime, ciprofloxacin, ofloxacin or levofloxacin have become the part of treatment plan.

54. C. A patient with gonorrhea is usually treated with dual antibiotics, e.g. ceftriaxone and azithromycin or doxycycline to treat coexisting chlamydial infection. If chlamydial infection is ruled out, patient may be treated with single dose of ceftriaxone or cefixime or ciprofloxacin. Coexisting syphilis is treated with same drugs used for gonorrhea. Combined antibiotics do not prevent reinfection. Penicillin resistant strains of gonorrhea are successfully treated with cephalosporin and do not require dual coverage if coexisting chlamydial infection is absent.

55. C. Two types of herpes simplex virus, type 1 and type 2 cause genital herpes but majority is due to type 2. Transmission of virus occurs through direct contact with skin or mucous membranes when an infected individual is symptomatic, or through asymptomatic viral shredding. Organism is also transmitted through fomites such as towel used by patient. The virus once entered remains in the individual life long. Symptomatic lesions usually heal spontaneously but recurrence is common. Antiviral medications such as acyclovir or famciclovir only suppress symptoms. Corneal ulcer leading to blindness is a complication of genital herpes.

56. D. Tingling, burning and itching at the site where the lesion will eventually appear are prodromal symptoms of recurrent herpes infection. These symptoms appear 30 minutes to 48 hours before the lesions appear. Headache, fever, regional lymphadenopathy, urinary retention and dysuria are the symptoms of primary infection. These symptoms may also occur with severity during recurrence of infection.

57. A. Stress, fatigue, sunburn and menses are common trigger factors for recurrent infection. So stress reduction may prevent recurrence of infection. Sexual activity should be avoided during outbreaks, and a condom should be used in between outbreaks as the woman can shed the virus although no visible lesion is present. As sunburn is a trigger factor for recurrence, the woman should not expose her to direct sunlight. Since an association has been observed with cervical cancer and herpes simplex virus infection, the woman should have yearly pelvic examination and Pap smear done.

58. D. Patient should be informed that this condition is caused by human papilloma (HPV) virus not a bacteria. The infection is transmitted by sexual contact. The lesion although painless, is not curable as no specific antiviral therapy is available. Visible lesions (infected tissues) are removed by a variety of chemical, mechanical and ablative technique, not the virus. HPV infection is associated with cervical and vulvar cancer in women and squamous cell carcinoma of the penis in men. So patient should be under long term follow up with yearly Pap test.

59. D. Pelvic inflammatory disease is an infectious condition of the pelvic cavity that may involve infection of the fallopian tubes (salpingitis), ovaries (oophoritis) and pelvic peritoneum (peritonitis). It is often the result of untreated cervicitis. The organism infecting the cervix ascends higher into the uterus, fallopian tubes, ovaries and peritoneal cavity.

60. B. Recent abdominal surgery is least likely to cause pelvic inflammatory disease. The organisms causing upper genital tract infections gain entrance most commonly during sexual intercourse, during or after childbirth, termination of pregnancy and during pelvic surgery. Other rare cause of pelvic inflammatory disease is systemic disease, e.g. tuberculosis and ruptured bowel.

61. C. A patient with the diagnosis of pelvic inflammatory disease (PID) is most likely to have a history of multiple sex partners. Because the most common organisms for PID, *Chlamydia trachomatis* and *Neisseria gonorrhea* are frequently found in women having multiple sex partners. Blood transfusion and multiparity are not associated with PID. Pulmonary tuberculosis rarely causes PID by travelling through blood.

62. B. The patient with pelvic inflammatory disease should be encouraged to be in semi Fowler's position in order to promote drainage of pus and other debris produced as a result of infection with *Chlamydia trachomatis, N. gonorrhea* and *Staphylococcal* organisms. Inadequate drainage will cause accumulation of pus in the peritoneal cavity resulting in to pelvic peritonitis or tuboovarian abscess, which is a common complication of PID. Thromboembolism, which is another complication of PID occurs due to thrombophlebitis caused by bacterial infection and not due to inadequate circulation. The position may relieve pain or ease breathing but these are not the important rationals in this situation.

63. C. The term endometriosis refers to the presence of normal endometrial tissue in sites outside the endometrial cavity, e.g. in or near the ovaries, the uterosacral ligaments, uterovesical peritoneum, or stomach, lungs, intestines and spleen. Endometriosis does not refer to inflammation, hypertrophy or metaplasia of endometrial tissue.

64. B. The most common manifestations of endometriosis are secondary dysmenorrhea, infertility, pelvic pain, dyspareunia and irregular bleeding. Dysuria, hematuria, painful bowel movements, rectal bleeding backach are usually less common manifestations of endometriosis.

65. A. Medical management of a patient with endometriosis experiencing distressing symptoms is to inhibit ovarian estrogen production and shrink the endometrial implants by various drugs, e.g. combined oral contraceptives, progestin agents, e.g. depo-provera. Patient is encouraged pregnancy, not avoid pregnancy, provided she has not completed her family. Amenorrhea produced during pregnancy results in shrinking of the endometrial implants. Patient with mild symptoms may be benefited with analgesics, emotional support, and teaching regarding the disease and coping strategies for pain management.

66. C. While planning care for a patient on hormonal therapy for endometriosis, the nurse should include teaching regarding the side effect of hormonal treatment to suppress ovulation. Danazol, a synthetic androgen is used in endometriosis to produce a pseudomenopause by ovarian suppression, which results in atrophy of ectopic endometrial tissue. The side effects of this drug include weight gain, acne, hot flashes and hirsutism. NSAIDs are not given as a long-term measure as they cause increased bleeding tendencies. Synthetic estrogen supplementation is not the modalities of care, rather estrogen production is inhibited by drugs. Similarly drugs (danazol) are used to inhibit anterior pituitary not stimulate anterior pituitary.

67. A. A 40-year-old African woman is at increased risk of developing leiomyomas since these tumors are more common among the African women, incidence being 30 percent. The incidence among the whites is 10 percent. These tumors are frequently seen in women approaching menopause. So, a 45-year-old white woman and 50-year-old Asian woman may also exhibit leiomyoma but risk in a 60-year-old Indian woman is less as these tumors undergo atrophy after menopause.

68. B. Most of the women with leiomyomas are asymptomatic. Of the women who develop symptoms the most common is abnormal uterine bleeding, which may be excessive in either amount or duration. Other manifestations are anemia, tiredness, weakness, lethargy, dysmenorrhea, urinary frequency and retention. Constipation, hydroureter, hydronephrosis, abdominal pain and dyspareunia are less common manifestations. Profuse vaginal discharge is not associated with leiomyomas.

69. C. The recommended medical management of 30-year-old woman with leiomyomas is myomectomy, i.e. removal of the tumor without removal of the uterus, as myomectomy preserves reproductive organ and reproductive capabilities. Hysterectomy is not the preferred method of management for a woman who wishes to have children. Use of NSAIDs or aspirin is discouraged in these patients because of its antiplatelet activity. Hormonal therapy to shrink tumor (GnRH agonist) is also not recommended in this case as hormone therapy results in hypoestrogenic state and amenorrhea, which may prevent pregnancy.

70. B. Dysplasia indicates an abnormal differentiation of dividing cells resulting in changes in the size, shape and appearance of the cells. Cervical dysplasia is a precursor of malignancy. An increase in the number of cells in a tissue is hyperplasia. This is a reversible process when stimulus is removed. A reversible transformation of one cell type in to another is metaplasia and an increase in the size of cells without cell division is hypertrophy.

71. A. The most important nursing action to include in the care plan of patient is observation of the amount and type of vaginal bleeding. The patient with incomplete abortion may have severe bouts of hemorrhage until all products of conception are expelled. The food and fluids per mouth need not be restricted. The patient needs nourishment and plenty of fluids. Emotional support and reassurance should be provided, however, observation of vaginal bleeding is most important. Patient should have limitation of activity, but lying flat in bed is not necessary.

72. C. Infection with human papilloma virus, causative organism of genital warts (condylomata acuminata) has been linked with cervical and vulvar cancer in women. Other risk factors associated with this disease are low socioeconomic status, early sexual activity, multiple sex partners, STDs, untreated chronic cervicitis, having a sexual partner with a history of penile or prostate cancer and smoking. Recurrent candidiasis, pregnancy before age 20 years and long history of oral contraceptives are not associated with increased incidence of cervical cancer.

73. D. Multiple sex partners and early age of first intercourse are important risk factors of cervical cancer. A high fat diet, menarche at age 12 years and occupational exposures to aromatic dye are not identified as risk factors for cervical cancer.

74. D. American Cancer Society recommends annual Pap test beginning with the onset of sexual activity. After 3 consecutive negative test results less frequent tests may be recommended by the health care provider.

75. B. There is no early manifestation of carcinoma *in situ* or early cervical cancer. Early cervical cancer is asymptomatic. Manifestations eventually occur with leukorrhea and vaginal bleeding. Initially discharge is thin, watery but becomes dark and foul smelling as the disease advances. Vaginal bleeding is initially usually spotting but becomes heavier and more frequent with enlargement of the tumor. Aching abdominal pain is a late symptom. Other late symptoms are weight loss, anemia and cachexia.

76. D. Pelvic exenteration, which involves hysterectomy and removal of all adjacent pelvic organs and structures does not preserve fertility. Conization, loop electrocautery excision procedure and laser therapy carried out for noninvasive cancer preserve fertility as only a small section of the cervical tissue is removed or destroyed.

77. D. Straining at stool and bowel movement could dislodge the applicator and the radiation source. So the patient is given an enema before the procedure to empty the bowel and a low residue diet during the procedure to prevent bowel movement. Feces in the bowel during radiation do not cause fecal impaction or contamination of the vagina. Applicators are placed under anesthesia in operating room. Preventing dislodgement of the applicator is the priority.

78. D. Bowel movement during treatment may dislodge the implant, so the patient is given low residue diet to prevent bowel movement. As a systemic reaction to the radiation patient may develop diarrhea. To prevent diarrhea antidiarrheal medication is administered. During treatment the patient should be on strict bed rest. Movement is restricted except deep breathing and leg exercises. A Foley's catheter is inserted for drainage of bladder. Visitors are restricted. She will be placed on bed in flat position. The head of the bed may be elevated to 20° only, as high, Fowler's position may cause the implant to move from its desired position.

79. B. To prevent deep vein thrombosis after hysterectomy the nurse should not place the patient in high Fowler's position. High Fowler's position cause stasis and pooling of blood promoting deep vein thrombosis. To prevent deep vein thrombosis the nurse should encourage change of positions, leg exercises, use of elastic stockings and avoiding use of pillow under the knees.

80. D. After hysterectomy the patient should avoid activities that may cause pelvic congestion, e.g. dancing, walking swiftly. All other statements, e.g. avoiding heavy lifting for 2 months, avoiding sexual activity for 4-6 weeks and swimming indicate adequate teaching.

81. D. A small percentages of patients with breast cancer exhibit unilateral nipple discharge, which may be clear or bloody. Other symptoms of breast cancer are hard, nonmobile, nontender, irregularly shaped lump, nipple retraction, and orange peel appearance of skin over breast, induration, infiltration and dimpling of the overlying skin. Breast enlargement, breast tenderness and darkening of nipple are not associated with breast cancer.

82. C. Breast conservation surgery also called lumpectomy involves removal of the entire tumor along with a margin of normal tissue. The entire tumor along with a margin of normal tissue is removed not only a portion, or only the whole tumor. Underarm lymph nodes are removed in axillary node dissection, which may or may not accompany lumpectomy.

83. C. A modified radical mastectomy involves removal of all breast tissue and axillary node dissection. Lymphedema occurs when remaining lymph channels do not adequately return flow of lymph to the circulation. Pneumonitis and rib fractures are mostly associated with irradiation to the breast. Compartment syndrome is not the complication of modified radical mastectomy.

84. A. Patient's affected arm should not be immobilized with a splint to prevent postoperative lymphedema as immobilization causes stasis of venous blood and lymph promoting venous thrombosis and lymphedema. Patient's affected extremity should be elevated to promote venous and lymphatic drainage. She should be instructed to squeeze a rubber ball to help promote circulation. Blood pressure cuff should not be applied on the arm of the affected side but on the opposite side to prevent lymphedema.

85. A. Breast self-examination involves both inspection of breasts before a mirror and a careful, systematic palpation of the breast tissue. Palpation of axillary lymph nodes, cervical lymph nodes and observing nipple discharge are the components of systematic palpation.

86. B. Breast self-examination should be done monthly at a regular time when the breasts are not tender. In premenopausal women the best time is 7 days after the start of menstruation. At this time hormonal stimulation of the breasts is at its lowest point and nodularity and tenderness will be minimum. If the women are on oral contraceptive they may perform the examination on the first day of opening a new package. But here there is no indication that the women are on oral contraceptive. Postmenopausal women or women with hysterectomies should perform the examination on a regular date, e.g. on the birthdate of each month.

87. D. The nurse, who is planning to teach breast self-examination (BSE) to a group of young women should include an opportunity to perform a return demonstration by all women of the group with individual guidance from the nurse. Lecture emphasizing the value of early detection of breast cancer, showing film on technique of BSE and live demonstration of BSE all are important but best learning and compliance may only be achieved by return demonstration with individual guidance by the nurse.

88. B. Fibrocystic changes in the breast is a benign condition characterized by development of excess fibrous tissue, hyperplasia of the epithelial lining of the mammary ducts, proliferation of mammary ducts and cyst formation. The cysts usually do not turn into cancer. So the teaching, that any lump in breast must be biopsied to rule out cancer is not appropriate. Biopsy in fibrocystic breast disease is indicated when the woman is a high-risk of breast cancer. All other teachings are appropriate.

89. A. Woman above 60 years is at greatest risk of developing breast cancer. Increasing age increases the risk of developing breast cancer.

After age 60 the incidence of breast cancer increases dramatically. Positive family history is an important risk factor, particularly when the affected woman was premenopausal and first degree relative. Risk of development of breast cancer using oral contraceptives and estrogen replacement therapy is controversial. Dietary fat intake is often related with breast cancer and is under study, but increasing age of a woman is at greatest risk.

90. B. The most important prognostic indicator in early stage breast cancer is the status of lymph node involvement. Absence of lymph node involvement indicates favorable prognosis and less chances of recurrence. Other prognostic indicators are the tumor size, estrogen and progesterone receptor status, DNA content analysis, cell proliferative indices and genetic marker HER-2/neu or c-erb-B2 status. A tumor size above 5 cm, estrogen-progesterone negative tumor indicate poor prognosis. Over expression of c-erb-B2 genetic marker also indicates poorer prognosis in breast cancer.

91. D. The nurse should inform the patient about the advantages, disadvantages and outcome of both the procedures. The most important factor in choosing the treatment options is the outcome of the procedure. The overall survival rate with lumpectomy and radiation is about the same as that with modified radical mastectomy. Lumpectomy with radiation involves a prolonged treatment course and not short treatment course. The treatment is costly as it involves both surgery and radiation. The procedure preserves breast but it changes the texture and sensitivity of the breast. The procedure may result in complications, e.g. lymphedema, impaired arm mobility as that of modified radical mastectomy. In addition patient is also at risk of complications associated with radiation therapy.

92. B. The patient after modified radical mastectomy is at risk of developing lymphedema for the rest of her life. The patient must be taught to protect her arm on the operated side from trauma- e.g. blood pressure readings, venipunctures, injections, pinprick and sunburn. Use of elastic bandages in the early postoperative period must be avoided as they inhibit collateral lymph drainage. Patient must perform regular arm exercises but lifting weight by the affected arm must be avoided.

93. C. The nursing diagnosis that should take priority when caring for a patient undergoing chemotherapy is fatigue. Chemotherapeutic agents cause bone marrow suppression giving rise to erythrocytopenia, leucopenia and thrombocytopenia. Erythrocytopenia or a reduction in red blood cell numbers may cause fatigue. Disturbed body image due to alopecia related to chemotherapy and altered sexuality pattern due to breast cancer and modified radical mastectomy are important nursing diagnoses but they would not take priority over fatigue. Impaired physical mobility is not usually associated with chemotherapy. It may be associated with pain due to modified radical mastectomy in the early postoperative period.

8 CHAPTER

Hematological System, Oncology and Immunology

Q1. The nurse is reviewing a laboratory report of complete blood count of a female patient. Which of the following she should recognize as an abnormal finding?

A. Red blood cell counts – 5 million/ cubic millimeter

B. White blood cell counts – 12,000/cubic millimeter

C. Platelets - 250,000/ cubic millimeter

D. Hematocrit - 45%

Q2. What diagnostic test for hematologic disorder measures the size of erythrocytes and the hemoglobin content?

A. Red blood cell counts

B. Hemoglobin level

C. Hematocrit level

D. Red blood cell indices

Q3. Which of the following blood components is deficient in anemia?

A. Erythrocytes

B. Hemoglobin

C. Hematocrit

D. All of the above

Q4. The underlying cause of all manifestations accompanying anemia is due to a tissue deficiency of which of the following substances?

A. Oxygen

B. Carbon dioxide

C. Hemoglobin

D. Iron

Q5. All of the following conditions can cause anemia *except*:

A. Gastritis

B. Cobalamine deficiency

C. G6PD deficiency

D. Herpes simplex infection

Q6. A patient with long-standing severe anemia is likely to exhibit which of the following symptoms?

A. Exertional dyspnea

B. Congestive heart failure

C. Pulmonary fibrosis

D. Arrhythmias

Q7. During assessment of a patient with microcytic hypochromic anemia the nurse would question the patient about:

A. Dietary intake of iron

B. A history of gastric surgery

C. A history of acute blood loss
D. A history of sickle cell anemia

Q8. A patient who is on ferrous sulfate for iron deficiency anemia takes antacid frequently for heartburn. The nurse is providing instructions regarding timing of administration of these two drugs. Which of the following instructions is appropriate?

A. Take ferrous sulfate and antacid together
B. Take ferrous sulfate followed by antacid at least after 1 hour
C. Take ferrous sulfate followed by antacid after 2 hours
D. Avoid taking antacid

Q9. Which of the following signs and symptoms are expected in a patient with iron deficiency anemia?

A. Itching, jaundice and fatigue
B. Fever, petechiae, and fatigue
C. Nausea, vomiting and anorexia
D. Pallor, tachycardia and dyspnea

Q10. Which of the following iron rich foods should the nurse encourage a patient with iron deficiency anemia requiring iron therapy to eat?

A. Milk and spinach
B. Liver and dry beans
C. Chicken and banana
D. Milk and apple

Q11. A patient with anemia is admitted in hospital. The laboratory results reveal hemoglobin of 5.8 g/dL. The nurse anticipates that the patient will be treated with:

A. Parenteral iron replacement therapy
B. Albumin intravenously
C. Packed red blood cells transfusion
D. Oral iron replacement therapy

Q12. A patient with severe anemia related to chronic kidney disease is admitted in the hospital. Which of the following nursing actions is appropriate?

A. Monitoring fluid intake and urine output
B. Instructing patient a high- iron diet
C. Monitoring urine for hematuria
D. Administering epoietin as prescribed

Q13. The nurse is assessing a patient with sickle cell anemia. During assessment she is expected to find all of the following manifestations *except*:

A. Paleness of hands and feet
B. Tachycardia and cardiomegaly
C. Petechia on abdomen and thigh
D. Bone pain

Q14. What is the only known cure for sickle cell anemia?

A. Bone marrow transplantation
B. Splenectomy
C. Exchange blood transfusion
D. Administration of hydroxyurea

Q15. Which of the following type of anemia is caused by the failure to absorb vitamin B_{12}?

A. Sickle cell
B. Microcytic hypochromic
C. Normocytic normochromic
D. Macrocytic normochromic

Q16. The nurse is assessing a patient with pernicious anemia. What sign and symptoms she is expected to find?

A. Pallor; sore, smooth and red tongue; paresthesias of the hands and feet
B. Pallor, bradycardia and decreased pulse pressure
C. Sore tongue, dyspnea and weight gain
D. Jaundice, anorexia and double vision

Q17. The nurse is teaching a patient with pernicious anemia regarding vitamin B_{12} therapy. Which of the following statement by the patient indicates effective teaching?

- **A.** 'I will require vitamin B_{12} therapy until sign and symptoms disappear'
- **B.** 'I need to take vitamin B_{12} supplementation for the next 6 months to 1 year'
- **C.** 'I will need to take tablet vitamin B_{12} for the rest of my life'
- **D.** 'I will require parenteral vitamin B_{12} therapy for the rest of my life'

Q18. The nurse is teaching a patient with pernicious anemia regarding vitamin B_{12} therapy. Which of the following regimen is the most usual dosage schedule for a patient with severe symptoms?

- **A.** Deep intramuscular injection of vitamin B_{12} 100 microgram each month
- **B.** Deep intramuscular injection of vitamin B_{12} 100 microgram every 3 months
- **C.** Deep intramuscular injection of vitamin B_{12} 100 microgram daily for 15 days followed by every 3 months
- **D.** Deep intramuscular injection of vitamin B_{12} 100 microgram daily for 2 weeks followed by weekly for several weeks and then monthly for life

Q19. The nurse is assessing a patient with polycythemia vera. During assessment, which of the following signs and symptoms she is expected to find?

- **A.** Hypertension, pruritus, thrombophlebitis, splenomegaly
- **B.** Hypotension, bradycardia, feeling of fullness, anginal pain
- **C.** Pallor, visual disturbances, vertigo, crepitation
- **D.** Fatigue, dyspnea, bone pain, splenomegaly, hypertension

Q20. The most frequent complication arising from hyperviscosity of polycythemia vera is:

- **A.** Thrombosis
- **B.** Cardiomyopathy
- **C.** Pulmonary fibrosis
- **D.** Leukemia

Q21. The nurse understands that the patient admitted with polycythemia vera would be treated by:

- **A.** Restriction of fluid to control hypervolemia
- **B.** Phlebotomy to reduce blood volume
- **C.** Iron supplementation to treat iron deficiency caused by therapeutic intervention
- **D.** Antiplatelet drugs to prevent thrombosis

Q22. Which of the following nursing interventions is not appropriate for a patient admitted with polycythemia vera?

- **A.** Teaching a patient about the side effects of myelosuppressive drugs
- **B.** Monitoring for fluid balance during hydration therapy
- **C.** Providing strict bed rest
- **D.** Encouraging patient to take adequate food intake

Q23. What is the life span of normal platelets?

- **A.** 1–3 days
- **B.** 3–6 days
- **C.** 8–10 days
- **D.** 8–10 weeks

Q24. A patient with immune thrombocytopenic purpura is admitted in the ward. Being aware of the potential risk of spontaneous intracranial hemorrhage the nurse monitors the patient's platelet count. Which of the following platelet counts predisposes a patient to intracranial bleeding?

- **A.** Below 20,000/cubic millimeter
- **B.** Below 50,000/cubic millimeter

C. Below 75,000/cubic millimeter
D. Below 1,50,000/cubic millimeter

Q25. The platelet count of a patient with mitral valve replacement surgery came down to 50,000/ cubic millimeter from 200,000/cubic millimeter on the third postoperative day. Which of the following conditions is suspected?

A. Immune thrombocytopenic purpura (ITP)
B. Thrombotic thrombocytopenic purpura (TTP)
C. Heparin-induced thrombocytopenia and thrombosis syndrome (HITTS)
D. Disseminated intravascular coagulation (DIC)

Q26. Which of the following signs and symptoms a patient with thrombocytopenia may exhibit?

A. Fatigue, weakness and dyspnea
B. Tachycardia, hypotension and fainting
C. Nausea, vomiting and dizziness
D. Epistaxis, gingival bleeding and petechiae

Q27. Concerned about the consequences of injury to a patient with thrombocytopenia, the nurse plans care to protect the patient from injury. Which of the following nursing actions is the best way to protect the patient from injury?

A. Restricting family members with upper respiratory infections
B. Teaching a patient deep breathing and coughing exercises
C. Practicing meticulous handwashing before caring for the patient
D. Avoiding intramuscular or subcutaneous injection

Q28. The nurse is preparing a patient with immune thrombocytopenic purpura for discharge. Which of the following statements by the patient indicates the need for further teaching?

A. 'I need to use a soft bristle tooth brush for brushing my teeth and an electric razor for shaving'
B. 'I need to take stool softeners daily and avoid Valsalva's maneuver'
C. 'I need to attend hospital monthly for platelet transfusion to keep my platelet count at normal limits'
D. 'I need to avoid aspirin and aspirin containing medications'

Q29. Which of the following drugs is used to manage the patient with immune thrombocytopenic purpura by improving platelet count?

A. Hydroxyurea
B. Corticosteroids
C. Vitamin K
D. Clopidogrel

Q30. A pregnant woman diagnosed with abruptio placenta is admitted in the hospital. Which of the following blood dyscrasias may occur to the patient?

A. Pancytopenia
B. Immune thrombocytopenic purpura
C. Heparin-induced thrombocytopenia and thrombosis syndrome
D. Disseminated intravascular coagulation

Q31. Which of the following statements accurately describes disseminated intravascular coagulation (DIC)?

A. DIC is a genetic disorder caused by defective or deficient coagulation factor that leads to abnormally initiated clotting in the vasculature
B. DIC is an acquired disorder where an underlying disease stimulates overproduction of clotting factors resulting in diffused thrombosis of the vasculature
C. DIC is a disorder in which an underlying disease initiates abnormally accelerated clotting resulting in depletion of clotting factors and ultimately lead to diffused hemorrhage
D. DIC is a syndrome where an underlying disease inhibits release of hemolytic factors leading to diffused microcoagulation and infarcts in the microvasculature

Q32. The nurse is taking care of a patient with crush trauma. Concerned about the development of disseminated intravascular clotting the nurse should monitor which of the following assessment parameters?

A. Blood count, bleeding time and clotting time
B. Platelet counts, prothrombin time and partial thromboplastin time
C. Platelet counts, Vitamin K level and fibrinogen level
D. Thrombin time, bleeding time and blood count

Q33. The nurse is caring for a patient with suspected diagnosis of disseminated intrvascular coagulation from metastatic cancer. To which nursing diagnosis should the nurse give highest priority?

A. Acute pain related to bleeding into tissues and disease process
B. Ineffective tissue perfusion (cerebral, cardiopulmonary, renal, gastrointestinal and peripheral) related to bleeding and sluggish blood flow secondary to thrombosis
C. Anxiety related to fear of unknown, disease process, diagnostic procedures and therapy
D. Activity intolerance related to weakness and malaise secondary to tissue hypoxia

Q34. A patient receiving chemotherapy for cancer develops marked granulocytopenia. Appropriate nursing intervention for this patient would be:

A. Meticulous handwashing and frequent temperature assessment
B. Inserting an indwelling catheter and monitoring hourly urine output
C. Monitoring lung sounds and administering packed cells as ordered
D. Relieving anxiety and encouraging visits from family members and friends

Q35. Acute leukemia is caused by:

A. Rapid growth of mature leukocytes
B. Block in the differentiation of cells in the hematopoietic cell line
C. Proliferation of increasing number of blasts in the bone marrow and blood
D. Unregulated proliferation of hematopoietic cells or disordered cell death

Q36. Which of the following types of leukemia is most common among the older adults in the United States and Europe but rarely seen in Asia?

A. Acute myelogenous leukemia
B. Acute lymphocytic leukemia
C. Chronic lymphocytic leukemia
D. Hairy cell leukemia

Q37. Multiple drugs are primarily used in combination to treat leukemia and lymphoma because:

A. There is decrease in drug resistance
B. Use of multiple drugs with varying toxicities minimize drug toxicity to the patient
C. They can interrupt cell growth at multiple points in the cell cycle
D. All of the above reasons are correct

Q38. A patient with leukemia on chemotherapy has developed neutropenia. Which of the following assessment the nurse should regularly perform?

A. Respiratory rate and breath sounds
B. Pulse rate and heart sounds
C. Abdominal pain and bowel sounds
D. Urine output and blood pressure

Q39. The risk factors associated with leukemia include all of the following *except*:

A. Genetics
B. Exposure to ionizing radiation and chemicals
C. Dietary factors
D. Congenital abnormalities

Q40. The goal of treatment in leukemia is complete remission with restoration of normal bone marrow function. This is achieved by:

A. Bone marrow transplantation
B. Radiation
C. Chemotherapy
D. Stem cell transplantation

Q41. The nurse is aware that the major difference between Hodgkin's disease (HD) and non-Hodgkin's lymphoma (NHL) is that:

A. Hodgkin's disease frequently originates outside the lymph nodes
B. Non-Hodgkin's lymphomas are less common and potentially curable
C. Biopsy specimen in Hodgkin's disease shows Reed-Sternberg cells
D. Non-Hodgkin's lymphomas are treated only with chemotherapy

Q42. Which of the following symptoms is most commonly an early indication of Hodgkin's disease?

A. Fatigue, weight loss, night sweats and recurrent pruritus
B. Fever, hypotension, bone pain, and jaundice
C. Anemia, hepatosplenomegaly, alcohol-induced pain
D. Dyspnea, cyanosis, dysphagia and hypothermia

Q43. Majority of the patients with stage I and stage II Hodgkin's disease are cured with:

A. Combination chemotherapy
B. Radiation therapy alone
C. Radiation therapy followed by chemotherapy
D. Surgical excision of the involved lymph glands

Q44. A 28-year-old patient with Hodgkin's disease has developed pancytopenia after being treated with combined chemotherapy and radiation therapy. Which of the following actions is appropriate and should be taken first when the nurse detects a temperature of 100.4°F in this patient?

A. Doing nothing as low-grade fever is a common manifestation of this disease
B. Administering aspirin to the patient
C. Informing the physician
D. Preparing patient to take cultures

Q45. Which of the following individuals is most at risk for developing multiple myeloma?

A. A 15-year-old white student
B. A 30-year-old Asian housewife
C. A 40-year-old nurse practitioner
D. A 60-year-old black farmer

Q46. The major manifestation of multiple myeloma is:

A. Enlargement of inguinal lymph nodes
B. Fever
C. Skeletal pain
D. Paraplegia

Q47. Which of the following diagnostic findings determines diagnosis of multiple myeloma?

A. X-ray showing distinct lytic areas of bone erosion
B. Bone marrow analysis showing significantly increased number of plasma cells in the bone marrow
C. Laboratory test detecting presence of a monoclonal antibody protein in blood and urine
D. All of the above

Q48. A patient with multiple myeloma has been admitted in hospital with the complaints of anorexia, nausea, drowsiness, confusion and disorientation. The nurse reviewing the laboratory reports anticipates evidence of which of the following conditions?

A. Hyperuricemia

B. Hypercalcemia
C. Hyperkalemia
D. Hypermagnesemia

Q49. A patient aged 55 years has been newly diagnosed with multiple myeloma. The nurse understands that the patient will be treated with:

A. Radiotherapy
B. Surgical excision of the bony lesion
C. Combination chemotherapy
D. Alpha Interferon

Q50. The nurse is teaching a patient with multiple myeloma regarding self-care. Which of the following instructions she should emphasize?

A. Maintain strict bed rest
B. Restrict fluid
C. Perform weight-bearing exercises
D. Keep lower extremity elevated while resting

Q51. Which of the following blood types is the most common?

A. A
B. B
C. AB
D. O

Q52. A patient has to receive a blood transfusion. Which of the following the nurse should keep in mind before the blood is transfused?

A. Verify the labels of the blood bottle carefully and check patient's own record and prescription with another nurse
B. Make sure that Ringer's lactate solution is administered before blood transfusion
C. Administer an antibiotic
D. Reassure the patient that the procedure is very simple and free from any untoward hazards

Q53. A patient who is receiving a blood transfusion develops acute hemolytic reaction. Which of the following interventions she should adopt?

A. Slow the transfusion, administer antihistamine, and inform physician
B. Immediately stop the transfusion, infuse 5% dextrose, and inform physician and blood bank
C. Immediately stop the transfusion, maintain a patent IV line with normal saline, and notify blood bank and physician
D. Stop the transfusion, administer 5% dextrose infusion, save blood bottle and tubing, inform physician

Q54. The nurse is encouraging a patient waiting for surgery about autologous transfusion to eliminate disease transmission and transfusion complications. The patient asks the nurse about how often he should donate blood. Which of the following responses by the nurse is appropriate?

A. 'Every 3 days if your hemoglobin remains at or above 11 g/dL'
B. 'Once every week if your hemoglobin level is 10 g/dL'
C. 'Once every 2 weeks if your hemoglobin level is 10 g/dL'
D. 'Once every month if your hemoglobin level is 11 g/dL'

Q55. The term cancer is used for a large group of diseases characterized by:

A. Rapid proliferation of cells
B. Production of toxins that alter cell morphology
C. Increasing differentiation of cells
D. Cell growth and proliferation that evades normal control and regulatory mechanisms

Q56. The major difference between a benign and malignant neoplasm is the:

A. Rate of cell growth and proliferation
B. Degree of differentiation
C. Ability to invade and metastasize
D. Ability to liberate toxins

Q57. Which of the following is not considered as carcinogen?

A. Tobacco
B. Ultraviolet rays

C. Viruses
D. Genes

Q58. Which of the following cancers is associated with ultraviolet radiation secondary to sunlight exposure?

A. Multiple myeloma
B. Melanoma
C. Leukemia
D. Non-Hodgkin's lymphoma

Q59. Which of the following neoplasms is benign?

A. Endothelioma
B. Lymphoma
C. Leiomyoma
D. Rhabdomyosarcoma

Q60. All of the following are benign neoplasm *except*:

A. Chondroma
B. Hemangioma
C. Glioma
D. Glioblastoma

Q61. Malignant tumor that arises in the bone marrow is a:

A. Multiple myeloma
B. Lymphosarcoma
C. Basal cell carcinoma
D. Hemangiosarcoma

Q62. During cellular reproduction DNA and protein of new chromosomes are synthesized in the:

A. G_1 phase
B. G_2 phase
C. S phase
D. M phase

Q63. Nurses' role in prevention and early detection of cancers include:

A. Instructing people to learn and practice self-examination
B. Instructing people to eat a low fiber and low fat diet
C. Teaching people to undergo annual screening test for all common cancers
D. Make use of peoples' natural fear of cancer and motivate them to eliminate or reduce exposure to carcinogens

Q64. The nurse is teaching a group of young women regarding the schedule of breast self-examination. Which of the following schedule is best for these women?

A. On the first day of the monthly period
B. On the last day of the menstrual period
C. Every day during shower
D. Seven days after menstrual flow

Q65. Mortality due to breast cancer could be reduced through early detection using screening mammography. According to American Cancer Society guidelines screening mammography should be done:

A. For all women every 3 years
B. For women above the age of 50 years every 2 years
C. For women above the age of 40 years annually
D. For women above the age of 40 years every 3 years

Q66. The nurse is teaching a group of young men regarding testicular self-examination. During teaching, which of the following statements made by her is appropriate?

A. Testicular cancer is very common in middle aged people
B. Testicular cancer is a very common type of cancer found in men
C. Testicular cancer is very difficult to treat
D. Testicular cancer is highly curable if detected early

Q67. The nurse is teaching a group of young men regarding risk factors of various cancers. Which of the following conditions if reported by a young man of 23 years would indicate high-risk for testicular cancers?

A. Measles

B. Crypto-orchidism
C. Hydrocele
D. Early onset of puberty

Q68. A young man of 35 years with family history of prostate cancer asks the nurse about ways to detect the disease early if at all occurs to him. Which of the following instructions by the nurse is appropriate?

A. 'Watch for urinary symptoms which occurs at an early stage of disease
B. "From the age of 40 years begin receiving a digital rectal examination as well as a blood test for prostate specific antigen (PSA)"
C. "Begin receiving a digital rectal examination from the age of 50 years"
D. "Test your blood for prostate specific antigen (PSA) now and every year onward"

Q69. Which of the following risk factors is associated with cervical cancer?

A. Increased age
B. Obesity
C. Early sexual activity
D. Family history of cervical cancer

Q70. A nurse is teaching a young woman regarding Pap (Papanicolaou's) test. Which of the following statements is appropriate?

A. All sexually active women should have Pap test done every 3 years
B. Women after the age of 40 years should have annual Pap test done
C. Pap test detects cancer as well as precancerous changes
D. Pap test results are 100% accurate

Q71. Which of the following biopsy method is used to obtain tissue from a small tumor of size 2 to 3 centimeter for diagnosis?

A. Excisional
B. Incisional
C. Subtotal
D. Fine needle aspiration

Q72. Which of the following statements regarding cancer treatment is appropriate?

A. Surgery is the single most effective treatment for cancer in early stage
B. Cancer treatment always aims at cure of cancer
C. A combination of treatment modalities are effective in the control of many cancers.
D. Cancer cure is rare, but treatment modalities improves quality of life for some time

Q73. In which of the following types of internal radiation therapy the radioactive material is administered systemically, e.g. by injection or orally?

A. Sealed source radiation therapy
B. Unsealed source radiation therapy
C. Intracavitary radiation therapy
D. Interstitial therapy

Q74. The nurse is caring for a patient with radioactive implants. She is aware that in order to protect herself from excessive radiation exposure she has to:

A. Maintain distance from the patient
B. Limit duration of time in direct care of the patient
C. Use a lead shield during direct care of the patient
D. All of the above are correct

Q75. The nurse explains to a patient scheduled for brachytherapy for treatment of cancer cervix. Which of the following statements is appropriate?

A. "You have to undergo simulation before the actual treatment"
B. "You have to stay in a private room where radiation precautions will be observed"
C. "You may experience skin changes on the abdomen or upper part of the thigh"
D. "You will remain radioactive for about a week after the treatment"

Q76. The nurse is teaching a patient before brachytherapy for treatment of cancer cervix. Which of the following statements by the patient indicates the need for further teaching?

A. "One of my family members may visit for short periods"

B. "I will need to ambulate daily"

C. "I will have a catheter in my bladder"

D. "I will need to take a low residue diet during the course of treatment"

Q77. A patient who is receiving internal radiotherapy with an intracavitary cesium insertion for uterine cancer discovers the implant accidentally comes out from its original position. What the nurse should do first?

A. Leave the room immediately and inform radiotherapy department

B. Cover the implant with heavy blanket and inform the radiotherapy department

C. Replace it in proper position and instructs the patient to restrict movement further

D. Using a long handled forceps pick up the implant and place it in a lead-lined container and inform the physician

Q78. The treatment effects and side effects of radiotherapy depend on which of the following factors?

A. The size of the treatment field

B. The total dose of radiation

C. The tumor location in relation to surrounding normal tissue

D. All of the above

Q79. The nurse is teaching skin care to a patient scheduled for radiation therapy. Which of the following instructions is appropriate?

A. Cover the irradiated area always with tight gauze dressing

B. If dryness apply a moisturizer without rubbing

C. Gently rinse the area with normal saline daily

D. Clean the area with a mild soap if needed

Q80. A patient who is receiving external radiation therapy for oral cancer has developed stomatitis. Which of the following instructions would be most helpful?

A. Gargle with a mouthwash and rinse thoroughly after each meal

B. Brush after each meal and rinse with saline

C. Drink a lot of ice-cold fluids and citrus juices

D. Discontinue use of brush and clean with finger after each meal

Q81. Treatment of cancers with chemotherapeutic drugs is a systemic intervention when:

A. The disease is wide spread

B. The risk of undetectable cancer is high

C. The tumor cannot be resected and is radiosensitive

D. All of the above

Q82. Which of the following parameters determines the doses of chemotherapeutic drugs?

A. Age of the patient

B. Sex of the patient

C. Body surface area in square meter

D. Body mass index

Q83. Which of the following routes is most commonly used for administration of chemotherapeutic drugs?

A. Oral

B. Intramuscular

C. Intravenous

D. Intra arterial

Q84. Chemotherapeutic drugs that are vesicants can be most effectively administered by:

A. Oral route

B. Intravenous route
C. Infusion pump
D. Central venous access device

Q85. Which of the followings is the most common side effect of chemotherapy?

A. Anorexia
B. Nausea and vomiting
C. Stomatitis
D. Constipation

Q86. The nurse is aware that when chemotherapeutic drugs are used in combination:

A. Drugs with different mechanism of action are used
B. Drugs that have different toxic side effects are used
C. Drugs that cause nadirs (lowest level of the peripheral blood cell counts that occur secondary to bone marrow depression) occurring at different time intervals are used
D. All of the above principles are followed

Q87. Which of the following nursing actions will best help the patient cope with chemotherapy?

A. Not tell the patient about the possible side effects of the drug administered
B. Tell only about the positive effects of the drugs
C. Give accurate information regarding the possible side effects of the drugs that may be experienced in advance
D. Tell the patient not to worry about chemotherapy since it is not his concern at all

Q88. When the patient is complaining about chemotherapy related alopecia, the nurse will:

A. Reassure the patient that hair loss is temporary and hair will grow again soon after chemotherapy is discontinued
B. Advise patient to shampoo hair frequently and comb hair at least 4 times a day
C. Advise patient to apply oil and massage scalp
D. Inform patient that hair loss is permanent and patient should use wigs

Q89. A patient with breast cancer has been prescribed cyclophosphamide, methotrexate, fluorouracil protocol. The nurse administering the drugs is aware that the patient is at risk of developing:

A. Cardiomyopathy
B. Hemorrhagic cystitis
C. Photosensitivity
D. Jaundice

Q90. A 35-year-old patient with leukemia is undergoing chemotherapy. The nurse should give priority to which of the following nursing diagnoses?

A. Risk for infection
B. Altered sexuality pattern
C. Body image disturbance
D. Impaired physical mobility

Q91. A 45-year-old patient is getting doxorubicine (adriamycin) as a part of chemotherapy regimen. Being aware that this drug may cause life threatening toxic effect the nurse monitors:

A. Pulse rate and blood pressure
B. Complete blood count
C. Lung sound
D. Serum bilirubin

Q92. The nurse is teaching a patient with breast cancer who is administered epirubicin regarding its adverse effects. Which of the following adverse effects is not related with this drug?

A. Alopecia
B. Constipation
C. Dysrhythmia
D. Infusion reactions

Q93. A patient with metastatic bone cancer is receiving continuous IV morphine for intractable pain. Which nursing assessment is appropriate?

A. Cardiac rhythm and rate
B. Rate and depth of respiration
C. Development of dependence
D. Diarrhea and dehydration

Q94. A patient with terminal lung cancer has been prescribed continuous morphine drip. Which of the following assessment findings suggests that the patient is experiencing an adverse effect of this drug?

A. The patient is awake and alert and requires minimum maintenance doses of medication for pain
B. The patient's urinary output is 350 mL/12 hour
C. Patient has not had a bowel movement for 5 days
D. Patient has an irregular heart rate of 80 beats/minute

Q95. A patient in terminal stage of lung cancer tells the nurse that if he had been given one more chance to live he would have given up smoking. Which of the following stages of grief does the person express?

A. Denial
B. Bargaining
C. Anger
D. Depression

Q96. A patient is prescribed cyclophosphamide tablets (endoxan) to be taken at home. Which of the following statements by the patient indicates patient has understood the instruction regarding self-care related to this drug?

A. "I need to report burning sensation in my hands and feet"
B. "I shall take the drug 1 hour after meals"
C. "I shall keep the extra drug in the refrigerator"
D. "I shall monitor my fluid intake and output and take lot of fluids"

Q97. In caring for a patient with cancer, which of the following psychological aspect the nurse should give priority?

A. Providing emotional support to the patient
B. Providing emotional support to the family
C. Promoting a positive self esteem
D. Helping patient cope with the consequences of the disease throughout the period of illness

Q98. Which of the following organs is part of the immune system?

A. Adrenal gland and kidneys
B. Thymus gland and bone marrow
C. Liver and spleen
D. Pharynx and tonsils

Q99. Which of the following statements best explains the role of thymus gland in immune system?

A. Thymus gland protects the body by filtering harmful pathogen from blood
B. Thymus gland is a reservoir for blood
C. Thymus gland functions in the differentiation and maturation of T lymphocytes
D. Thymus gland plays part in the differentiation and maturation of B lymphocytes

Q100. T lymphocytes are essential for which of the following types of immune response?

A. Humoral immune response
B. Antibody mediated immune response
C. Immune complex reactions
D. Cell mediated immune response

Q101. Which of the following is one of the functions of cell mediated immunity?

A. Production of antibody
B. Formation of antigen antibody complexes

C. Destruction of cancer cells
D. None of the above

Q102. Which of the following immunoglobulins are transmitted to the infants from mother's breast milk and colostrum and produces passive immunity?

A. IgG **B.** IgM
C. IgA **D.** IgE

Q103. Which of the following antibodies are produced in an allergic disorder?

A. IgA
B. IgE
C. IgM
D. IgD

Q104. The initial symptoms of a possible anaphylactic shock in a hypersensitive person after a intramuscular injection of penicillin would be:

A. A wheal and flare reaction at the injection site
B. Edema and itching at the injection site
C. Sneezing and chest tightness
D. Tachycardia and hypotension

Q105. After receiving a dose of penicillin, a client develops dyspnea and hypotension. The nurse suspects the client is experiencing anaphylactic shock. What should the nurse do first?

A. Call an anesthesiologist and prepare for intubation.
B. Administer IV fluid as ordered and continue to monitor patient's vital signs
C. Administer epinephrine as ordered and prepare for intubation if necessary
D. Insert an indwelling catheter and monitor urine output every hour.

Q106. Which of the following agents most commonly causes anaphylaxis?

A. Drugs
B. Foods
C. Insect venom
D. All of the above

Q107. Allergic reactions caused by environmental allergens is known as:

A. Anaphylactic reactions
B. Atopic reactions
C. Cytotoxic reactions
D. Immune-complex reactions

Q108. All of the following diagnostic tests are commonly performed allergy test *except*:

A. Skin test
B. Pulmonary function test
C. Cardiac function test
D. Radioallergosorbent test (RAST)

Q109. A patient with allergic rhinitis is prescribed loratadine. The nurse is teaching the patient about this drug. Which of the following is not appropriate?

A. This drug produces antihistamine action without sedation
B. The drug should be taken once a day in empty stomach
C. The drug is equally effective in acute asthma
D. The drug causes photosensitivity

Q110. Which of the following conditions is an example of delayed hypersensitivity reactions?

A. Contacts dermatitis
B. Allergic rhinitis
C. Acute glomerulonephritis
D. Drug induced hemolytic anemia

Q111. A patient has been admitted in hospital emergency department with anaphylactic shock following an insect bite. The nurse anticipates that the patient will be treated with all of the following *except*:

A. Ensuring patent airway and oxygen therapy
B. Administering intravenous fluids and volume expanders as ordered
C. Administering epinephrine 1:1000, 0.5 mL cutaneously at 20 minute intervals
D. Administering epinephrine 1:10,000, 0.5 mL IV at 5–10 minute intervals

Q112. The physician has recommended immunotherapy for a patient with severe allergies. The nurse explains the patient about immunotherapy. Which of the following statements about immunotherapy is appropriate?

A. Immunotherapy aims at suppressing the immune system so that hypersensitivity reactions in response to allergen is controlled

B. Immunotherapy aims at first detecting the offending allergen and then administering the allergen extract in small titers and in increasing strengths until hyposensitivity to the allergen is achieved

C. Immunotherapy usually requires 6 months to 1 year time for maximal therapeutic effect

D. Immunotherapy though costly, completely protects a person against anaphylaxis

Q113. A patient attends hospital clinic to get his biweekly dose of immunotherapy. The nurse administering the dose will take which of the following measures?

A. Check records for date and amount of last dose

B. Keep ready emergency equipment and drugs to treat anaphylaxis reaction before administering the dose

C. Instruct patient to wait for 30 minutes after the injection before leaving the clinic

D. All of the above

Q114. All of the following conditions are examples of autoimmune diseases *except*:

A. Systemic lupus erythematosus (SLE)

B. Thyroiditis

C. Goodpasture's syndrome

D. Parkinson's disease

Q115. The incidence of systemic lupus erythematosus (SLE) is more in:

A. Asian women than black

B. Elderly women above the age of 50 years

C. Family members of a person with SLE

D. All of the above

Q116. Which of the following statements made by a patient with systemic lupus erythematosus indicates that she needs further teaching regarding factors causing exacerbation of her disease?

A. "I need to use an umbrella or sunscreen to protect myself from exposure to sunlight"

B. "I should avoid any kind of infections as much as possible"

C. "Hard work and mental happiness will keep me healthy"

D. "I should avoid oral contraceptives and use some other contraceptive methods"

Q117. The nurse is assessing a patient with systemic lupus erythematosus (SLE). Which of the following clinical findings she is expected to find?

A. Weight gain, lethargy, photosensitivity and arthralgia

B. Weight loss, fever, polyarthralgia, facial erythema

C. Fatigue, alopecia, hypotension, ankle edema

D. Bradycardia, bradypnea, syncope, blurred vision

Q118. Which of the following laboratory test results confirms SLE?

A. Negative antinuclear antibody (ANA) titer

B. Elevated anti-DNA (Deoxyribonucleic acid) levels

C. Elevated erythrocyte sedimentation rate (ESR)

D. Decrease CRP(C-reactive protein) level

Q119. Recent studies have demonstrated strong association between human leukocyte antigen (HLA) type and susceptibility to certain diseases. Which of

the following diseases is found to be associated with HLA antigens?

- **A.** Degenerative diseases
- **B.** Infectious diseases
- **C.** Malignant diseases
- **D.** Autoimmune diseases

Q120. Which of the following is the most important aim in the treatment of SLE?

- **A.** Encouraging physiotherapy to promote muscular strength and joint function
- **B.** Use of drugs to suppress end-organ inflammation and prevent progressive loss of function
- **C.** Use of drugs to boost natural immunity so that acute exacerbation is prevented
- **D.** Maintaining proper nutrition to prevent disease related disabilities

Q121. Which of the following drugs is effective to manage cutaneous and musculoskeletal features of SLE?

- **A.** Methylprednisolone
- **B.** Methotrexate
- **C.** Hydroxychloroquine
- **D.** NSAIDs

Q122. A patient with systemic lupus erythematosus who is on steroid therapy receives information from the nurse regarding self-care. Which of the following statements if made by a patient would indicate understanding regarding the therapy?

- **A.** "I will limit carbohydrate in my diet"
- **B.** "I will avoid individuals who have infections"
- **C.** "I will take the medication before meals"
- **D.** "I will stop the medication when my symptoms subside"

Q123. Which of the following individuals is most at risk for developing rheumatoid arthritis?

- **A.** A 20-year-old American woman
- **B.** A 35-year-old Asian woman
- **C.** A 45-year-old African man
- **D.** A 50-year-old woman who smokes

Q124. The nurse is assessing disease manifestations of a patient with suspected rheumatoid arthritis. The assessment data noted by the nurse will commonly include:

- **A.** Symmetrical joint swelling of three or more joints
- **B.** Increasing stiffness at the end of the day with activity
- **C.** Muscle weakness
- **D.** Appearance of tender subcutaneous nodules seen in wrist, knee and elbow joints

Q125. Rheumatoid arthritis can affect nearly every system in the body. Which of the following is the most common extra-articular manifestation of rheumatoid arthritis?

- **A.** Rheumatic nodule
- **B.** Sjögren's syndrome
- **C.** Felty syndrome
- **D.** All of the above

Q126. Ocular problems are commonly associated with connective tissue disorder, rheumatoid arthritis. The most common ocular problem seen in rheumatoid arthritis is:

- **A.** Sjögren's syndrome
- **B.** Felty syndrome
- **C.** Caplan's syndrome
- **D.** Vasculitis

Q127. Which of the following diagnostic tests detects rheumatoid arthritis in an early stage?

- **A.** X-ray
- **B.** Bone scan
- **C.** Rheumatoid factor
- **D.** Erythrocyte sedimentation rate

Q128. Which of the following drugs will be prescribed first in the early stages of rheumatoid arthritis?

A. Antibiotic
B. Antihistamine
C. Calcium
D. NSAIDs

Q129. The goals of drug therapy in the treatment of rheumatoid arthritis is to:

A. Stimulate normal immune system
B. Reduce inflammation and halt the progress of disease
C. Increase bone density and prevent bone erosion
D. All of the above

Q130. Disease modifying antirheumatic drugs (DMARD) are now being used in the treatment of rheumatoid arthritis (RA) instead of aspirin or NSAIDs to lessen the permanent effects of RA, e.g. joint erosion and deformity. Which of the following drugs does not belong to DMARD?

A. Hydroxychloroquine
B. Sulfasalazine
C. Methotrexate
D. Celecoxib

Q131. Which of the following adverse reactions is to be reported by a patient, who has been prescribed aspirin for rheumatoid arthritis?

A. Lethargy
B. Tinnitus
C. Bradypnea
D. Convulsion

Q132. A patient with rheumatoid arthritis has been on prednisolone with other DMARDs to control the symptoms of the disease. During follow-up visits the nurse is expected to find which of the following side effects of prednisolone?

A. Fluid retention and weight gain
B. Anorexia and weight loss
C. Lethargy and confusion
D. Hypotension and bradycardia

Q133. The nurse is teaching a group of patient with rheumatoid arthritis. To promote optimal functioning in these patients which of the following instructions she should emphasize?

A. Take as much rest as possible to prevent fatigue
B. Immobilize painful joints
C. Take pain medication as prescribed to decrease pain and increase functioning
D. Perform daily exercises as prescribed by the physiotherapist

Q134. Which of the following exercises should be performed daily by an elderly woman with rheumatoid arthritis?

A. Walking
B. Active range of motion
C. Isometric
D. Resistive

Q135. The nurse is planning teaching for a patient with rheumatoid arthritis who is on multiple drug therapy. Which of the following information she should include in her teaching plan?

A. Use aspirin only to get relief from acute pain
B. Stop tking prednisolone as soon as symptoms are relieved
C. Get a 12 lead ECG done every 6 months while on hydroxychloroquine.
D. Have frequent laboratory monitoring while taking methotrexate

Q136. The nurse is teaching a patient with rheumatoid arthritis regarding the disease process. Which of the following sentences indicates that the patient understands disease process?

A. "My bone will gradually become brittle"
B. "It will get better and worse again"
C. "Overuse of my joints caused this problem"
D. "I will definitely have to have surgery for this"

Q137. Which of the following factors most commonly causes immunodeficiency?

A. Drugs
B. Stress
C. Increasing age
D. Malnutrition

Q138. Which of the following assessment findings in a patient indicates that his immune system is functioning adequately?

A. Absence of fever
B. Elevated eosinophil level
C. Elevated IgE levels
D. Positive skin test

Q139. A nurse caring for a postoperative patient formulates a nursing diagnosis of high-risk for infection related to immunodeficiency. Which of the following laboratory findings supports this diagnosis?

A. Decreased leukocyte counts
B. Increased eosinophil counts
C. Increased lymphocyte counts
D. Decreased serum globulin levels

Q140. To which of the following classifications does human immunodeficiency virus belong?

A. Reovirus
B. Rhabdovirus
C. Retrovirus
D. Rotavirus

Q141. The most common mode of transmission of HIV from an infected person to another occurs by:

A. Sexual contact
B. Blood transfusion
C. Transplacental
D. Contact with contaminated articles

Q142. Which of the following blood test is done first to detect the presence of HIV infection in an individual?

A. Complete blood count
B. CD4+T cells count
C. Enzyme-linked immunosorbent assay (ELISA)
D. Western blot

Q143. The diagnosis of acquired immunodeficiency syndrome (AIDS) is made when an individual with HIV infection has:

A. CD4+T cell count below 200 cells/ microliter
B. CD4+T cell count below 500 cells/ microliter
C. A high level of HIV in the blood
D. CD4+ to CD8+ cells ratio gradually increases

Q144. Screening test for HIV involves detection of HIV-specific antibodies in blood. Which of the following time periods is usually required in order to detect the antibody in blood after initial infection?

A. 2 weeks
B. 4 weeks
C. 6 weeks
D. 8 weeks

Q145. What is the time interval between untreated HIV infection to the development of acquired immunodeficiency syndrome?

A. 1 year
B. 5 years
C. 5-8 years
D. 10 years

Q146. A nurse is reviewing the laboratory test results of a patient and finds his enzyme-linked immunosorbent assay test positive. She understands that:

A. The patient is immune to the acquired immunodeficiency syndrome
B. The patient is having antibodies to the human immunodeficiency virus in his blood
C. The patient is having human immunodeficiency virus or antigen in his blood
D. The patient is having immune deficiency virus or antigen in his plasma

Q147. What changes in the laboratory test values are found as the untreated HIV infection progresses?

A. Platelet count increases
B. CD4+T cells count decreases
C. Detectable HIV viral load decreases
D. Cholesterol level increases

Q148. A parson infected with human immunodeficiency virus is prescribed zidovudin. The nurse explains to the patient the action of zidovudin. Which of the following explanation is appropriate?

A. The drug stimulates immune system
B. The drug kills the viruses by changing the composition of cellular protein
C. The drug prevents viral replication by blocking viral DNA chain formation
D. The drug attaches with viral body thus preventing entry of virus to healthy cells

Q149. The nurse is taking care of a patient with acquired immunodeficiency syndrome (AIDS) on antiretroviral therapy with zidovudin. Which of the following laboratory tests to be conducted frequently?

A. Serum bilirubin level
B. Blood sugar level
C. Serum creatinine level
D. Complete blood count

Q150. The nurse is teaching a person who has been recently tested positive for human immunodeficiency virus. Which of the following instructions is appropriate?

A. To take rest as much as possible to prevent fatigue
B. To keep separate the person's eating utensils and other belongings from others
C. Limiting close contact with children
D. To practice safe sex

Q151. The nurse is teaching a patient with HIV infection regarding development of AIDS. Which of the following statements by the patient indicates that the patient understands the disease process?

A. "I can expect to develop AIDS in a short time"
B. "I may remain healthy for a number of years"
C. "Due to the advances in medical technology I may recover from this infection"
D. "I know that I have to make frequent trips to hospital off and on"

Q152. A patient with HIV infection has been prescribed antiretroviral drugs. The nurse is explaining the rational for treatment with antiretroviral drugs. Which of the following explanations is appropriate?

A. Antiretroviral drugs cure acute infection with HIV
B. Antiretroviral drugs will prevent AIDS
C. Antiretroviral drugs delay the development of HIV-related symptoms
D. Antiretroviral drugs cure the opportunistic infections associated with HIV infections

Q153. The nurse is caring for a patient with HIV infection. Which of the following standard precautions she should follow to protect herself when performing a venipuncture?

A. Ask the physician to perform venipuncture on patient, as it is not nurses' duty
B. Put on a mask, gown and gloves
C. Put on gloves
D. Put on gloves and mask

Q154. A hospitalized patient with acquired immunodeficiency syndrome has a CD4+T cell count of 150/microliter. While planning care for the patient, the nurse should give priority to which of the following measures?

A. Maintaining standard precautions to protect her and other staff

B. Implement reverse isolation technique
C. Monitoring body temperature
D. Instituting strict hygienic measures

Q155. A patient with AIDS is being treated with zidovudin. To check for adverse effects of the drug the nurse should monitor which of the following laboratory tests?

A. Complete blood count
B. Serum sodium level
C. Serum bilirubin level
D. Serum creatinine level

ANSWERS AND RATIONALS OF HEMATOLOGICAL SYSTEM, ONCOLOGY AND IMMUNOLOGY

1. **B.** The nurse will recognize the white blood cell counts of 12,000/cubic millimeter as abnormal. The normal value of white blood cell counts is 4000–9000/cubic millimeter. The values of red blood cell counts, platelet counts and hematocrit percentages are within normal limits.

2. **D.** Red blood cell indices are measures of erythrocyte size and hemoglobin content. Red blood cell count measures the number of RBCs per cubic millimeter of blood. Hemoglobin level measures the hemoglobin content of erythrocytes by measuring the number of grams of hemoglobin per 100 milliliter (mL) of blood and hematocrit level is a measure of the volume of RBCs in whole blood expressed as a percentage.

3. **D.** Anemia is a deficiency in the number of erythrocytes, the quantity of hemoglobin and/or the hematocrit (volume of packed RBCs).

4. **A.** All manifestations accompanying anemia is due to a tissue deficiency of oxygen or tissue hypoxia. Hemoglobin is lacking or the number of erythrocytes is too low to carry adequate oxygen to tissues and hypoxia develops. When tissue hypoxia develops, the amount of carbon dioxide will be more, rather than deficient due to impaired perfusion. Hemoglobin is a component of blood, and iron is a component of hemoglobin and not of tissue.

5. **D.** Anemia is caused by decreased erythrocyte production, e.g. cobalamine deficiency, chronic blood loss, e.g. gastritis, and increased erythrocytes destruction due to G6PD deficiency. It is not caused by herpes simplex infection.

6. **B.** Patient with severe anemia exhibits many clinical manifestations involving multiple body systems. Cardiopulmonary manifestations of severe anemia result from additional attempt by the heart and lungs to provide adequate amounts of oxygen to the tissues. If the heart is overworked for an extended period of time congestive heart failure may develop. Patient with mild anemia will exhibit exertional dyspnea. Patient with severe anemia will develop pulmonary congestion not pulmonary fibrosis. Arrythmias are not directly associated with anemia.

7. **A.** Microcytic, hypochromic anemia is iron deficiency anemia. So the nurse would like to question the patient regarding dietary intake of iron. Gastric surgery would result in inadequate vitamin B_{12} absorption due to deficient intrinsic factor. The anemia due to lack of vitamin B_{12} is macrocytic, normochromic. Anemia resulting from acute blood loss is normocytic and normochromic and in sickle cell anemia the RBC will be elongated and sickle shaped.

8. **C.** The nurse should instruct to take ferrous sulfate followed by antacid at least 2 hours apart, because antacids bind with iron in gastrointestinal tract, decrease the rate and extent of absorption of iron. So antacids should not be taken with ferrous sulfate or within an hour of taking ferrous sulfate.

9. D. Signs and symptoms of iron deficiency anemia include pallor, tachycardia and dyspnea. Patient may also exhibit fatigue, headache, irritability, cheilitis, glossitis and burning sensation of the tongue. Itching, jaundice and fatigue are the symptoms of hemolytic anemia. Fever, petechiae and fatigue are the symptoms of aplastic anemia and nausea, vomiting, and anorexia are not associated with anemia.

10. B. The nurse should encourage the patient to eat liver and dry beans, as they are rich sources of iron. Other rich sources of dietary iron are egg yolk, dry fruits, wheat germs and yeast. Milk is a poor source of iron. Chicken, meat, fish, banana, apple are medium sources of iron.

11. C. The nurse will anticipate administration of packed red blood cells transfusion. Blood transfusion or packed red blood cells transfusion benefits acute or chronic severe anemia of hemoglobin less than 6 g/dL. Oral or parenteral iron replacement therapy is indicated in patients with mild to moderate forms of anemia. Hemoglobin level would not be affected by intravenous albumin.

12. D. Appropriate nursing action for a patient with severe anemia related to chronic kidney disease is administration of epoietin as prescribed, as erythropoietin a hormone necessary for erythropoiesis is deficient in chronic kidney disease and must be supplemented to treat anemia. Monitoring fluid intake and urine output does not help in the treatment of anemia. Patients with chronic kidney disease are usually given oral iron supplementation as most of the rich sources of dietary iron is restricted in these patients. Anemia associated with chronic kidney disease is not due to loss of blood through hematuria but due to deficient erythropoietin.

13. C. The nurse is expected to find all of the above symptoms except petechia on abdomen and thigh, as bleeding tendencies, e.g. bruising or petechia is not a common manifestation of the disease. Sickling of red blood cells causes increased viscosity or stasis in the peripheral vasculature, resulting in infarction, not bleeding. Since sickle cell anemia is common in dark skinned individual, paleness of skin is most obvious in palms of hands and soles of feet. Tachycardia occurs to compensate low hemoglobin level, which ultimately results in cardiomegaly and heart failure. Infarction of bone results in bone pain.

14. A. Bone marrow transplantation is the only available treatment that can cure some patients with sickle cell anemia. Splenectomy is not indicated in this disease. Repeated exchange transfusion is helpful in the management of symptoms but not cure. Administration of hydroxyurea is also helpful in the management of the disease but offer no cure.

15. D. Failure to absorb vitamin B_{12} results in pernicious anemia. This type of anemia is morphologically classified as macrocytic normochromic anemia. Sickle cell anemia is due to inherited disorder of hemoglobin synthesis. Microcytic hypochromic anemia is due to iron deficiency and normocytic normochromic anemia results from acute blood loss.

16. A. Pallor; sore, smooth and red tongue; tachycardia; paresthesias of the hand and feet are characteristic manifestations of pernicious anemia. Other clinical manifestations being anorexia, nausea, vomiting, abdominal pain, weight loss, ataxia, confusion, and dementia. Manifestations listed in other options are not characteristic symptoms of pernicious anemia.

17. D. Since patients with pernicious anemia lacks intrinsic factor, oral vitamin B_{12} cannot be absorbed. So parenteral vitamin B_{12} is recommended and required for life.

18. D. The dosage and frequency of injection vitamin B_{12} varies depending upon the condition of the patient. But a typical dosage schedule for a patient with severe symptoms is 100 microgram daily for 2 weeks and then followed by weekly for several weeks and then monthly for life.

19. A. The nurse is expected to find hypertension, pruritus, thrombophlebitis and splenomegaly in a patient with polycythemia vera. Other signs and symptoms of the disease include angina, congestive heart failure, intermittent claudication, petechia, ecchymoses, epistaxis, GI bleeding, plethora (ruddy complexion) and hyperuricemia.

20. A. The most frequent complication of polycythemia vera is stroke due to thrombosis. Cardiomyopathy and pulmonary fibrosis are not related to polycythemia vera. A very low incidence of leukemia and lymphomas develop in some patients with polycythemia vera, which may be due to chemotherapeutic agents used in the treatment or secondary to a disorder in the stem cell that progresses to erythroleukemia.

21. B. The treatment of polycythemia vera involves phlebotomy to diminish blood volume until the desired hematocrit level is reached. From the time of diagnosis about 300 to 500 mL of blood may be removed every other day until hematocrit is reduced to normal level. Later on phlebotomy is done every 2 to 3 months. To reduce blood's viscosity hydration therapy is used, not restriction of fluids. Although repeated phlebotomy results in deficiency of iron, iron supplementation is avoided. Use of antiplatelet medication to prevent thrombosis is controversial because of increased irritation of gastric mucosa resulting in gastrointestinal problems including bleeding. Other treatment measure involves use of myelosuppressive drugs to reduce bone marrow activity.

22. C. The patient with polycythemia vera is at risk of developing thrombus formation due to relative immobility imposed by hospitalization, so patient must be encouraged active or passive leg exercises and ambulation whenever possible instead of providing strict bed rest.

23. C. The life span of normal platelets is 8–10 days. But in immune thrombocytopenic purpura (ITP) formerly known as idiopathic thrombocytopenic purpura, the life span is only 1–3 days.

24. A. The patient with a platelet count below 20,000/cubic millimeter is at increased risk of intracranial bleeding. A count of 75,000/cubic millimeter is less than normal however prolonged bleeding from trauma or injury does not usually occur until platelet counts are less than 50,000/cubic millimeter. The platelet count of 1,50,000/ cubic millimeter is normal.

25. C. Heparin-induced thrombocytopenia and thrombosis syndrome may occur after valve replacement surgery due to heparin use during surgery. All other conditions may lower platelet count but neither is common after valve replacement surgery.

26. D. Manifestations of thrombocytopenia are usually mucosal and cutaneous bleeding. Mucosal bleeding is manifested as epistaxis and gingival bleeding and cutaneous bleeding is exhibited as petechiae or superficial ecchymoses. Fatigue, weakness and dyspnea are the manifestations of anemia. Tachycardia, hypo-tension and fainting may be the symptoms of internal bleeding, which may result from any invasive procedure, e.g. IM injection to a patient with thrombocytopenia. Nausea, vomiting and dizziness are not related to thrombocytopenia.

27. D. Intramuscular or subcutaneous injections should be avoided in patients with thrombocytopenia. If unavoidable, a small-bore needle should be used and after injection direct pressure to be applied for at least 5–10 minutes to prevent prolonged bleeding. Patient should not be taught coughing technique as coughing increases intracranial pressure and risk of intracerebral hemorrhage. Restricting visitor with upper respiratory infection and practicing hand washing does not protect a patient with thrombocytopenia.

28. C. Platelets are rarely transfused prophylactically to patients with immune thrombocytopenic purpura, because the cells are destroyed prematurely, providing little therapeutic benefit. All other statements by the patient indicate adequate learning.

29. B. Corticosteroids suppress the phagocytic response of splenic macrophages and alters the spleen's recognition of platelets and increases the life span of platelets. They also suppress antibody formation. Hydroxyurea causes thrombocytopenia. Vitamin K is used to prevent or treat bleeding from warfarin overdose. Clopidogrel inhibits platelet function.

30. D. Abruptio placenta is a cause of disseminated intravascular coagulation (DIC) because of activation of the clotting - cascade after hemorrhage. Pancytopenia results from decreased bone marrow production. Immune thrombocytopenic purpura (ITP) is an autoimmune disease and cannot be caused by abruptio placenta. Patient with abruptio placenta is not advised heparin so heparin-induced thrombocytopenia and thrombosis syndrome cannot occur from abruptio placenta.

31. C. Disseminated intravascular coagulation is a serious hemorrhagic disorder caused from abnormally initiated and accelerated clotting. The abnormal clotting mechanism ultimately leads to depletion of clotting factors and platelets with resultant severe hemorrhage. An underlying disease or condition always causes the disorder. It is not a genetic disorder. Neither it is caused by overproduction of clotting factors or hemolytic factors or due to deficiency of clotting factors.

32. B. The nurse should closely monitor platelet counts, prothrombin time and partial thromboplastine time for the development of DIC, which will be prolonged in this disorder. Other assessment parameters are history of the patient, activated partial thromboplastine time, thrombin time, fibrinogen level, etc. Vitamin K level, blood count and bleeding time are not used for the diagnosis of DIC.

33. B. The nurse should give highest priority to the diagnosis of ineffective tissue perfusion (cerebral, cardiopulmonary, renal, gastrointestinal, and peripheral) related to bleeding and sluggish blood flow secondary to thrombosis, since the risk of cerebral, cardiopulmonary, gastrointestinal and peripheral hemorrhage pose the greatest risk to the physiological integrity of the patient. All other nursing diagnoses are appropriate but are not priority.

34. A. Persons with granulocytopenia are at increased risk of infection from pathogenic and even nonpathogenic bacteria that constitute normal flora. So strict hand washing with antiseptic solution for all persons in contact with patient is extremely important. Because low granulocyte count depresses normal phagocytic response and pus formation, and masks some of the signs and symptoms of infection, the presence of even a low-grade fever is of great significance in the early detection of infection. For these patients invasive procedure like catheterization should be avoided. Administration of packed cells is not indicated in these patients, instead hematopoietic growth factor is administered if possible. Visitors need to be restricted and screened because of danger of potential transmission of harmful pathogens to patient. Monitoring hourly urine output is not necessary. Monitoring lung sounds and relieving anxiety are required.

35. B. Acute leukemia is caused by blocking in the differentiation of cells in the hematopoietic cell line or blood cell precursors. This results in accumulation of undifferentiated or leukemic cells in the blood and bone marrow. These cells then proliferate and compete with normal cellular proliferation. So acute leukemia is termed as accumulation disorder as well as proliferation disorder. Rapid growth of mature leukocytes is leukocytosis. Unregulated proliferation of hematopoietic cells or disordered cell death occurs in chronic leukemia. Proliferation of increasing number of blasts in the blood and bone marrow known as blasts crisis occur in patients with chronic myelogenous leukemia.

36. C. Chronic lymphocytic leukemia is a common malignancy of older adults. Two-thirds of all patients are older than 60 years at the time of diagnosis. It is the most common form of leukemias in the United States and Europe but is rarely seen in Asia.

37. D. Combination chemotherapy is the mainstay of treatment for leukemia. The purposes for using multiple drugs are to decrease drug resistance, minimize the drug toxicity to the patient by using multiple drugs with varying toxicities and interrupt cell growth at multiple points in the cell cycle.

38. A. The nurse should regularly assess respiratory rate and breath sounds in order to detect respiratory infections early. Pneumonia both viral and fungal is a common cause of death among neutropenic patients. So regular assessment is required. Although other assessment parameters are important but they do not reveal early signs of infection in a neutropenic patient.

39. C. Dietary factors, e.g. deficiency or excess of any nutrient so far have not been implicated in the development of leukemia. All other factors listed are associated with leukemia. Another factor, presence of primary immunodeficiency, and infection with the human T-cell leukemia virus type1 (HTLV-1) is also associated with leukemia.

40. C. Chemotherpy is the mainstay of the treatment of all kinds of leukemias. Chemotherapy is given to destroy the malignant cells of the bone marrow so that normal function of bone marrow may be restored. Radiation therapy is given as an adjunct to chemotherapy when leukemic cells infiltrate the CNS, skin, rectum and testes. Bone marrow transplantation and stem cell transplantation are treatment modalities used to cure the disease in selected patients and in certain kinds of leukemias.

41. C. Hodgkin's disease is characterized by proliferation of abnormally large giant multinucleated cells, called Reed and Sternberg cells. These cells are seen in biopsy specimen and are diagnostic. Hodgkin's disease originates in lymph nodes in most of the patients (90%) and not outside lymph nodes. Non-Hodgkin's lymphomas are seven times more common than Hodgkin's disease and have variable prognosis. The low grade lymphomas are considered to be incurable. Non-Hodgkin's lymphomas are treated by both chemotherapy and radiotherapy.

42. A. The early symptoms of Hodgkin's disease are enlargement of cervical, axillary or inguinal lymph nodes. The patient may notice fatigue, weight loss, night sweats and recurrent generalized pruritus without skin lesion. In addition patient may have fever, chills, weakness, tachycardia and alcohol-induced pain at the site of the enlarged lymph node. As the disease progresses and with additional node involvement patient may complain bone pain, jaundice, anemia, hepatosplenomegaly, dyspnea, cyanosis and dysphagia. Hypotension and hypothermia are not associated with Hodgkin's disease.

43. B. Majority (95%) of the patients with Hodgkin's disease in stage I and stage II are cured with radiation therapy for 4–6 weeks. Combination chemotherapy is used in some patients in early stages who are believed to have resistant disease or have more chances of relapse. Stage IIIA disease is treated by both chemotherapy and radiation therapy. With advancement of therapy some of the stage IIIB and IV diseases are treated with high dose chemotherapy followed by bone marrow or stem cell transplantation. Surgical excision of the involved lymph nodes is not included in the treatment plan of Hodgkin's disease.

44. C. The appropriate nursing action, which should be taken at first is informing the physician, and then preparing patient for taking cultures, as it is expected that the physician would order for cultures. A temperature of 100.4°F is not normal for a patient with pancytopenia and may lead to sepsis if not treated early. Aspirin is contraindicated in these patients as it may lead to gastrointestinal bleeding due to low platelet counts, which exist in pancytopenia.

45. D. A 60-year-old black farmer is at increased risk of developing multiple myeloma because the disease is twice as common in men as in women and develops after 40 years of age, with an average age of 65 years. The disease occurs more commonly in black men than in whites. Other risk factors associated with multiple myeloma are exposure to radiation, organic chemicals, herbicides and insecticides.

46. C. Symptoms of multiple myeloma usually appears when the disease is advanced. The major symptoms being skeletal pain. Pain at the pelvis, spine and ribs are particularly common. Other manifestations being diffuse osteoporosis, pathologic fractures, collapse of vertebra resulting into spinal cord compression and hypercalcemia due to bony degeneration. Fever and enlargement of inguinal nodes are not associated with multiple myeloma. Paraplegia may occur due to spinal cord compression, which results from destruction of vertebra in some patients. But skeletal pain is more common.

47. D. The diagnosis of multiple myeloma involves radiologic, bone marrow and laboratory examinations. X-ray reveals generalized thinning of bones, lytic areas of bone erosion and/or fractures. Bone marrow analysis shows significantly increased number of plasma cell in bone marrow. Laboratory tests for blood and urine detect presence of a monoclonal antibody protein. Beside this pancytopenia, hypercalcemia, and presence of Bence Jones protein and elevated serum creatinine are possible findings.

48. B. While reviewing the laboratory report of the patient with multiple myeloma admitted in a state of confusion and disorientation, the nurse would anticipate a finding, which indicates hypercalcemia. Because calcium is released when bone is destroyed it will cause an increase in serum calcium level. Multiple myeloma does not affect potassium and magnesium levels. Although in multiple myeloma hyperuricemia occurs but it does not cause drowsiness, confusion and disorientation.

49. C. Chemotherapy using a combination of drugs is usually the first treatment recommended for multiple myeloma. It is used to reduce the number of plasma cells. A variety of drugs given together affects rapidly dividing cells of different stages of cell division. Radiation therapy may be done in later stage to treat localized vertebral lesions. Surgical excision of any single lesion is not effective as multiple diffuse lesions appear in this disease. Treatment with alpha Interferon may be done following chemotherapy; it is not the first treatment.

50. C. The patient with multiple myeloma should be encouraged to perform weight bearing exercises and other activities that place stress on the long bones if he is able. The stress on long bones helps to increase resorption of calcium. The patient need to be ambulated as much as possible and not be in strict bed rest as immobility causes calcium loss from bones. Patient must not restrict fluids instead drink at least 3 liters of fluid in order to attain an urinary output of 1.5–2 liter per day. Patient need not keep lower extremity elevated while resting.

51. D. The majority of people 45 percent possess blood type O. So blood type O is the most common. The next common type is A, which is about 41percent. Type B is only 10 percent and type AB is only 4 percent.

52. A. Before administering blood, the nurse will verify the prescription, patient's records about grouping and cross matching and the label of the blood bottle carefully with another nurse. Checking and verifying with another nurse reduces the risk of administering incompatible blood by mistake. Lactated Ringer's solution or 5 percent dextrose should never be infused with blood or prior blood transfusion, as it may cause hemolysis. Normal saline should be given. Antibiotics are usually not given before blood transfusion. Blood transfusion procedure is not free from hazards. Patient should be explained about these hazards before transfusion and no false reassurance should be given.

53. C. If a patient develops acute hemolytic reaction, the nurse should immediately stop the transfusion, maintain a patent IV line with normal saline, and notify the blood bank and physician. Other nursing actions are rechecking identification of patient and label of blood bottle, monitoring vital signs and urine output, obtaining blood and urine samples for laboratory analysis, providing proper documentation and carrying out symptomatic treatment as advised. Antihistamine may be ordered for a mild allergic reaction. Dextrose solution should not be administered with blood products as it may cause hemolysis.

54. A. Autologous donations can be made every 3 days if the donor's hemoglobin remains at or above 11 g/dL. For the blood to be maintained in a liquid state, donations should begin within 5 weeks of the transfusion date. So donation is not made every month. Depending upon the amount of blood expected to require the frequency of blood donation is determined, e.g. every 3 days or less frequently, provided the hemoglobin remains at or above 11 g/dL.

55. D. Under normal conditions all cells of a tissue are controlled by a intracellular mechanism that determines when cellular growth and proliferation is necessary. Normally cellular growth and proliferation is activated only in the presence of cellular death or degeneration or when the body has a physiologic need for more cells. In cancer this normal control and regulatory mechanism is absent. Cancer cells proliferate at the same rate as the normal cells of the tissue from which they originate. The difference is that proliferation of the cancer cells is continuous and without any physiological need. No toxins are known to cause alteration in cellular morphology. Increasing differentiation or well-differentiated cells are present in benign neoplasms whereas cancers range from differentiated from undifferentiated.

56. C. The major difference between a benign and malignant neoplasm is the ability to invade and metastasize. The rate of cell growth and proliferation is usually same as that of their normal counterpart. Benign tumor is usually well differentiated, but malignant tumors range from well differentiated to undifferentiated. No toxin is known to be liberated by any of these type of tumor.

57. D. Carcinogens are agents that are capable of causing cancers. Genes are not considered as carcinogens. Genes or genetic susceptibility increase an individual's susceptibility to development of certain cancers.

58. B. Ultraviolet radiation secondary to sunlight exposure is linked with melanoma. Multiple myeloma is associated with exposure to radiation, organic chemicals, herbicides and insecticides. Leukemia is associated with ionizing radiation and chemical agents and nonHodgkin's lymphoma is associated with virus.

59. C. Leiomyoma is the benign tumor of smooth muscle. Endothelioma is the malignant tumor of the endothelium. Lymphoma is the malignant tumor of the lymphoid tissue and rhabdomyosarcoma is the malignant tumor of the striated muscle.

60. D. Glioblastoma is the malignant neoplasm originating from glial cells, but glioma is a benign tumor originating from the same glial cells. Chondroma is the benign tumor originating from cartilage and hemangioma is the benign tumor originating from blood vessels.

61. A. Malignant tumor that arises in the bone marrow is multiple myeloma. Others are Ewing's sarcoma and leukemia. Lymphosarcoma arises from lymphoid tissue, basal cell carcinoma from glandular tissue and hemangiosarcoma arises from blood vessels.

62. C. The cell's replication cycle is divided into G_0, G_1, S, G_2 and M phase. The letter G stands for gap- the interval separating cell division, S stands for synthesis and M stands for mitosis. The synthesis of both DNA and proteins of new chromosomes occur in S phase. In G_1 phase RNA and protein are synthesized. In G_2 phase synthesis of some RNA and other biochemical processes take place in preparation for mitosis. In M phase actual division of cell (mitosis) occurs.

63. A. Nurses' role regarding prevention and early detection of cancer includes educating the public to learn and practice self examination e.g. breast self examination and testicular self examination; to eat a balanced diet that includes vegetables, fresh fruits, whole grains and adequate amounts of fiber (not low fiber) and low fat, preservatives and smoked and salt cured meats. People aged 20–40 years should undergo a cancer related check up every 3 years and every year for people aged 40 years and older. The check up includes health counseling, and depending upon the person's age and sex, examinations and screening test for specific cancers. When teaching people regarding cancer, care is taken to reduce the fear of cancer and not increase fear. The goal of public education is to motivate the learner to change the pattern of behavior as necessary to achieve and maintain an optimal state of health.

64. D. The best time for the young women or the premenopausal women to perform breast self-examination is one week after the start of menstruation since this time breasts are less congested. On the first day and last day of menstruation the breasts remain congested. Breast self-examination is done monthly not daily.

65. C. American Cancer Society recommends that all women above the age of 40 years should have mammography annually. Women having high-risk of breast cancer, e.g. strong family history should have mammography earlier.

66. D. Testicular cancer is highly curable. If detected early, about 95 percent of patients obtain complete remission. Testicular cancer is a rare type of cancer accounting for 1 percent of all cancers found in men. However it is common in younger men aged 15 to 35 years and not in middle aged men.

67. B. Crypto-orchidism (undescended testes) commonly associated with testicular cancer. Other risk factors include a history of orchitis, mumps, inguinal hernia in childhood, maternal use of diethylstilbestrol in pregnancy, and family history of testicular cancer. Measles, hydrocele and early onset of puberty are not related to testicular cancer.

68. B. According to American Cancer Society's guidelines every man with high-risk of prostate cancer, e.g. African American, family history of prostate cancer and exposure to cadmium should undergo screening test with digital rectal examination and blood test for prostate specific antigen (PSA) annually, starting at age of 40 years. Others may start receiving screening test from 50 years onwards. 35 years is too early, as the disease commonly occurs at old age. Prostate cancer is asymptomatic in the early stage. Occurrence of urinary symptoms usually indicate the disease is present for some time.

69. C. Early sexual activity is one of the most common risk factors of cervical cancer. The other risk factors include low socioeconomic status, multiple sexual partners, infection with human papiloma virus and smoking. Increased age, obesity and family history is most commonly associated with breast cancer.

70. C. Pap (Papanicolaou's) test detects cancer as well as precancerous changes. So by treating precancerous lesions progression to cervical cancer can be prevented. All sexually active women irrespective of their age should have Pap test done every year. After 3 negative Pap tests, it may be done less frequently. Pap test results are not 100% accurate. There are problems of false-positive and false-negative reports.

71. A. When the suspected tumor is small (2-3 cm) the entire tumor is excised for examination, this is called a total or excisional biopsy. If the tumor is large, only a part of the tumor is excised. This process is called an incisional or subtotal type of biopsy. In fine needle aspiration biopsy cells are withdrawn from the tumor with a needle and syringe.

72. C. The goal of cancer treatment can be cure, control or palliation. These goals are achieved through the use of four treatment modalities for cancer—surgery, radiation therapy, chemotherapy and biologic therapy. These therapies can be used alone or in any combination in the treatment of cancer. For many cancers two or more of the modalities are used in combination to achieve the goal of cure or control for a long period of time.

73. B. In unsealed source of radiation therapy, the radioactive material is in the form of colloid suspension and is administered orally, intravenously or by direct instillation into body cavities. For example iodine 131 is given orally to treat thyroid cancer. In sealed sources of internal radiation, the radioisotope is completely enclosed by nonradioactive material. These sealed sources are then placed in the desired location through applicator or by needles, beads, seeds, ribbons or catheters. Intracavitary therapy and interstitial therapy are two different kinds of sealed source of radiation therapy.

74. D. The key principles the nurse should follow to protect herself and also others from excessive radiation exposure are 1) distance, 2) time, 3) shielding. The greater the distance from the radiation source, the less the exposure dose of ionizing rays. Nurses should aim to limit the exposure time to 30 minutes per 8-hour shift. Care for the client should be rotated among available nursing staff to limit exposure for each nurse. The use of shielding devices whenever possible reduces radiation exposure. The dose of X-rays and gamma rays is reduced as the thickness of the lead shield is increased.

75. B. The nurse should explain to the patient scheduled for brachytherapy for treatment of cancer cervix that patient has to be treated in a private room where all other radiation precautions will be observed. Radiation precaution includes principles of distance, time and shielding. Patient does not have to undergo simulation before brachytherapy. Simulation is used before teletherapy. With brachytherapy the patient does not experience external skin reactions. Brachytherapy for cervical cancers uses sealed source of radioactive material. So patient ceases to be radioactive as soon as the source is removed after treatment.

76. B. Brachytherapy for cervical cancer involves insertion of an applicator with the radioactive material in the cervical canal. The patient remains on absolute bed rest (not ambulatory) during the treatment to prevent displacement of the applicator. So patient needs further teaching regarding ambulation restrictions. Patient's visitors will be restricted. No visitors who are pregnant or under age 18 will be allowed. Patient will have an urinary catheter and a low residue diet to prevent frequent bowel movements, which may cause dislodgement of applicator.

77. D. The nurse should immediately pick up the implant with a long handled forceps and place it in a lead-lined container to prevent exposure to the patient and herself. Leaving the room or covering it with blanket does not reduce exposure from harmful radiation. The nurse must not try to replace the implant in proper place. The physician or the radiotherapist is the proper person to place an implant in the diseased area. Inaccurate placement can cause irreparable harm to the patient.

78. D. The size of the treatment field, total dose of radiation, and tumor location all influences the effects and side effects of radiation therapy. If a small area is treated patient can tolerate a larger dose of radiation than the effect of treatment of a larger area. Side effects a patient may experience are related to the total dose of radiation. Dose is higher usually when the goal is curative and less for palliation. Patient experiences more side effects when receiving curative dose (5000 cGy) than receiving palliative dose (2000cGy) in the same treatment field. Tumor location in relation to surrounding normal tissue affects both treatment effects and side effects. Certain normal tissues like spinal cord, gastrointestinal tract, myeloproliferative system, etc are at greatest risk for damage.

79. D. Irradiated area should be cleaned with water alone or with a mild soap and water. Care has to be taken not to rub the area. After cleaning, the area need to be pat dried gently with a soft towel. The irradiated area does not need to be covered with dressing. Normal saline or any type of lotion should never be used on the irradiated area. Cream, powder, moisturizer, after-shave and deodorant spray all are contraindicated.

80. D. Patient with stomatitis should discontinue use of toothbrush and clean mouth with finger in order to prevent further irritation of the oral mucosa. Patient should rinse thoroughly after each meal and every 2–3 hours with water or normal saline, but not use any commercial mouthwashes until prescribed. Commercial mouthwashes citrus juice may cause further irritation. Too hot or too cold drinks should also be avoided for the same reason.

81. D. Unlike surgery and radiotherapy, treatment of cancers by chemotherapy is systemic and appropriate when the disease is widespread; the risk of undetectable disease is high; and the tumor cannot be resected or radioresistant. The objective of chemotherapy is to destroy all malignant tumor cells without excessive destruction of normal cells. The goals of chemotherapy can be cure, control or palliation of manifestations.

82. C. The doses of chemotherapeutic drugs are determined by body surface area in square meters, which is calculated by patient's height and weight. The dosage can also be determined by weight of the patient also. Once the decision for chemotherapy is taken age and sex of the patient is not a deciding factor in determining dosage. Body mass index also is not used in dosage calculation.

83. C. Chemotherapeutic drugs may be administered by various routes. Most common being the intravenous and oral routes. Other routes being intracavitary, intrathecal, perfusion, continuous infusion, subcutaneous and topical.

84. D. Vesicant drugs most effectively are administered by a central venous access device. Central venous access devices are placed in large vessels, so the chances of extravasation are rare. Vesicants are not administered orally. They are frequently administered by intravenous route but chances of extravasation also run high. Infusion pumps are used primarily for the continuous infusion of chemotherapy by subcutaneous, intravenous, intra-arterial and epidural routes. They do not increase the effectiveness of drug administration related to extravasation.

85. B. Nausea and vomiting is the most frequently occurring side effect of chemotherapy. Most of the patients experience this side effect with most of the drugs. Anorexia, stomatitis and constipation are less commonly experienced with certain chemotherapeutic drugs.

86. D. In order to have maximum cancer cell kill but minimum toxic side effects combination chemotherapy is used. The drugs chosen for combination are based on all of the principles mentioned. The other principles of combination include 1) the drugs used are effective against the cancer being treated and 2) when drugs are given in combination, a synergistic effect occurs.

87. C. The patient will best cope with chemotherapy when the nurse gives accurate information about what to expect during the course of treatment in advance. Pretreatment teaching regarding possible side effects to be experienced by the patient relieves anxiety and fears, which is often associated with chemotherapy. Withholding information regarding side effects and telling only the positive effects will result in unnecessary fear and anxiety when the patient experiences troublesome side effects. Telling the patient not to worry is also not correct, as patient must learn to manage the problems actively when they occur with the help of the supportive care available from therapeutic team.

88. A. The nurse will reassure the patient that hair loss is temporary and that hair will grow soon after the treatment is discontinued. Patient should avoid frequent shampooing and combing as these actions hastens hair loss. Patient should use a wide toothed comb for combing hair. Hair loss is not permanent. Patient may use some alternatives, e.g. wigs, scarf or hat, etc. during the period of temporary baldness.

89. B. The nurse is aware that the patient getting cyclophosphamide is at increased risk of developing hemorrhagic cystitis. Hemorrhagic cystitis is a common side effect of cyclophosphamide. The risk diminishes with high intake of fluid. None of the prescribed medications will cause cardiomyopathy, photosensitivity or jaundice.

90. A. The nursing diagnosis that should receive priority when caring for a patient undergoing chemotherapy is risk for infection. Chemotherapy results in leukemia and a depressed immune system. So nurse should protect the patient from exposure to microorganisms. Sexual functioning, fertility and body image may be affected by chemotherapy, but they would not receive priority over risk for infection. Impaired physical mobility is not usually associated with chemotherapy. Fatigue and lethargy may be seen due to decrease in red blood cells and may result in inability to carry out activities of daily living but not impaired physical mobility.

91. A. Life threatening toxic effect that is unique to adriamycin is cardiotoxicity. Patient may develop irreversible cardiomyopathy manifested as dysrhythmias (tachycardia, heart block, premature ventricular contractions), high blood pressure, congestive heart failure. So nurse should assess patient's cardiac status by monitoring pulse for rate, rhythm, character; blood pressure and ECG.

92. B. Administration of epirubicin may cause diarrhea not constipation. Alopecia, infusion reactions, fatigue, nausea, vomiting commonly occurs with epirubicin. Dysrhythmia due to cardiomyopathy is an occasional adverse effect of epirubicin.

93. B. The adverse effect of morphine is respiratory depression. So the nurse should frequently assess the rate and depth of respiration of a patient who is on a continuous IV infusion of morphine. Cardiac rhythm is not altered by morphine although there may be bradycardia. Long-term administration may lead to dependence, but it is unlikely in a patient with cancer experiencing intractable pain. Morphine causes constipation as its side effect. So development of diarrhea and dehydration is unlikely.

94. C. The nurse will recognize constipation as common side effects of morphine. Other common side effects are sedation, nausea, vomiting and respiratory depression. Patient is awake and alert and requires minimum maintenance doses of medication means effective pain relief. Urinary output of 350 mL/ 12 hour means fluid deficit and irregular heartbeat of 80/minute signals cardiac problem, and not adverse effects of morphine.

95. B. The nurse recognizes patient's reaction as bargaining. In the bargaining stage the person promises to make amendments for previous wrongs that may have occurred. In denial stage the individual can not believe that he is in terminal stage of cancer. In the anger stage the individual is angry about his situation and in the depression stage the individual realizes that he is dying and experiences a great sense of loss.

96. D. Cyclophosphamide causes renal irritation and cystitis. Patient should take lot of fluids and he should monitor intake and output. Burning sensation in the hands and feet is not a usual side effect of cyclophosphamide. The drug should be stored in closed container in room temperature. Endoxan should be taken in empty somach. If nausea and vomiting is trouble some it may be taken after food.

97. A. The most valuable intervention a nurse can offer a patient with cancer is providing emotional support to the patient. The nurse presents herself to the patient as caring person, conveys verbal expressions of empathy, positive regard and practical support. Emotional support to the family, promoting positive self-esteem and helping patient cope with the consequences of the disease are all important aspects of care, but providing emotional support to the patient is most important and priority.

98. B. Thymus gland and bone marrow constitute the central lymphoid organs. The peripheral lymphoid organs are the tonsils, gut, genital, bronchial and skin associated lymphoid tissues; lymph nodes and spleen. Adrenal gland is part of endocrine system, kidneys are organs of renal system. Liver is an accessory organ of digestion and pharynx is an organ of digestive system.

99. C. Thymus gland secretes hormones, including thymosin that stimulate the maturation and differentiation of T lymphocytes. B lymphocytes are produced, matured and differentiated as beta cells in the bone marrow. Spleen, not thymus, filters foreign substances from the blood, and thymus does not store blood.

100. D. T lymphocytes are essential and responsible for cell mediated immune response. This type of immune response is initiated through specific antigen recognition by T cells. Humoral immune response or antibody mediated immune response is produced by B cells or plasma cells. Immune complex reaction is a type of hypersensitivity reactions and is an example of humoral immune response.

101. C. Destruction of cancer cells is one of the function of cell mediated immunity. The other functions are: 1) immunity against pathogens that survive inside of cells, e.g. mycobacterium; 2) immunity against fungal infections; 3) rejection of transplanted tissues; 4) contact hypersensitivity reactions and 5) tumor immunity. Production of antibody and formation of antigen antibody complexes, which activates the complement system in type II hypersensitivity reactions, are functions of humoral immunity.

102. C. Infants get passive immunity through IgA from their mother's breast milk and colostrum. IgA lines mucous membrane and protects body surfaces. IgG is the only immunoglobulin which crosses placenta and provides the newborn with passive acquired immunity for at least 3 months. IgM and IgE immunoglobulins are not passed to the newborn.

103. B. The key intermediate in allergic disorder is the IgE antibody. The production of IgE in response to an allergen results in allergic or hypersensitivity reaction in an individual. IgA antibody lines mucous membrane and protects body surfaces. IgM is responsible for primary immune response and IgD assists in the differentiation of B-lymphocytes.

104. B. Initial symptoms of anaphylactic shock are edema and itching at the site of exposure to the allergen. Wheal and flare reaction occurs in anaphylactic reaction when the mediators remain localized. Tachycardia, hypotension, chest tightness or dyspnea are late signs of anaphylactic shock. Sneezing is a symptom of allergic rhinitis.

105. C. To resuscitate the patient from shock the nurse should first administer epinephrine, a potent bronchodilator as prescribed. The patient will also be treated with antihistamines and corticosteroids as advised by the physician. If these medications do not relieve respiratory distress patient should be prepared for intubation.

106. D. The most common causes of anaphylaxis are exogenous pollen e.g. drugs, foods, insect bites and stings. Various drugs may cause anaphy-laxis. Penicillin is the most common. Common foods are peanut, tree nuts, shellfish, eggs, seafood etc. Insect venom of honeybees, wasps frequently cause anaphylaxis in sensitive individuals. Other common allergens are latex, antisera, vaccines, blood and blood products, iodinated contrast media, etc.

107. B. Allergic or hypersensitivity disorder caused by environmental allergens is known as atopic reactions. Allergic rhinitis, asthma, atopic dermatitis, urticaria, and angioedema are examples of atopic reactions. Anaphylactic reactions occur when allergens are released systemically. Cytotoxic reactions occur with blood or blood product transfusion and immune-complex reactions occur with extracellular fungus, virus or bacteria.

108. C. Cardiac function test is not performed to diagnose allergy. Skin testing is generally used to confirm specific sensitivity for suspected allergens. Pulmonary function test is performed when asthma is suspected. Radioallergosorbent test is performed to detect elevated levels of allergen-specific IgE associated with atopy.

109. C. Loratidine a second generation anti histamine is used in allergic rhinitis. It is contraindicated in acute asthma attack. The drug binds to peripheral histamine receptors, providing antihistamine action without sedation. It should be taken in empty stomach. The drug causes photosensitivity so exposure to sun should be avoided.

110. A. Contact dermatitis is an example of delayed hypersensitivity reactions (type IV). Other examples of delayed hypersensitivity reactions are transplant rejection and microbial hypersensitivity reaction, e.g. body's defense against tubercle bacillus. Allergic rhinitis is an example of atopic reactions (type I). Acute glomerulonephritis is an example of immune complex reactions (type III) and drug-induced hemolytic anemia is an example of cytotoxic reactions (type II).

111. C. The nurse anticipates that the patient in anaphylactic shock will be treated with IV epinephrine, diluted 1:10,000 at 5–10 minute intervals and other measures required for a patient in shock. Epinephrine is not given cutaneously.

112. B. Immunotherapy involves administration of small titers of an allergen extract in increasing strengths until hyposensitivity to the specific allergen is achieved. The allergen administered are chosen by skin testing with a panel of allergens found in the local geographical area. Immunotherapy does not aim in suppressing the immune response but it aims in gradual desensitization against a specific allergen. The therapy usually requires 1–2 years time to reach maximum therapeutic effect, but it may be continued about 5 years. For patients with severe allergies or sensitivity to insect stings maintenance therapy should be continued indefinitely. Patient should continue to avoid the allergen whenever possible because complete desensitization is not possible.

113. D. The patient who is scheduled to get a dose of immunotherapy is at risk of developing anaphylactic reactions. So the nurse should keep ready all emergency equipment and drugs necessary to treat an anaphylactic reactions. She must check previous records for date and amount of last dose and record of patient's reaction if any. The patient should be instructed not to leave the clinic before 30 minutes and also watch for delayed hypersensitivity reactions.

114. D. Parkinson's disease is a degenerative disease and involves degeneration of dopamine-producing cells in the substantia nigra. In systemic lupus erythematosus autoantibodies cause widespread tissue damage throughout the body. In thyroiditis autoantibodies are directed against thyroid tissue only and in Goodpasture's syndrome autoantibodies destroy the basement membrane of the lungs and kidneys leading to diseases in these organs.

115. C. Systemic lupus erythematosus (SLE) has a familial tendency. When a twin has the disease, the incidence is 25 to 50 percent greater in the other twin than in the general population. The disease is more common in African Americans, followed by Asians and then whites. It is a disease of younger women between ages of 15 and 40 years and not of women above the age of 50 years.

116. C. Physical and emotional stress may exacerbate systemic lupus erythematosus. So patient should avoid hard work which may lead to physical stress and fatigue. Patient should plan frequent rest periods in between activity to avoid physical stress. All other statements indicate understanding of patient regarding factors that may exacerbate the disease, e.g. sunlight, infection and hormones.

117. B. Since SLE is an autoimmune disease involving the connective tissue, various clinical manifestations occur. Common clinical manifestations are fever, weight loss, arthralgia, excessive fatigue, polyarthralgia, facial erythema, butterfly rashes on face, alopecia. It may also cause pleuritis, pericarditis, hypertension, hypercholesterolemia, protinemia, glomerulonephritis, etc. Weight gain, hypotension, ankle edema, bradycardia, bradypnea, syncope and blurred vision are not associated with SLE.

118. B. Laboratory test results specific of SLE is above normal levels of anti-DNA and positive not negative anti-nuclear antibody (ANA) titer. Because high levels of anti DNA are rarely found in any condition other than SLE, this test is more specific and confirms SLE. Elevated erythrocyte sedimentation rate and C-reactive protein (CRP) are not diagnostic but are used to monitor disease activity.

119. D. Most of the HLA–associated diseases are classified as autoimmune diseases, e.g. 1) HLA-B27 is associated with ankylosing spondilitis, 2) HLA-DR2 and HLA-DR3 with SLE and 3) HLA-DR3 and DR4 with diabetes mellitus. Degene-rative diseases, infectious diseases and malig-nant diseases have not yet been found to be associated with HLA antigens.

120. B. Treatment of SLE involves management of acute and chronic diseases. The most important aim is to control progressive disease activity or exacerbation that may involve any organ system, by using drugs that help suppress active inflammation secondary to SLE. The other important aim is to prevent disease related disability and complications from therapy by encouraging the patient to maintain a healthy lifestyle, preventing physical and emotional stress, promoting proper nutrition, etc. Proper nutrition is important but not enough to prevent disease related disabilities. Treatment of SLE may require use of immunosuppressive drugs and not drugs to boost immunity. Promotion of muscular strength and joint function is not important aim in the treatment of SLE but most important is to halt the inflammatory process.

121. C. Antimalarial medications like hydroxychloroquine are effective for managing musculoskeletal, cutaneous and mild systemic features of SLE. Corticosteroids, e.g. methylprednisolone is reserved for severe disease. Methotrexate is used as an alternate to steroid therapy. NSAIDs are helpful for arthritis but not for cutaneous management.

122. B. The patient should avoid individuals with known infectious diseases due to immunosuppression secondary to the use of corticosteroids. The patient receiving steroids should have high protein, high potassium and low sodium diet. Steroids irritate gastric mucosa and should be taken with meals or milk and the patient should be cautioned that withdrawal of steroids must be carried out slowly and under supervision to avoid adrenal insufficiency.

123. D. Rheumatoid arthritis occurs at any age of life, but it is more common between age 40 and 60 years. Women are affected two to three times more frequently than male till the age of 65 years, after that, men are affected equally. Smoking appears to be associated with the disease development and severity. Rheumatoid arthritis affects globally, no ethnic groups are particularly susceptible.

124. A. Patients presenting with manifestations suspected of rheumatoid arthritis will commonly have the characteristic manifestation of joint swelling involving three or more symmetrical joints, e.g. wrist, proximal interphalangeal (PIP) or metacarpophalangeal (MCP) joints. Other manifestations include morning stiffness lasting for at least an hour with inactivity, not evening stiffness with activity; appearance of non-tender subcutaneous nodules commonly seen in wrist, carpal, knee elbow, proximal interphalangeal (PIP) and metacarpophalangeal (MCP) joints. Positive results on tests for rheumatoid factor (RF) and erosion or bony decalcification seen in X-ray of hand.

125. D. Clinical manifestation of rheumatoid arthritis is divided into 1) articular and 2)extra-articular. Extra-articular manifestation can occur in nearly all system of the body. The three most commonly occurring extra-articular manifestations are: rheumatic nodules (occur in 25% of all patients with RA), Sjögren's syndrome (seen in 10–15% of patients with RA) and Felty syndrome occurs most commonly in patients with severe nodule forming rheumatoid arthritis.

126. A. The most common ocular problem seen in rheumatoid arthritis is Sjögren's syndrome. It involves decrease in lacrimation and salivation caused by obstruction of the secretory ducts by immune complexes. People with Sjögren's syndrome exhibit dry eyes and a dry mouth. Other ocular problems seen in patients with rheumatoid arthritis are episcleritis and scleritis. Episcleritis produces redness in the eyes and some discomfort but no pain. In scleritis there may be pain, corneal ulcer, glaucoma, and blindness.

127. B. Bone scans are helpful in detecting early joint changes and confirming a diagnosis so that treatment of rheumatoid arthritis is initiated early. X-rays may be inconclusive during the early stage of disease and are not specifically diagnostic of rheumatoid arthritis. Test for rheumatoid factor (RF) is diagnostic of rheumatoid arthritis but it may be positive only in 25% of people within 3 months of onset of clinical symptoms. After 1 year about 80% of patients are found to have positive RF. Erythrocyte sedimentation rate (ESR) is a general indicator of active inflammation. It is used to evaluate progress of the disease.

128. D. The treatment of rheumatoid arthritis begins with a balanced program of pharmacologic therapy with non-steroidal anti-inflammatory drugs (NSAIDs), education, physical therapy, occupational therapy and psychosocial therapy. Aspirin and other NSAIDs are used to control the local inflammatory process. Antibiotics are not used in rheumatoid arthritis, as it is not an infectious disease. Antihistamine is used in allergic disorder and calcium supplementation is required in osteoporosis.

129. B. The primary objective of drug therapy in rheumatoid arthritis is to reduce inflammation, which will result in control of local inflammatory process in the joints as well as control of systemic involvement. Rheumatoid arthritis being an autoimmune disease and not an immunodeficiency disease, drug therapy often aims in immunosuppression. The disease causes bone erosion at joints and not osteoporosis. Medications are not available to prevent bone erosion.

130. D. Celecoxib belongs to Cox-2 inhibitor. It does not belong to DMARD. Cox-2 inhibitor is the newer generation NSAIDs and is effective against both rheumatoid arthritis and osteoarthritis. Hydroxychloroquine, sulfasalazine and methotrexate all belong to disease modifying antirheumatic drugs. Hydroxychloroquine is an antimalarial drug, sulfasalazine is an anti-inflammatory drug and is primarily used in ulcerative colitis. Methotrexate, an antineoplastic drug has prominent immunosuppressant and anti-inflammatory property. These drugs can suppress the rheumatoid process and bring about a remission but do not have nonspecific anti-inflammatory or analgesic action. Other drugs used as DMARDs are gold salts, dpenicillamine, leflunomide, azathioprine and cyclosporine.

131. B. Aspirin given at a dose of 4–6 g/day in rheumatoid arthritis may produce the syndrome called salicylism, which is exhibited by tinnitus, dizziness, vertigo, and reversible impairment of hearing and vision. Other symptoms associated with salicylism are excitement and confusion not lethargy, hyperventilation, not bradypnea and electrolyte imbalance. The dose has to be adjusted to one, which is just below that producing these symptoms. Occurrence of tinnitus indicates the need for adjustment of dose. Convulsion is associated with acute salicylate poisoning.

132. A. The important side effects of prednisolone are fluid retention and weight gain. Anorexia, loss of weight, lethargy, confusion, hypotension and bradycardia are not associated with prednisolone. Instead patient may experience increased appetite, mild euphoria, gradual rise of blood pressure.

133. D. Individualized exercise to maintain joint motion and optimal functioning is an integral part of the management of patients with rheumatoid arthritis. The physiotherapist determines limitation of joint movement and effect on function to establish a baseline and then plan and execute an individualized exercise program to maintain and promote joint function. Patient should maintain a balance between activity or exercise and rest. Immobilization of joints when painful is important but does not promote function. Patient can schedule pain medication before performing exercises, which is vital for optimal functioning of joints.

134. B. The woman should perform active range of motion of her affected joints as well as unaffected joints. Isometric exercises strengthen muscles but may be too strenuous for an elderly lady. So isometric exercises and resistive exercises should be avoided. Walking, stationery bicycle and aquatic exercises all increase joint motion, flexibility and endurance, but active range of motion exercises promote greater mobility and prevent joint destruction.

135. D. The patient taking methotrexate should be advised to have frequent blood count done as the drug causes pancytopenia. Aspirin given in rheumatoid arthritis reduces inflammation and pain. Discontinuing medication will have recurrence of inflammation. Prednisolone should be discontinued with supervision, as it should be tapered because of danger of suppresion of adrenal gland function. Patient taking hydroxychloroquine should get ophthalmoscopic examination done every 6 months as it may cause irreversible retinal degeneration. There is no indication of doing 12 lead ECG done every 6 months while on hydroxychloroquine.

136. B. The patient with rheumatoid arthritis needs to understand that it is a somewhat unpredictable disease characterized by periods of exacerbation and remission. Patient with RA does not have brittle bones. Brittle bones are found in osteoporosis and with prolonged treatment with steroids, which is avoided as much as possible with the use of DMARDs. The cause of osteoarthritis may be overuse or trauma of joints. The cause of rheumatoid arthritis is unknown. Drug therapy, physical therapy and education often control the disease. Surgery is indicated only in some patients, but not always.

137. A. Various factors are responsible for causing immunodeficiency. Among them most common is drug-induced immunosuppression. Immunosuppressive drugs are frequently used to treat autoimmune diseases and to prevent transplant rejection. Immunodeficiency is a common side effect of antineoplastic drugs, which cause leukocytopenia. Stress, increasing age and malnutrition all cause immunodeficiency but not as common as drug induced immunodeficiency.

138. D. One can determine if a patient's immune system is functioning properly if the patient has a positive reaction to a skin test after exposure to a disease agent. Absence of fever indicates that the patient is not having an infection. Elevated IgE levels and elevated eosinophil level is found in allergic diseases, which is a disordered immune mechanism.

139. A. The laboratory finding which supports the nursing diagnosis of high-risk for infection related to immunodeficiency is a decreased leukocyte count. Individual with immunodeficiency will have decreased lymphocyte counts and an increased, serum globulin level not decreased. Eosinophil counts is increased in allergic reactions.

140. C. Human immunodeficiency virus (HIV) is a ribonucleic acid (RNA) virus and is called a retrovirus as it replicates in a backward manner or going from RNA to deoxyribonucleic acid (DNA). HIV does not belong to the other classes.

141. A. The most common mode of transmission of HIV from an infected person to another is by sexual contact. The frequency of transmission by other routes is much less.

142. C. Diagnosis of HIV infection is done by detecting HIV specific antibodies in blood by means of ELISA test. ELISA is the first screening for HIV. If the blood is ELISA positive more specific test, western blot test is done to confirm the diagnosis. CD4+T cell count is done to monitor the progression of HIV infection. Complete blood count is not diagnostic of HIV infection but it is decreased in untreated HIV infection.

143. A. The diagnosis of acquired immunodeficiency syndrome (AIDS) is established when a HIV infected person has a CD4+T cell count of less than 200 cell/microliter. CD4+T cell counts drop to below 500 cell/microliter in intermediate chronic infection. A high level of HIV may be found during acute infection and a CD4+ to CD8+ ratio, which is usually 2:1 gradually reverses in AIDS not increases.

144. D. In order to detect antibody after the person is exposed to the virus, a minimum of 8 weeks or 2 months time period is required. This is called window period, and before this time an infected individual will not test HIV antibody positive.

145. D. The median interval between untreated HIV infection and a diagnosis of AIDS is about 10 years.

146. B. A positive ELISA test indicates that the patient is having HIV antibodies in his blood. This test does not detect HIV virus or antigen in the blood or plasma. There is no known immunity to the human immunodeficiency virus that causes acquired immunodeficiency syndrome (AIDS).

147. B. As the effects of HIV infection progresses CD4 lymphocyte count decreases. Other laboratory findings include leukopenia, thrombocytopenia, anemia, increased sedimentation rate and altered liver function tests and increased viral load.

148. C. Zidovudin inhibits deoxyribonucleic acid (DNA) synthesis in HIV, thus preventing viral replication. The drug does not stimulate immune system, kills viruses or prevent entry of viruses into the healthy cells.

149. D. Frequent monitoring of complete blood count should be done for the patient who is on zidovudin therapy to detect anemia and leukopenia, which are its important adverse effects. Other adverse effects of this drug are nausea, vomiting, myopathy, fatigue and headache. Serum bilirubin is tested to detect jaundice, blood sugar for diabetes mellitus and serum creatinine is tested to detect kidney function, which are not indicated during zidovudin therapy.

150. D. The nurse should teach the person to practice safe sex, as sexual transmission is the most common mode of transmission of HIV. The person should continue to carry out his normal activities with rest periods in between activities to prevent fatigue and not take prolonged rest. HIV infected person can share living rooms and other household goods as long as basic hygienic practice is good. But he should not share razors, toothbrushes or other household goods that may contain blood or other body fluids. The infected person should avoid crowd and person with upper respiratory infections and need not avoid contact with healthy children.

151. B. The nurse should make the patient understand that the diagnosis of HIV infection does not necessarily mean that the patient has developed AIDS. AIDS is the last stage of disease process. The median time interval between HIV infection and development of AIDS may take 10 years or more and during this time patient may remain healthy. Although new knowledge regarding treatment and cure of AIDS is coming up, till now there is no cure for AIDS and patient should not assume that he will recover from the infection. With medical supervision, modification of lifestyle and hygienic health practices patient may remain healthy and need not visit hospital off and on.

152. C. The nurse should explain that antiretroviral drugs delay the development of HIV-related symptoms, including a wide range of opportunistic diseases. The other rationals for treatment with antiretroviral drugs are 1) decrease HIV RNA levels to less than 50 copies/microliter, 2) maintain or raise CD4+T cell counts to greater than 200 cells/microliter. Antiretroviral drugs do not cure acute infection, will not prevent AIDS, and do not cure opportunistic infections.

153. C. According to universal precaution a nurse should always wear gloves whenever she is coming in contact with patient's blood and body fluids. Mask is to be worn when nurse is anticipating airborn droplets of blood and body fluids. A gown is needed only for anticipated contact with splashes of blood or body fluids. The nurse needs to know the hospital policy regarding carrying out invasive procedures. In most of the health care facilities the nurses are required to perform venipuncture for patients.

154. B. The patient's immune system is severely depleted (CD4+T cell count of 150/microliter) and the patient is at high-risk for opportunistic infections. So reverse isolation technique should be maintained for such an immunosuppressed patient. The nurse needs to maintain standard precautions to protect her and others while giving care to every patient. Monitoring of body temperature and instituting strict hygienic measures are all important for the patient but practicing reverse isolation is the priority.

155. A. Adverse effect of zidovudin is pancytopenia. So nurse should monitor complete blood count every alternate week. If the count is low the treatment may be withheld, and restarted after hematologic recovery. Zidovudin is not known to be associated with retention of sodium, hepatotoxicity and nephrotoxicity.

9
CHAPTER

Musculoskeletal System

Q1. While obtaining subjective data related to the musculoskeletal system, which of the following informations is least important?

A. Lifestyle data
B. Past health history
C. Family history
D. Vital signs

Q2. All of the following are major functions of bone *except:*

A. Voluntary movement
B. Blood cell production
C. Mineral storage
D. Hormone storage

Q3. Which of the following bone cells is the basic bone forming cells?

A. Osteons
B. Osteoblasts
C. Osteocytes
D. Osteoclasts

Q4. During physical examination a woman aged 60 years asks the nurse 'why am I only 5' now but was 5'2" when I got married'. The nurse's best response would be to say:

A. 'Let me check it once more, since you disagreed'
B. 'The last time you measured, it was with a different instrument'
C. 'It seems you were not standing as straight as you could have been when I measured your height'
D. 'The intervertebral disc in your backbone is becoming thinner as you are aging'

Q5. A patient has undergone arthroscopy following an injury to the right knee. After the procedure the nurse should place patient's affected leg in which of the following position?

A. Flexed position by placing a pillow under the knee
B. Elevated and knee extended
C. Flat on bed
D. Elevated and knee flexed

Q6. A patient who has developed paresthesia in lower limbs is scheduled for an electromyogram. What the nurse need to do to prepare the patient for this procedure?

A. Keep the patient nothing per oral (NPO) for 6 hours before the procedure
B. Reassure patient that the procedure is not painful

C. Omit any scheduled sedative or caffeinated drink 24 hours before procedure

D. Inform the patient that a radiopaque dye will be injected during the procedure

Q7. Which of the following statements about osteoarthritis is true?

A. Osteoarthritis is a rare form of arthritis commonly affecting younger women

B. Osteoarthritis is a slowly progressive noninflammatory disorder of the synovial joints

C. Osteoarthritis damages multiple small joints of the body

D. Osteoarthritis is characterized by the recurrent inflammation of joints leading to the destruction of joint srtuctures

Q8. Which of the following factors are associated with the development of idiopathic osteoarthritis?

A. Increased age, strenuous exercise, obesity

B. Increased age, lack of regular moderate exercise, lack of estrogen

C. Trauma, obesity, increased age

D. Congenital skeletal deformity, elderly women, obesity

Q9. The nurse is assessing a patient complaining of joint pain. Which of the following findings suggests the diagnosis of osteoarthritis?

A. Fever and malaise

B. Tender swollen joints

C. Morning stiffness generally resolves within 30 minutes

D. Morning stiffness lasting more than a hour

Q10. Diagnostic test finding noted by the nurse in the patient with osteoarthritis commonly includes:

A. Elevated blood uric acid level

B. Elevated erythrocyte sedimentation rate

C. X-ray showing osteophyte formation

D. Increased white blood cells count in the synovial fluid

Q11. During assessment of a patient sign of osteoarthritis is noted. Which of the following findings indicates osteoarthritis?

A. Symmetrical involvement of metacarpophalangeal joints

B. Increase in joint pain and stiffness after inactivity

C. Heberden's nodes on the distal interphalangeal joints

D. Multiple subcutaneous nodules

Q12. The nurse is reviewing the findings of synovial fluid analysis of a patient complaining of pain in the left knee joint. Which of the following findings suggests osteoarthritis?

A. Gray colored synovial fluid

B. Below normal glucose content of the synovial fluid

C. White blood cells count in the field exceeds 25,000/microliter

D. Clear yellow colored synovial fluid

Q13. Which of the following instructions should be included in the teaching of a patient with osteoarthritis?

A. To keep the affected joint immobilized with splints and braces

B. To maintain a careful balance between rest and exercise

C. To consume a high carbohydrate, high protein and low fat diet

D. All of the above

Q14. A middle aged housewife with osteoarthritis of both knees is expressing her concern regarding the inability to carry out household activities. The nurse is teaching the lady to get adjusted with

the disease and daily activities. Which of the following is most helpful?

- **A.** Try to complete all your household activities in the morning when pain and stiffness is absent
- **B.** Do the household activities after performing the exercises taught to you
- **C.** Do the activities in the evening when pain and stiffness is usually less
- **D.** Schedule the activities throughout the day in such a way that you can rest in between the activities

Q15. An elderly patient with osteoarthritis frequently takes ibuprofen, (NSAIDs) for pain relief. The nurse should warn the patient about which of the following adverse effects?

- **A.** Hypotension and dizziness
- **B.** Sodium retention and hypertension
- **C.** Injury to articular cartilage and increased pain in joints
- **D.** Diminished vision

Q16. Which of the following methods helps to restore the elasticity and viscosity of the synovial fluid in an osteoarthritic joint?

- **A.** Dietary supplementation of vitamin C
- **B.** Intra-articular administration of hyaluronic acid
- **C.** Application of capsaicin cream
- **D.** Alternate heat and cold application

Q17. A patient who has been diagnosed with osteoarthritis of knees asks the nurse 'what is wrong with my knees?' The nurse's appropriate response would be:

- **A.** 'You have infection in your knees'
- **B.** 'Your right knee has become shorter than the left knee'
- **C.** 'Your weight bearing joints are damaged'
- **D.** 'Beside the knees many organs of your body are also inflamed'

Q18. Which of the following objectives of care is most appropriate for an elderly patient with osteoarthritis?

- **A.** Establishing effective breathing pattern to prevent respiratory complications related to immobility
- **B.** Providing adequate nutrition to increase body weight
- **C.** Helping to achieve independence in self-care
- **D.** All of the above

Q19. A nurse is teaching a patient with osteoarthritis to use a cane. Which of the following instructions regarding the use of cane is appropriate?

- **A.** To use the cane during acute pain only
- **B.** To hold the cane on the affected side
- **C.** To hold the cane on the unaffected side
- **D.** Not to use the cane when at home

Q20. Which of the following factors are involved in the development of osteoporosis?

- **A.** Heredity, late menopause, vigorous physical activity
- **B.** Heredity, low body weight, early menopause
- **C.** Cigarette smoking, inadequate physical activity, late menopause
- **D.** Excessive consumption of alcohol, low intake of calcium, above normal levels of serum vitamin D

Q21. All of the following medical conditions can give rise to osteoporosis *except:*

- **A.** Thyrotoxicosis
- **B.** Hypoparathyroidism
- **C.** Long-term use of corticosteroids
- **D.** Long-term use of anticonvulsant

Q22. Which of the following conditions is the most common complication of osteoporosis?

- **A.** Fragility fractures
- **B.** Damage of synovial joints of the body
- **C.** Renal stone
- **D.** Bone cancer

Q23. The nurse is teaching a group of woman regarding prevention of osteoporosis. Which of the following instructions she should emphasize to reduce the risk for the development of osteoporosis?

A. To avoid caffeinated drinks
B. To take part in the regular weight bearing exercises like walking and stair climbing
C. To reduce exposure to sunlight
D. To take a high protein diet

Q24. The nurse should provide which of the following dietary instructions for a patient with osteoporosis?

A. Reduce fat intake to lower body weight
B. Increase consumption of fruits and vegetables
C. Increase consumption of dietary dairy products
D. Increase consumption of sodium

Q25. Recommended calcium intake for a postmenopausal woman is:

A. 500-800 mg
B. 800-1000 mg
C. 1000-1200 mg
D. 1500 mg

Q26. All of the following drugs are used in preventing and treating osteoporosis *except:*

A. Estrogen
B. Alendronate
C. Raloxifene
D. Human parathyroid hormone

Q27. Which of the following mechanisms is involved in the development of gout?

A. Increased purine synthesis
B. Decreased renal excretion of purine
C. Increased consumption of purine
D. All of the above

Q28. The nurse is assessing a patient diagnosed with gout. Which of the following symptoms she is expected to find?

A. Involvement of single joint
B. Appearance of tophi on the elbows and feet
C. Appearance of Bouchard's nodes around the interphalangeal joints of hands
D. Appearance of rheumatic nodules on elbows

Q29. A patient with an acute attack of gout has been prescribed colchicine 1 g orally followed by .25 mg 1-3 hourly till pain is relieved or diarrhea starts. The nurse reassures the patient that his pain will disappear after:

A. 1 to 2 hours
B. 2 to 4 hours
C. 8 to 12 hours
D. 12 to 48 hours

Q30. The nurse administers colchicine to a patient with an acute attack of gout. The nurse understands that colchicine relieves pain in acute gout by:

A. Reducing inflammation
B. Controlling the infection
C. Inhibiting the synthesis of uric acid
D. Promoting excretion of the uric acid

Q31. A patient with chronic gout has been prescribed allopurinol (zyloprim). The nurse undertands that this drug is being given to:

A. Inhibit renal tubular reabsorption of urates
B. Block the production of uric acid
C. Promote urate diuresis
D. A and C only

Q32. A patient with gout is being treated with probenecid. Which of the following tests should be performed periodically to determine the effectiveness of therapy?

A. X-rays of involved joints
B. Serum calcium level
C. Serum uric acid level
D. Serum creatinine level

Q33. A 60-year-old patient comes to the hospital emergency with acute gouty arthritis. An immediate nursing intervention would be to:

A. Relieve pain
B. Demonstrate crutch walking
C. Teach dietary modification
D. Promote diuresis by administering diuretics

Q34. The nurse is teaching a patient with gout. Which of the following instructions is appropriate?

A. Avoid high calorie and high fat diet
B. Drink plenty of fluids
C. Take indomethacin on an empty stomach to increase absorption
D. Monitor white blood cells count regularly

Q35. Which of the following persons is at greatest risk for developing low back pain?

A. A 60-year-old clerk who walks regularly
B. A 25-year-old lady dance teacher who weighs 45 kg
C. A long distance bus driver
D. A 30-year-old nurse who works in critical care unit

Q36. A patient with acute low back pain is being treated with indomethacin, diazepam and bed rest for 2 days. The purpose of prescribing diazepam in this situation is to:

A. Reduce anxiety associated with sudden onset of low back pain
B. Suppress the acute inflammatory process
C. Enhance the analgesic action of indomethacin
D. Decrease muscle spasm

Q37. Which of the following positions during sleeping should be recommended by the nurse to a patient with low back pain?

A. Sleeping in a prone position
B. Sleeping on sides with legs straight
C. Sleeping in a supine position on a firm mattress
D. Sleeping in a side-lying position with the knees and hips flexed

Q38. Which of the following conditions is responsible for the herniation of an inter-vertebral disc?

A. Degeneration of disc with aging
B. Degeneration of vertebra with aging
C. Repeated stress to the spine
D. All of the above

Q39. The most common sites of herniation of an intervertebral disc is the:

A. L1-L2 and L2-L3
B. L4-L5 and L5-S1
C. C5-C6 and C6-C7
D. C3-C4 and C4-C5

Q40. A patient has a herniated disc in the region of the 4th and 5th lumbar vertebra. Which of the following sign and symptoms the nurse is expected to find in the patient?

A. Severe lower back pain radiating down the buttocks to dorsum of foot and big toe
B. Severe lower back pain radiating down the buttocks to inner calf
C. Shortness of breath
D. Weakness and atrophy of the arm muscles

Q41. Which of the following tests may be used to diagnose a herniated nucleus pulposus?

A. X-rays
B. Lumbar puncture
C. Myelography
D. Bone biopsy

Q42. A patient complains to the nurse of severe low back pain radiating down to the heel. Which of the following actions would the nurse take first?

A. Teach back strengthening exercises
B. Assess sensation of the lower extremities

C. Enforce strict bed rest

D. Administer pain-relieving drugs as prescribed

Q43. The immediate treatment of acute herniated disc includes all of the following *except:*

A. Drugs, e.g. analgesics, NSAIDs and muscle relaxants

B. Physical therapy, e.g. ultrasound and massage

C. Application of heat or cold

D. Back strengthening exercises

Q44. The most common and traditional surgical procedure for lumbar disc disease is:

A. Diskectomy

B. Percutaneous laser diskectomy

C. Laminectomy

D. Spinal fusion

Q45. After laminectomy which of the following nursing actions should be included in the nursing care plan?

A. Keeping the patient on absolute bed rest for at least 72 hours after the operation

B. Maintaining a 45° angle at head end.

C. Keeping the knees flexed by placing a pillow under them always

D. Using log roll technique while turning patient from side to side

Q46. A nurse caring for a patient who has undergone laminectomy for herniated disc observes that the patient has not voided for last 8 hours after operation. Which of the following actions the nurse should carry out first?

A. Assess bladder for distension

B. Increase the flow rate of intravenous fluid

C. Help the patient to use a bedside commode

D. Report physician and obtain an order for catheterization

Q47. A patient has undergone spinal fusion for intractable low back pain. Postoperatively the nurse assesses for which of the following complications?

A. Paralytic ileus

B. Frequency of urination

C. Paresthesia of upper extremities

D. Flank pain

Q48. The nurse is preparing a patient who has undergone the lumbar laminectomy for the discharge. Which of the following instructions she should include in her teaching?

A. Sleep on a bed with a soft mattress

B. Do not sit or stand for prolonged time

C. Limit fluid intake to control frequency of urination

D. Use an abdominal binder to support the incision

Q49. During assessment of a 65-year-old lady the nurse observes a severely increased thoracic curve or hump back. She documents her observation as:

A. Lordosis

B. Scoliosis

C. Kyphosis

D. Ankylosis

Q50. The school health nurse is assessing a 14-year-old girl. Which of the following assessment findings indicates scoliosis?

A. Head in alignment with gluteal fold

B. Unequal shoulder and scapula height

C. Equal leg length

D. Symmetry in the flank area

Q51. A nurse is teaching a teenaged boy who is being treated for scoliosis with a Milwaukee brace regarding self-care. Which of the following instructions is appropriate?

A. To wear the brace continuously for 24 hours, 7 days a week

B. To wear the brace directly over the bare body for perfect fit

C. To remove the brace during sleeping
D. To remove the brace for 1 hour, only during swimming and bathing

Q52. Which of the following mechanisms most commonly causes osteomyelitis?

A. Blunt trauma
B. IV drug abuse
C. Immunosuppression
D. Pelvic surgery

Q53. A patient is admitted in the orthopedic ward with the diagnosis of osteomyelitis. The nurse expects that the patient will be treated by the surgical debridement followed by the high dose of parenteral antibiotics for a period of 4-8 weeks then by oral antibiotics of another 4-8 weeks. Which of the following rationals best explains the expected therapeutic regimen of long-term use of antibiotics?

A. Bone has poor circulation so blood borne antibiotics inadequately reach the area of infection
B. Organisms responsible for the osteomyelitis are usually resistant to usual antibiotics
C. The pus and necrotic bone material formed in the osteomyelitis absorbs most of the antibiotic leaving very less to actually act on the infecting organisms
D. All of the above are correct

Q54. Which of the following represents the correct sequence of the stages of bone healing?

A. Inflammatory, callous formation, ossification, fibrocartilage formation, consolidation, remodelling
B. Hematoma, fibrocartilage, ossification, callous formation, consolidation, remodelling
C. Inflammatory, fibrocartilage formation, callous formation, scar formation, consolidation
D. Inflammatory, fibrocartilage formation, callous formation, ossification, consolidation, remodelling

Q55. The clinical manifestations of the fracture include:

A. Tingling, coolness, loss of pulses
B. Coolness, heaviness, paresthesias
C. Edema, pain, ecchymosis
D. Pain, deformity, loss of function

Q56. When the fracture line occurs at 90° angle to longitudinal axis of long bone, the fracture is known as which of the following types?

A. Linear
B. Longitudinal
C. Oblique
D. Transverse

Q57. What is a Colle's fracture?

A. Fracture at the distal radius
B. Fracture at the distal fibula
C. Fracture at the distal tibia
D. Fracture at the distal ulna

Q58. The nurse is assessing a patient with fractured tibia. Assessment data includes pain, tenderness and swelling at the site of injury. The patient is in which stage of bone healing?

A. Inflammatory
B. Fibrocartilage formation
C. Callous formation
D. Ossification

Q59. A patient attends the hospital emergency with a suspected fracture in his right humerus. During initial assessment the patient complaints of numbness in his right hand. The nurse anticipates that the numbness may be due to:

A. Pressure on the ulnar nerve
B. Ischemia
C. Muscle spasm
D. Fear and anxiety

Q60. An elderly woman is admitted in the hospital with fracture pelvis. The nurse caring for the patient is particularly aware of fat embolism. Which of the

following symptoms indicates fat embolism?

A. Chest pain, dyspnea, nausea, vomiting
B. Tachypnea, dyspnea, mental confusion, petechial rash
C. Bradycardia, bradypnea, chest pain, hypothermia
D. Tachycardia, tachypnea, hypotension, oliguria

Q61. A short leg weight-bearing cast has been applied on a patient with synthetic casting material. The nurse would allow the patient to walk with the cast after:

A. 30 minutes
B. 2 hours
C. 6 hours
D. 24 hours

Q62. A long arm cast has been applied to an 80-year-old lady for the fracture of humerus. While the cast is drying, which of the following assessment findings should be reported to the physician?

A. Mild edema of the fingers
B. Pain on movement of the fingers
C. Capillary refill is greater than 3 seconds
D. Patient complains of cold

Q63. A few hours after a long leg cast is applied, the patient complains of tingling sensation in her casted leg and foot. Which of the following actions the nurse should take?

A. Reassure the patient that these feelings are common during drying of the cast
B. Elevate the casted leg over a pillow
C. Instruct the patient to exercise her fingers to increase the circulation
D. Inform the physician

Q64. All of the following are the purposes of applying a traction *except:*

A. To keep injured bones and joints aligned
B. To prevent and treat deformity
C. To provide comfort
D. To decrease muscle spasms

Q65. A patient with fracture is being treated with a balanced suspension traction. Which of the following nursing interventions is appropriate?

A. Assess pin site and perform pin site care
B. Assess distal neurovascular status daily
C. Maintain elevation of head of bed at 45°
D. Perform activities of the daily living for the patient as the patient is immobilized

Q66. A patient with fracture femur on a balanced skeletal traction is required to visit X-ray department for X-rays. Which of the following nursing interventions during transport of the patient is not appropriate?

A. Explain the procedure to the patient
B. Offer a bedpan or urinal as required
C. Administer pain medication 30 minutes before transport as ordered
D. Remove weight of the traction before transferring to the radiology department

Q67. A young lady is being treated with a pelvic traction for a minor fracture in the lower spine. Nursing care should include assessment of which of the following?

A. Assessment of pin site every shift for infection
B. Checking for skin irritation over iliac crests and in the intergluteal cleft because of irritation from the pelvic belt
C. Assessment of peripheral pulses for decreased volume due to pressure on femoral artery
D. Checking for the ankle edema due to immobility

Q68. A young adult is placed in the Buck's traction following a fracture femur. The nurse explains to the patient that the purpose of Buck's traction is to:

A. Immobilize fractured limb

B. Prevent contractures
C. Promote circulation
D. Relieve pain

Q69. A nurse is caring for a patient who has balanced skeletal traction applied to his femur. Which of the following findings requires immediate intervention?

A. The foot end of the bed is elevated 30°
B. The traction cord is touching the edge of the bed
C. Patient's leg is suspended above the bed
D. The overhead trapeze is above the patient's chest

Q70. The nurse is caring for a patient whose left leg is in skeletal traction. Which of the following assessment should a nurse include in the patient's care plan?

A. Noting capillary refill time
B. Checking femoral pulses of both extremities for equality
C. Checking patellar reflex for nerve damage
D. All of the above

Q71. A Buck's traction has been applied on the right leg of a patient as a temporary measure. Which of the following range of weights should be applied for the traction?

A. 2-3 pounds
B. 3-5 pounds
C. 5-7 pounds
D. 7-10 pounds

Q72. A patient with fracture of the hip is placed on a Buck's traction as a temporary measure before surgery for internal fixation. To apply countertraction in the traction system the nurse should:

A. Elevate the foot end of the bed
B. Elevate the head end of the bed
C. Increase the weight of the traction
D. Decrease the weight of the traction

Q73. A patient has come to the hospital emergency with a compound fracture of tibia following an automobile accident. Which of the following actions by the nurse is appropriate?

A. Splint the leg in its present position
B. Irrigate the wound with normal saline
C. Apply pressure directly over the wound to stop bleeding
D. All of the above

Q74. A patient with fracture humerus has a temporary splint applied by an elastic bandage. The nurse caring for the patient suspects compartment syndrome when the patient experiences:

A. Pain at the fracture site
B. Severe edema of the limb
C. Twitching of the fingers
D. Pain when the nurse passively extends the fingers

Q75. Permanent damage of muscles and nerve may occur due to ischemia secondary to compartment syndrome within:

A. 1-2 hours
B. 2-4 hours
C. 4-12 hours
D. 24 hours

Q76. A patient has developed an acute compartment syndrome following a supracondylar fracture of the humerus. Appropriate treatment strategies for acute compartment syndrome include:

A. Amputation
B. Fasciotomy
C. Bivalving of the cast
D. Elevation of the extremity

Q77. The most frequent candidates of amputation of the lower extremities are the:

A. Young adults with an automobile accidents
B. Adolescents with bone cancer

C. Defense personnel with gunshot injuries
D. Elderlies with peripheral vascular diseases

Q78. Which of the following factors should be considered in deciding the levels of amputation?

A. Circulation in the parts
B. Functional usefulness of the residual limb
C. Possibility of preserving knee and elbow joints
D. Both A and B

Q79. Which of the following levels of amputation is called a Syme's amputation?

A. Hip disarticulation
B. Knee disarticulation
C. Ankle disarticulation
D. Wrist disarticulation

Q80. Which of the following methods of amputation will be adopted for a patient with gas gangrene following a gunshot wound of the right lower limb?

A. Closed amputation
B. Flap amputation
C. Guillotine amputation
D. Amputation with the immediate fitting of prosthesis

Q81. A nurse is caring for a patient with left above the knee amputation. Which of the following measures is appropriate on the first postoperative day?

A. Helping the patient to stand beside the bed with crutches
B. Helping the patient to lie prone in the bed
C. Making the patient to sit on the bed in high Fowler's position
D. Elevating the stump with a pillow placed under it

Q82. A nurse is educating a patient scheduled for an above the knee amputation of the left leg about phantom limb sensation. Which of the following information about phantom limb sensation is not correct?

A. Phantom limb sensation are feelings that the amputated limb is still present
B. Majority of the patients experiences this symptom after amputation for a varying period of time
C. Phantom limb sensation are always painful and distressing
D. Phantom sensation is due to the intact peripheral nerves proximal to the amputation site that is used to carry messages between the brain and the now amputated part.

Q83. A nurse is caring for a patient with an above knee amputation for traumatic injury. Which of the following actions should the nurse include in the postoperative care plan?

A. To monitor for post-traumatic stress disorder
B. Maintaining the patient for complete bed rest for the first 3 days
C. Keeping the residual limb elevated for the first 48 hours
D. Encouraging the patient to sit in high Fowler's position during waking hours from the first postoperative day onwards

Q84. A patient with above the knee amputation is being fitted with a cast after the amputation. 6 days after amputation the cast dressing accidentally comes off. What the nurse will do first?

A. Inform the surgeon
B. Reassure the patient that the incident commonly happens
C. Try to refit the cast
D. Wrap the residual limb with an elastic compression bandage immediately

Q85. The nurse was demonstrating stump-wrapping technique to a patient with below knee amputation before dis-

charge. When asked about the purposes of the procedure, the nurse's best response would be:

A. Stump wrapping would control pain
B. Stump wrapping would prevent injury
C. Stump wrapping would stimulate circulation
D. Stump wrapping would decrease edema

Q86. The nurse is taking care of a patient following open reduction with internal fixation of a hip fracture. Which of the following nursing actions she should include in the plan of care?

A. Monitoring peripheral circulation of the affected extremity
B. Instructing patient to perform extension and flexion of knee
C. Limiting fluid intake
D. Maintaining patient on strict bed rest for 72 hour postoperatively

Q87. A patient has undergone the hip replacement surgery following a complicated fracture of the hip. Postoperatively the nurse should place the patient's hip in which of the following positions?

A. Elevated with a pillow placed under the affected extremity
B. Abducted with a pillow placed in between the knees
C. Adducted with 2 pillows placed on both sides of the patient's legs
D. Flexed by placing a bolster under the affected leg

Q88. The nurse knows that after surgery on the left hip joint the affected extremity should be maintained in anatomical position but the patient is seen to keep the extremity externally rotated. To prevent external rotation the nurse should:

A. Place a pillow under the affected extremity
B. Place a sandbag on the outside of the ankle of the affected extremity
C. Place a pillow at the side of the knee of the affected extremity
D. Place a bolster under the knee of the affected extremity

Q89. The patient who has undergone open reduction and internal fixation for a hip fracture should be instructed to perform which of the following exercises in the immediate postoperative period?

A. Passive leg raising
B. Flexion and extension of the knee
C. Quadriceps and gluteal isometrics
D. Dorsiflexion, extension and plantiflexion of the ankle

Q90. The nurse is preparing a patient for discharge after a total hip replacement surgery. Which of the following statements if made by the patient indicates the need for further teaching?

A. I need to elevate my toilet seat
B. I should not sit with my legs crossed at the knee
C. Someone has to help me to put on my shoes
D. I do not need to sleep with a pillow in-between my legs any more

Q91. A patient has undergone a total knee replacement to treat degenerative joint disease of the right knee. During the immediate postoperative period the nurse should assess for which of the following conditions?

A. Restlessness, dyspnea and petechia
B. Redness and edema at the incision site
C. Fever and headache
D. Fecal impaction and abdominal pain

Q92. A patient admitted with the spinal cord injury complains of acute severe headache. The nurse understands that this is a symptom of:

A. Spinal shock
B. Autonomic hyperreflexia
C. Increased intracranial pressure
D. Meningitis

Q93. A victim of car accident has been brought to the emergency department.

The physician is suspecting spinal cord injury. Which of the following actions the nurse should take?

A. Elevating the patient's head at 30° angle to decrease the intracranial pressure
B. Placing the patient flat in bed with head turned to one side
C. Stabilizing patient's neck in a neutral position
D. Apply a head halter traction as ordered.

Q94. A patient with spinal cord injury complains of pounding headache. Anticipating patient's complain as a symptom of autonomic hyperreflexia the nurse should immediately assess:

A. Bladder distension
B. Breath sounds
C. Peripheral pulses
D. Body temperature

Q95. A patient with a total hip replacement of the left side is instructed to adopt which of the following techniques during turning in bed?

A. Turn while supporting affected leg with the unaffected leg
B. Flex both knees together and then turn to the unaffected side
C. Place a pillow in between the legs while turning to sides
D. Maintain flexion of the knee of the affected leg while turning

Q96. The nurse while taking care of a patient with cervical level spinal cord injury should give priority to which of the following nursing diagnoses?

A. Risk for hypotension
B. Ineffective airway clearance
C. Ineffective thermoregulation
D. Impaired physical mobility

Q97. A patient with fracture of the spine at the thoracic level has undergone instrumentation (stabilization of spine with internal fixation), and is on strict bed rest. Which of the technique the nurse should follow while repositioning the patient?

A. Do not reposition as the patient is on strict bed rest
B. Instruct the patient to cross right leg over left and turn on left side and vice versa
C. Instruct the patient to turn head to one side and then turn holding the side-rail of the bed
D. Get enough assistance and log- maneuver roll for the patient

Q98. The nurse is taking care of a young patient who has undergone open reduction for compound fracture of tibia. To which of the following nursing diagnoses she should give priority?

A. Impaired physical mobility related to surgery
B. Altered nutrition less than body requirement related to immobility
C. Boredom related to activity intolerance secondary to weight bearing limitations
D. Risk for infection related to the effects of trauma and surgery

Q99. A young boy aged 20 years who is rehabilitating after sustaining a fracture of the femur followed by open reduction with internal fixation is advised crutch walking with non-weight bearing on the affected leg. Which of the following observations by the nurse indicates further teaching on crutch walking?

A. He is using 3-point gait
B. He is placing crutches about 8-10 inches in the front and to the side of his toes
C. He is walking with his back straight
D. He is bearing weight on the axilla

Q100. The nurse is teaching a patient with a long leg cast to climb stairs with crutches. She should tell the patient to:

A. Advance both legs first
B. Advance unaffected leg first
C. Advance affected leg first
D. Advance both crutches first

ANSWERS AND RATIONALES OF MUSCULOSKELETAL SYSTEM

1. **D.** Obtaining information regarding vital signs is least important while assessing the status of musculoskeletal system. Musculoskeletal history consists of biographical and demographical data, chief complaints, past health history, psychosocial history, lifestyle history and review of systems.

2. **D.** Bones do not store any hormone. The major functions of bone are support, protection of internal organs, voluntary movement, blood cell production and mineral storage.

3. **B.** Osteoblasts are the basic bone-forming cells who synthesize organic bone matrix or collagen. Osteons are the structural units of compact bone and not bone cells. They are also known as haversian systems. Osteocytes are the mature bone cells. Osteoclasts are the cells that remove (resorb) damaged or old bone cells during the period of growth or repair.

4. **D.** The nurse should explain to the woman that with aging the intervertebral disc get narrowed due to loss of water from them resulting in disc compression and loss of height. Another cause of reduction in height in elderly women may be decrease in bone density due to osteoporosis resulting in vertebral compression. Other statements by the nurse are not appropriate.

5. **B.** After arthroscopy the nurse should place the affected limb elevated and the knee extended. This will reduce swelling and pain. To reduce swelling a compression dressing will also be applied.

6. **C.** The nurse should not administer any sedative or caffeinated drink 24 hours before the procedure since both affects muscle tone. Electromyography involves insertion of small gauze needles into the muscles to be examined. These are then connected to needle probes, which are attached to the leads that feed information about the electrical activity of the muscles to EMG machine and graphical records obtained. Patient feels discomfort from needle insertion, which should be explained beforehand. Patient need not remain nothing per oral (NPO) before the procedure. No radiopaque dye is used in this test.

7. **B.** Osteoarthritis is a slowly progressive noninflammatory disorder of the synovial joints. The disease was previously known as a degenerative disease but it is now known to involve new joint tissue formation in response to articular cartilage destruction. It is a most common form of arthritis, not rare, occurring in elderly persons, and not young persons. The primary osteoarthritis affects women more than men. It primarily affects the large and weight bearing joints of the body. It is a noninflammatory disease. Recurrent inflammation leading to destruction of joint occurs in the rheumatoid arthritis.

8. **B.** A number of factors have been identified for the development of idiopathic (formerly known as primary) osteoarthritis, e.g. increased age, lack of regular moderate exercise, and lack of estrogen after menopause. Mechanical stress, e.g. strenuous exercise like sports activities, trauma, e.g. fractures and dislocations, congenital skeletal deformity are the

causative factors of secondary osteoarthritis.

9. C. The characteristic symptom of osteoarthritis is the joint stiffness occurring after a period of rest or static position. Morning stiffness is a common manifestation. Morning stiffness usually resolves within 30 minutes with activity. Fever, malaise, tender swollen joints and morning stiffness lasting more than an hour is the manifestations of rheumatoid arthritis, a systemic inflammatory disease.

10. C. In the X-ray of a patient with osteoarthritis the nurse will note the formation of osteophytes, joint space narrowing and bony sclerosis. Elevated blood uric acid is found in the gout. Elevated erythrocyte sedimentation rate and increased white blood cells count in synovial fluid is found in rheumatoid arthritis.

11. C. One characteristic sign of osteoarthritis is the occurrence of Heberden's nodes appearing on distal interphalangeal (DIP) joints as an indication of osteophyte formation and loss of joint space. Similarly, Bouchard's nodes may appear on the proximal interphalangeal (PIP) joints. Osteoarthritis usually affects the joints asymmetrically, not symmetrically. Patient complains of increasing pain on activity, not after rest. Multiple subcutaneous nodules are present in, rheumatoid arthritis.

12. D. In osteoarthritis synovial fluid analysis shows a clear yellow colored synovial fluid with little or no sign of inflammation. Gray colored fluid, below normal glucose content and a white blood cells count above 25,000/ microliter is found in the presence of infection, i.e. septic arthritis.

13. B. The patient with osteoarthritis should be taught to maintain a careful balance between rest and exercise. Exercise helps in weight loss, increases muscle tone and enhances joint stability. Patient should be taught to rest the affected joint when it is painful and inflamed. Affected joints should be rested with splints or braces if necessary. But immobilization should not exceed more than 1week, because of the risk of joint stiffness with inactivity. Patient should be taught to consume a well balanced diet and not a high caloric diet to maintain a healthy body weight. If the patient is overweight she should consume a low caloric diet.

14. D. Osteoarthritis is a chronic and disabling disease. The most common symptom of the disease is deep aching joint pain especially in the morning and after weight bearing activities. As rest usually reduces the pain the nurse should instruct the patient to rest frequently particularly after activities.

15. B. Sodium retention and hypertension is one of the adverse effects of ibuprofen. Other adverse effects are gastrointestinal bleeding, injury to articular cartilage, renal and hepatic damage. Hypotension, increased pain in joints and diminished vision are not associated with ibuprofen. Dizziness and hearing loss are associated with salicylates.

16. B. Intra-articular administration of hyaluronic acid is effective in treating the pain and functional impairment of ostoarthritic knee by restoring the elastoviscosity of the synovial fluid. Application of capsaicin cream and hot and cold application is effective in the treatment of osteoarthritis

but their action do not restore elastoviscocity of the synovial fluid of the knee joint, neither vitamin C has any effect on the treatment of osteoarthritis.

17. C. Osteoarthritis is a non-inflammatory disease of the joints that particularly affect the weight bearing joints. It is not due to infection. Non-inflammatory changes of osteoarthritis causes thinning of articular cartilage resulting in narrowing of joint spaces and shortening of limbs. Extra-articular systemic involvement occurs in rheumatoid arthritis not in osteoarthritis.

18. C. Nursing management of an elderly patient with osteoarthritis should be aimed in helping the patient to achieve independence, as these patients has joint stiffness resulting in impaired functional ability and range of motion. These problems coupled with old age severely impair self-care capacity of the patient. Osteoarthritis does not cause ineffective breathing pattern; neither the patient should remain immobile in bed, so the objective of establishing effective breathing pattern is not appropriate. Providing adequate nutrition to increase the body weight is also not appropriate, as the patient needs to reduce weight.

19. C. The nurse should instruct the patient to hold the cane on the unaffected side. In normal walking, the opposite leg and arm move together (reciprocal motion) and this motion has to be carried through in walking with a cane. A patient with osteoarthritis should always use a cane whether at home or outside. The use of cane or any other assistive device, e.g. walker or crutches takes weight and stress off joints.

20. B. Heredity, low body weight and early menopause are involved in the development of osteoporosis. Other factors involved are inadequate physical activity, low intake of dietary calcium, suboptimal levels of serum vitamin D, not above the normal levels, cigarette smoking, and excessive alcohol consumption.

21. B. Osteoporosis can result from many underlying medical conditions. All of the conditions mentioned here can result in the osteoporosis except hypoparathyroidism. Hyperparathyroidism may cause osteoporosis. Other associated conditions are anorexia nervosa, Cushing's syndrome, and long-term use of thyroid hormone and furosemide.

22. A. The most common complication of osteoporosis is the fragility fractures or osteoporotic fractures. Damage of synovial joints occurs in the osteoarthritis. Renal stone may occur in the patients with osteoporosis but it is not that common as osteoporotic fractures. Bone cancer is not related to osteoporosis.

23. B. The nurse should emphasize regular physical activity and weight bearing exercises like walking, stair climbing, dancing, etc. as exercises decrease bone resorbtion and stimulates bone formation. Inactivity produces the rapid bone loss. Consumption of caffeine promotes calcium excretion, but consuming extra calcium may offset the negative effects of caffeine. Exposure to sun provides vitamin D which is necessary for the metabolism of calcium. Osteoporosis may be prevented by the high calcium intake in diet not protein.

24. C. The dietary instruction to a patient with osteoporosis should include increased consumption of dairy products for an adequate amount of calcium in the diet. Dairy products provide about 75% of the calcium in the average daily diets. Reducing fat intake and increasing consumption of fruits and vegetables do not help a patient with osteoporosis. Patient should not consume high sodium in diet. High sodium consumption increases calcium excretion.

25. D. The daily calcium intake for postmenopausal woman should be 1500 mg. Less than this would be inadequate for a postmenopausal woman.

26. D. Human parethyroid hormone is not used in the prevention or treatment of osteoporosis. Parethyroid stimulates bone resorption so that it will develop osteoporosis, not prevent or treat. All drugs used in the prevention and treatment of osteoporosis inhibit bone resorption thereby increasing bone mineral density (BMD) and total bone mass. The drugs used are estrogens, calcitonin, biphosphonates (alendronate) and selective estrogen receptor modulators (SERM).

27. D. Gout is caused by an increased purine synthesis, decreased excretion of purine or increased consumption of purine in diet.

28. B. In chronic gout, the nurse is expected to find the appearance of tophi (visible deposits of sodium urate crystals) on the ears, hands, elbows, feet and knees. Chronic gout is characterized by the multiple joint involvement. Bouchard's nodes appear in the osteoarthritis and rheumatic nodules appear as extra-articular manifestation of rheumatoid arthritis.

29. D. After oral administration of colchicine dramatic pain relief occurs usually after 12 to 48 hours. Pain may be relieved within 4 to 12 hours of intravenous administration.

30. A. Colchicine controls the pain in acute gout by relieving the sudden onset of severe inflammation. The drug inhibits granulocyte migration into the inflamed joints and thus interrupts inflammation initiated by the deposition of urate crystals in the synovial fluid. Gout is not associated with infection. The drug does not regulate serum uric acid levels. So treatment with colchicine may be continued for 4-8 weeks with maintenance doses in which time control of hyperuricemia is achieved with other drugs.

31. B. Allopurinol given in the chronic gout, acts by blocking the production of uric acid and thus maintains normal uric acid level in the blood. Probenecid inhibits renal tubular reabsorption of urates and losartan an angiotensin II receptor antagonist promotes urate diuresis and is helpful in the elderly patients with hypertension.

32. C. To determine the effectiveness of the therapy with probenecid or any other drug the serum uric acid level should be checked regularly. Although X-ray are diagnostic in the late stages of gout but not done periodically to monitor the effectiveness of treatment. Serum calcium level is not related to gout. Serum creatinine level is checked before initiation of therapy with probenecid as the drug is ineffective in the presence of kidney damage. So serum creatinine level is required to determine the effectiveness of therapy before initiation of treatment with the drug but not during treatment.

33. A. Immediate nursing intervention for a patient with acute gouty arthritis would be to relieve pain. Bed rest; relieving pressure and injury from affected joint; immobilization of affected joint and administering drugs like colchicine or NSAIDs may relieve the pain. Crutch walking may be taught during ambulation if needed. It is not an immediate intervention. After the initial attack of pain subsides the patient should be taught self- care measures which include adhering to treatment program, modification of diet, encouraging ample fluid intake, etc. as it is a chronic problem. Administration of diuretics to promote diuresis is not a method of treatment of acute gouty arthritis.

34. B. A patient with gout should be instructed to drink plenty of fluids to promote uric acid excretion. Dietary modification is not essential in the treatment of gout. Some physician may recommend avoiding red and organ meats. Patient should avoid excessive alcohol consumption. High calorie and high fat diet should be avoided for the gradual weight reduction if the patient is overweight. If indomethacin is prescribed for pain relief, it should be taken with food and not on empty stomach, to reduce gastric irritation. Patient's blood should be periodically examined for serum uric acid level and not for white blood cells count, to check the effectiveness of treatment.

35. C. Prolonged period of sitting is a risk factor for low back pain. Regular walking, ideal body weight and young age are at low-risk of developing low back pain.

36. D. Diazepam is prescribed for a patient with acute low back pain to decrease muscle spasm. Diazepam is an antianxiety drug and is used to relieve anxiety but in this situation the purpose is to reduce muscle spasm. Diazepam does not have any action in inflammatory process neither it enhances analgesic action of indomethacin.

37. D. Patient with low back pain should be advised to sleep in a side-lying position with his knees and hips flexed. Patient may also sleep in supine position with a lift under the knees and legs. These positions with knees and hips flexed prevent unnecessary pressure on support muscles, ligamentous structures and lumbosacral joints. Sleeping in side-lying position or supine position with legs straight should be avoided for the same reason. Patient should avoid sleeping in prone position as it produces excessive lumbar lordosis resulting in excessive stress on the lower back.

38. D. Herniation of an intervertebral disc can be the result of natural degeneration of the disc or vertebra with age or repeated stress and trauma to the spine. Strenuous activity or degeneration of the disc or vertebra can allow the disc to move from its normal position and results in herniation.

39. B. Herniation of intervertebral disc may occur at any level but most common sites of herniation are the L4-L5 and L5-S1.

40. A. The patient with herniated disc at the region of 4th to 5th lumbar vertebra is likely to experience severe lower back pain that radiates down the buttocks to dorsum of foot and big toe along the distribution of sciatic nerve as a result of compression of the spinal nerve roots. Herniation of the disc at the region of L3 to L4 will have severe lower back pain radiating down the buttocks to inner calf. Herniation of disc at lumbar region is not associated with the shortness of breath. Weakness and atrophy of leg muscles, not arm muscles, may appear at the later stage of the disease.

41. C. A herniated nucleus pulposus can be diagnosed with a myelography. Other tests to diagnose this condition include CT scan, MRI. X-rays and lumbar puncture cannot diagnose this condition.

42. B. The nurse should first assess the sensation of lower extremities by asking whether there is paresthesia or numbness in the involved limb. The nurse will enforce bed rest for 1-2 days, administer pain medication as prescribed and teach back strengthening exercises only after thorough assessment of the patient to identify his actual needs.

43. D. Back strengthening exercises are not initiated in the acute stage. Once the acute symptoms subside back strengthening exercises are begun twice a day and are encouraged for a lifetime. In addition to back strengthening exercises the patient is taught principles of good body mechanics, and to avoid extremes of flexion and torsion.

44. C. The most common and traditional surgical procedure for lumbar disc disease is laminectomy. Diskectomy is the another common type of surgical procedure. Percutaneous laser diskectomy and microdiskectomy are the other versions of standard diskectomy where a microscope is used for better visualization and a laser is used on the herniated portion of the disc respectively. Spinal fusion is also performed for disc disease but are less common.

45. D. To avoid twisting the spine or hips when turning a patient on to the side, the nurse should use the log roll technique. After surgery the nurse should not put anything under the knees or place the patient in the semi-Fowler's position as these actions increase the risk of deep vein thrombosis. The patient should be out of bed on the first or second postoperative day.

46. A. The nurse should first assess the bladder for distension. If the bladder is distended, then she should obtain an order for catheterization. If the bladder is not distended she should assess hydration of the patient and increase the flow rate of intravenous infusion if needed. After spinal surgery, the patient usually remains on flat bed rest for 1-2 days depending on the amount of surgery. So helping the patient to use a commode on the day of operation would not be an appropriate action by the nurse.

47. A. Postoperatively the nurse should assess for the development of paralytic ileus which may result due to lack of peristalsis from a sudden loss of parasympathetic function innervating the bowels. Postoperatively the patient may have the retention of urine due to difficulty in bladder emptying, not frequency of urination. Patient may develop paresthesia of lower extremities, not upper extremities. Flank pain is associated with kidney problem not a complication of spinal surgery.

48. B. After lumbar laminectomy, the patient should be instructed not to sit or stand for a prolonged time. The patient should sleep on the bed with a firm, not soft mattress. He should drink plenty of water and high fiber food in order to prevent constipation and straining on stools. Frequency of urination is usually not associated with the spinal surgery. Patient does not need an abdominal binder to support the incision after laminectomy.

49. C. The nurse will document her observation as kyphosis (an increased roundness or convexity of the thoracic spinal curve). Kyphosis is frequently seen in elderlies who are experiencing osteoporosis. Other causes of kyphosis are poor posture, tuberculosis, arthritis and growth disturbance of vertebral epiphyses. Lordosis is the exaggeration of the concave portion of the thoracic spine, and is normal in toddler and pregnant women, but considered abnormal in other populations. Scoliosis is a lateral curving of the thoracic spine. Scoliosis may be congenital, idiopathic or due to injury or osteomalacia.
Ankylosis is scarring within a joint leading to the stiffness or fixation due to chronic joint inflammation.

50. B. Scoliosis is a lateral curvature or S shaped curvature of the thoracic and lumbar spine. Unequal shoulder and scapula height usually indicates scoliosis. Other assessment findings include head not in alignment with gluteal fold, unequal leg length and asymmetry in the flank area.

51. D. The nurse should instruct the patient to wear the brace continuously for 23 hours a day, 7 days a week. The brace may be removed during bathing or swimming for 1 hour only. The brace should not be worn over bare body as it may give rise to skin irritation. It should be worn over one shirt.

52. A. In osteomyelitis, microorganism can invade bone, bone marrow or surrounding tissue by direct or indirect mechanisms. Blunt trauma or any other penetrating injury is most commonly responsible for osteomyelitis. IV drug abuse and immunosuppression are not the cause of osteomyelitis, but people with IV drug abuse and immunosuppression are at higher risk of developing osteomyelitis. Pelvic surgery is not likely to cause osteomyelitis, but the presence of foreign body such as an implant or an orthopedic prosthetic device may cause osteomyelitis.

53. A. Bone has very poor blood circulation making it difficult to treat an infection in the bone. This requires long-term use of parenteral antibiotics in order to eradicate the infection. Pus and necrotic bone material does not absorb antibiotic but they cause pressure in the affected area, further compromising the blood circulation. So surgical debridement and drainage prepares the area so that circulation is promoted and antibiotics may work more effectively. Organisms responsible for osteomyelitis most commonly are *Staphylococcus aureus, Escherichia coli, Pseudomonas, Klebsiela, Salmonella,* etc. are sensitive to many available antibiotics.

54. D. The correct sequence of stages of bone healing are inflammatory stage or hematoma stage, fibrocartilage formation, callous formation, ossification, consolidation and remodelling. Likeother tissues, bone healing does not take place by the scar formation.

55. D. Clinical manifestations of fracture include pain and tenderness, deformity, loss of function. Other sign and symptoms include edema and swelling, muscle spasm and ecchymosis. Edema, pain and ecchymosis occur in the sprain also. Tingling, coolness and loss of pulses are the signs of vascular insufficiency. Coolness, heavyness and paresthesia are the signs of neurological impairment.

56. D. When the fracture line occurs at the 90° angle to longitudinal axis of long bone, the fracture is called a transverse fracture. A linear fracture has an intact fracture line. In oblique fracture, the fracture line is at 45° angle across the longitudinal axis of the bone and in logitudinal fracture, fracture line extends in the direction of the bone's longitudinal axis.

57. A. A colles' fracture is the fracture of the distal radius and is a very common fracture of the adults. The styloid process of the ulna may also be involved along with the radius.

58. A. The patient is experiencing the inflammatory stage of the bone healing process. During this stage there is bleeding into the injured tissue and the formation of a hematoma. White blood cells begin debridement of dead cells. Fibrocartilage formation stage occurs within 314 days of injury. Fibrin strands begin to form and the interrupted blood supply is recreated, cartilage and fibrous connective tissue develop. The callous formation stage occurs as minerals are deposited in the fibrocartilage formed on each bone fragment. The gap created by the fracture begins to close. After approximately 3-4 weeks the fractured bone fragments will be united. The ossification stage is identified by the formation of bone substance within the callous and continued unification of the fracture. The process may take 3-6 months after the fracture. The final remodelling of the affected bone may take additional months to years depending upon the injury, the bone and the general healing process.

59. A. Numbness complained by the patient is most probably due to pressure on the ulnar or median nerve by the fracture hematoma or due to the damage of the nerves by the broken fragments of bone. Ischemia would have caused coolness and cyanosis of the hand and fingers. Muscle spasm would give rise to pain not numbness. Fear and anxiety usually causes exaggeration of pain sensation, not numbness.

60. B. Symptoms of fat embolism are tachypnea, dyspnea, mental confusion and petechial rash. Chest pain, dyspnea, nausea, vomiting may be the symptoms of myocardial infarction. Bradycardia, bradypnea, hypothermia, chest pain are not associated with the fat embolism. Tachycardia, tachypnea, hypotension, oliguria are the symptoms of shock.

61. A. The nurse would allow the patient to walk with the cast after 30 minutes as synthetic cast takes 30 minutes to set completely and allow weight bearing depending on the nature of injury and the physician's order.

62. C. The nurse should immediately report capillary refill is greater than 3 seconds which indicates vascular compromise or pressure from the cast. Mild edema is usually present after injury and is seen in the dependent uncasted fingers and need not be reported. Severe edema indicates the pressure from the cast and should be reported. Some pain immediately after injury is usually present which should lessen after the fracture is reduced and immobilized. Increasing pain should be reported. An elderly lady of 80 years may feel cold due to heat lost by evaporation during drying of the cast and is normal and need not be reported.

63. D. The physician should be informed immediately since tingling sensation in the leg and foot indicates too tight cast is causing neurovascular compromise. Tingling sensation during drying of the cast is not an usual symptom. Patient's symptoms indicate arterial insufficiency so elevation of the limb is not recommended. Exercise of the fingers does not allow increased circulation.

64. C. Traction is not applied for comfort. In fact traction is rather uncomfortable. Other purposes of traction are the to reduce a fracture, reduce a dislocation, immobilize extremity and provide rest.

65. A. The appropriate nursing intervention for a patient in balanced suspension traction is to assess the pin site and perform pin site care, as balanced suspension traction is a form of skeletal traction. The nurse should assess the distal neurovascular status of the affected extremity every 4 hourly, not daily. The head of the bed should not be elevated more than 25° as it may cause continued movement toward the foot of bed. Patient should be encouraged self-help in activities of daily living and movement in bed with the help of trapeze.

66. D. Traction weight should never be removed or changed without the order of the physician. The nurse should maintain the traction constantly and not interrupt the weight applied to the traction. All procedures should be explained to the patient. Offering bedpan or urinal before transport is appropriate, as the patient may have to wait in radiology department for sometime. A pain medication the 30 minutes before transport helps to relieve pain associated with the transfer to trolley from bed and vice versa.

67. B. Nursing care of a patient with pelvic traction should include checking for skin irritation over iliac crests and in the intergluteal fold due to irritation by the pelvic belt or girdle. Pelvic traction is applied by the pelvic belt or girdle and no pin is inserted. Exerting pressure on the deep femoral artery by pelvic traction belt is very unusual. Ankle edema is also not associated with the pelvic traction or immobility. It may occur if the patient has concurrent heart disease or renal disease.

68. A. Buck's traction provides a straight pull on the affected extremity and is used to immobilize a limb temporarily until the skeletal traction or surgery is possible. The traction is also a means to maintain alignment, assist in reduction and helps diminish the muscle spasms in the injured extremity. Buck's traction does not prevent contractures, but it may be used to correct hip and knee joint contractures. Buck's traction does not promote circulation. By reducing muscle spasm, relieving pressure on nerves by fractured bone and immobilizing, it may lessen pain but it is not used for the purpose of reliving pain.

69. B. When a patient is in traction, the nurse should check the traction apparatus in each shift. The traction cord attached with the weight should hang freely and not touch the edge of the bed. Foot end should be elevated 30° to augment countertraction. In balanced suspension traction patient's leg is suspended, this allows raising of the buttocks off the bed for bedpan use and skin care. The overhead trapeze should be above the patient's chest.

70. A. While caring for a patient in traction the nurse should assess patient regularly for neurovascular complications. Capillary refill time should be checked daily to detect the arterial insufficiency. Femoral pulses are proximal to the traction, hence equality of femoral pulses would not indicate vascular impairment due to traction. Nurse should palpate posterior tibial and dorsalis pedis for the same. To check for nerve damage, functioning of the peroneal and tibial nerves should be assessed by the dorsiflexion and plantar flexion, not the patellar reflex.

71. D. In a Buck's traction, traction weight should not be more than 7- 10 pounds because of skin's intolerance to pressure.

72. A. Elevating the foot end of the bed helps gravity to work on the weight of the patient and thus increases countertraction.

73. A. The nurse will first immobilize the limb before the patient is transferred to the orthopedic department. Adequate splinting is essential to prevent further soft tissue damage. No attempt should be made to reduce the fracture or to correct the alignment. The wound should be covered with a sterile dressing to prevent contamination of deeper tissue. Pressure should not be applied directly on the wound.

74. D. One of the manifestations of the compartment syndrome is pain on passive stretch of muscle traveling through the compartment. Other manifestations are pain distal to the injury, paresthesia, increased compartment pressure, pallor, paralysis and pulselessness. Pain at the fracture site, severe edema of the limb, twitchings of the fingers do not indicate the compartment syndrome.

75. C. Ischemia can occur within 4-12 hours after onset of compartment syndrome. So early recognition and treatment are essential to avoid permanent damage to muscles and nerve due to ischemia.

76. B. Treatment strategies for acute compartment syndrome include surgical decompression or fasciotomy of the involved compartment. Amputation is not a treatment of compartment syndrome. A functionally useless extremity resulting from compartment syndrome may be amputated. Timely bivalving of a constricted cast may prevent compartment syndrome. Elevation of the extremity above the heart level is contraindicated in a patient with suspected compartment syndrome as elevation reduces arterial perfusion.

77. D. Elderlies with peripheral vascular diseases are the most frequent candidates for the lower limb amputation. Traumatic injuries among the young are also a common cause of amputation.

78. D. Amputation is performed at the most distal point that will heal successfully. The most favorable site is determined by the two factors. 1. Circulatory status in the parts as adequate muscle and skin perfusion is essential for the proper healing and 2. Functional usefulness, i.e. the length of the residual limb which meets the requirement of prosthesis. Preservation of knee and elbow joints are desirable but most important is circulatory status of the part.

79. C. Ankle disarticulation is known as Syme's amputation.

80. C. For the patient with gas gangrene or any other infection or potential to infection guillotine amputation or open amputation is performed. In this type of amputation, a surface on the residual limb is left that is not covered with the skin flap in order to allow the wound to drain freely. When the infection is totally eradicated the patient undergoes another operation for stump closure. This method of amputation is also called staged amputation. Closed amputation and the flap amputation are the same procedure and are done when there is no evidence of infection. Amputation with immediate fitting of prosthesis is also not indicated in the patient with infection.

81. B. The nurse should help and encourage the patient to lie in the prone position for 20-30 minutes for 3-4 times a day. Lying in the prone position with extension of the hip will prevent flexion contracture which, if develops will delay rehabilitation. The patient does not use crutches until he has stable balance. An amputee usually begins ambulation with parallel bars. Patient should not sit in the high Fowler's position or on the wheelchair for more than 1 hour. Sitting for prolonged time will promote flexion contracture. Elevating the stump on pillow also promotes flexion contracture.

82. C. Although phantom limb sensation are often referred to as phantom pain, not all of the sensations are painful. The patient may describe sensations of cold, warmth, itching or pain especially in the amputated fingers or toes. Phantom sensation often are felt immediately after surgery and gradually decrease over the next 2 years.

83. A. The postoperative care of a patient with above knee amputation for traumatic injury should include monitoring for post-traumatic stress disorder because the patient had no time to get prepared or perhaps even participate in the decision to have a limb amputated. The residual limb should remain elevated for only 24 hours. Longer than this will cause flexion contracture. Maintaining the patient in complete bed rest for first 3 days will cause complications due to immobility.

84. D. If the rigid dressing or cast comes off accidentally, the nurse must immediately wrap the residual limb with an elastic compression bandage. If not, excessive edema will develop in a short time, resulting in a delay in rehabilitation. The nurse then notifies the surgeon so that another cast can be applied. Only reassuring does not help the patient. Trying to refit the cast also not helpful. The cast may not fit as the stump tends to shrink as it heals and a loose cast will not provide adequate compression. Usually the rigid dressing (cast) is changed 3-4 times before an application of a permanent prosthesis.

85. D. Wrapping a stump with an elastic compression bandage reduces edema and shapes the residual limb in a firm conical form for the prosthesis. Stump wrapping is not done for the purpose of stimulating circulation, controlling pain, or preventing injury.

86. A. Monitoring peripheral circulation of the affected extremity must be included in the postoperative care plan of a patient with the hip surgery. A comprehensive evaluation of peripheral circulatory status of the affected extremity by frequently checking peripheral pulses, edema, capillary refill color, temperature of extremity is absolutely important as the patient is at the risk for peripheral neurovascular dysfunction. Patient is not instructed to perform flexion and extension of knee because postoperatively an abduction pillow is placed in between the knees which will interfere with flexion and extension of knee. Adequate fluid is administered to the patient to prevent increased blood viscosity and development of deep vein thrombosis. To prevent complication of immobility, the patient should be ambulated on the first or the second post-operative day.

87. B. After a total hip replacement the patient's hip and leg should be placed in a position of abduction. This position of abduction will help the prosthesis to remain within the acetabulum. The affected leg is not placed elevated or flexed. Placing a bolster under the knee will facilitate deep vein thrombosis which must be avoided. External rotation of the hip to be avoided by placing a trochanter roll.

88. C. Prevention of external rotation is a function of the hip joint. During the postoperative period support must be provided by placing a pillow or a sandbag outside the knee of the affected limb.

89. D. The patient after hip surgery is at high-risk of developing deep vein thrombosis. So the patient should be instructed to perform dorsiflexion, extension and plantiflexion of the ankle as soon as he is alert. One day postoperatively the patient should begin exercises to restore strength and tone of the hip muscles by gluteal and quadriceps isometrics, active leg raising.

90. D. The patient after total hip replacement surgery should maintain the hip in a position of abduction. He should continue to use a pillow in between the legs when lying supine or on the good side for the first 8 weeks postoperatively. All other statements indicate adequate teaching.

91. A. Patients with total knee replacement surgery are at high-risk for fat embolism during the first 24-72 hours after surgery. Symptoms of fat embolism include anxiety, chest pain, dyspnea, tachypnea, restlessness, confusion and petechia. Redness and edema at the incision site and fever and headache indicates infection which is usually not present in the immediate postoperative period. Fecal impaction may occur in the postoperative period but assessment of fecal impaction in the immediate postoperative period is not a priority.

92. B. Autonomic hyperreflexia is a life-threatening syndrome resulting from exaggerated sympathetic response to a noxious stimulus below the level of the cord lesion which is above the T 6 level. Symptoms of autonomic hyperreflexia are hypertension, a pounding headache, diaphoresis, bradycardia, restlessness, nausea, dilated pupils and blurred vision. Spinal shock is characterized by the paralyzed and flaccid muscles, loss of autonomic reflexes, hypotension, loss of temperature control mechanism. Patients with increased intracranial pressure and meningitis also complains of headache, but these are not associated with the spinal cord injury.

93. C. The nurse should stabilize the neck of the injured person in neutral position without flexion or extension until a fixed immobilizing device can be applied. No part of the body should be twisted or turned. Cervical traction should not be applied without X-ray film to guide movements as the spinal cord may be injured.

94. The manifestations of autonomic hyperreflexia result from an exaggerated sympathetic response to a noxious stimuli. The stimuli are commonly bladder and bowel distension. So the nurse should immediately assess for bladder distension. The other stimuli which may precipitate autonomic hyperreflexia are pressure ulcers, spasms, pain and pressure on the penis or uterine contractions, excessive rectal stimulation, etc. Breath sounds, peripheral pulses and body temperature are not the priority assessment for autonomic hyperreflexia.

95. C. A patient with total hip replacement should be instructed to place a pillow in between the legs while turning on sides in order to maintain the abduction. Care should be taken to maintain the hip extended and abducted. All other methods promote adduction and must be avoided.

96. B. Cervical level spinal cord injuries are mostly associated with a high-risk of respiratory compromise. So the priority nursing diagnosis is ineffective airway clearance. All other nursing diagnoses are appropriate but not priority as compared to ineffective airway clearance.

97. D. The patient should be repositioned by using log-rolling maneuver to maintain proper bony alignment after surgery. Twisting movements may cause indwelling instruments to twist the spine which must be avoided. Other techniques mentioned will cause twisting movements of the spine. The patient should be repositioned every 2 hourly.

98. D. A compound fracture has a break in the skin over the bone injury and is open to the environment. Because the wound communicates with the external environment the risk of infection is high. The risk increases with surgical repair of the fracture. So the priority nursing diagnosis should be risk for infection related to the effects of trauma and surgery. All other nursing diagnoses are appropriate but not priority over the risk of infection.

99. D. The patient should not bear weight on the axilla. He should support weight on the hand pieces. If weight is borne on the axilla, the constant pressure on the brachial plexus nerve may cause crutch paralysis. The boy needs further teaching on this area. The other observations about crutch walking are correct.

100. B. The nurse should teach the patient to advance unaffected leg first ('up with the good'). While climbing stairs body weight is first transferred to the crutches. Unaffected leg is then advanced to the stair. Body weight is then shifted to the unaffected leg. The affected leg together with the crutches is then advanced. The process is repeated with other steps.

10 CHAPTER

Integumentary System and Burns

Q1. The innermost layer of the epidermis is:

A. Stratum corneum
B. Stratum germinativum
C. Stratum lucidum
D. Stratum granulosum

Q2. The eccrine glands secrete:

A. Melanine
B. Sebum
C. Sweat
D. Hormones

Q3. The most important function of the skin is :

A. Absorption of medication
B. Protection of underlying tissues
C. Sensory perception for environmental stimuli
D. Production of vitamin

Q4. The most important contributing factor for the wrinkling of skin of the aged is:

A. Heredity
B. Poor nutrition
C. Ill health
D. Chronic exposure to ultraviolet (UV) rays

Q5. Which of the following would the nurse expect to find in an elderly patient's skin?

A. Increased sweat production
B. Increased nail growth
C. Increased awareness of pain
D. Diminished rate of wound healing

Q6. During the physical examination of a patient's skin the nurse would:

A. Have a private examination room with good daylight
B. Inspect skin to determine skin turgor
C. Examine specific lesion first followed by a general inspection
D. Palpate areas of bruising for the possible blanching

Q7. Patient comes to the outpatient department with skin lesions. The nurse finds the skin lesions as the elevated, sharply defined, less than 1cm in diameter and filled with serous fluid. The nurse documents her observation as:

A. Papule
B. Vesicles
C. Cysts
D. Pustules

Q8. The skin lesions that are found by the nurse during physical examination of a patient and described as firm, edematous and irregularly shaped areas of varying diameter are called:

A. Macules
B. Papules

C. Wheals
D. Pustules

Q9. The technique of obtaining the skin specimen for the histological assessment include:

A. Shave biopsy
B. Punch biopsy
C. Surgical excision
D. Any of the above

Q10. During physical examination of a patient's skin and fingernails, the nurse notes a linear brown streak in the nail plate. When documenting this finding the nurse should use which of the following terms?

A. Beau's line
B. Splinter hemorrhage
C. Clubbing
D. Paronychia

Q11. Which of the following ingredients makes a sunscreen most effective?

A. Parsol (Avobenzone)
B. Salicylates
C. Cinnamates
D. Benzophenones

Q12. A patient with severe impetigo should be treated with:

A. Warm saline soaks followed by soap and water removal of crusts
B. Topical antibiotics
C. Systemic antibiotics
D. All of the above

Q13. To treat a patient with severe acne vulgaris, the physician is most likely to prescribe which of the following pharmacological agents?

A. Erythromycin
B. Pyrimethamine
C. Miconazole
D. Acyclovir

Q14. A patient has developed cellulitis in the right leg. There is a swelling above the ankle and below the knee. The nurse will teach the patient:

A. A range of motion exercises to prevent contractures
B. To apply elastic bandage to reduce the swelling
C. To apply warm moist compresses frequently
D. To immobilize the limb by applying splint to the affected leg

Q15. A patient is getting IV gentamicin sulphate for severe cellulitis of the right leg. The nurse teaches the patient to report if he experiences:

A. Double vision
B. Disturbances in hearing
C. Hoarseness of voice
D. Tightness in the chest

Q16. A patient with herpes zoster has come to a medical ward for the admission. Where the nurse should place the patient?

A. Isolation room with negative pressure airflow
B. Private cabin
C. Room shared by one patient with COPD
D. Room shared by a patient with diabetes having previous history of chickenpox

Q17. The nurse anticipates that a patient who is diagnosed with herpes zoster will be treated by:

A. Tetracycline
B. Famciclovir
C. Liquid nitrogen
D. Miconazole

Q18. A patient with herpes zoster has been prescribed famciclovir 500 mg 8 hourly. The nurse should inform the patient that this drug may cause:

A. Hypotension
B. Burning urination

C. Diarrhea
D. Palpitation

Q19. An elderly woman with the complain of pruritus and skin rash in submammary folds attends the hospital clinic. On examination the nurse finds diffuse papular erythematous rash with pinpoint satellite lesions around the edges of the affected area. The nurse suspects that the patient may be suffering from:

A. Moniliasis
B. Tinea corporis
C. Scabies
D. Herpes zoster

Q20. Which of the following terms refers to a fungal infection of the foot?

A. Tinea corporis
B. Tinea pedis
C. Tinea capities
D. Tinea curis

Q21. The nurse is examining a child's scalp for the presence of lice. Which part of the patient's scalp the nurse should especially examine?

A. Top of the head
B. Behind the ears
C. Back of the neck
D. All except A

Q22. A patient admitted in the medical ward is found to have scabies. What the nurse should do to prevent the scabies infection in other patient?

A. Practice meticulous handwashing
B. Place the patient on enteric precaution
C. Isolate patient's bed linen until the patient is no longer infectious
D. Apply pediculicide to the patient's scalp

Q23. The physician has prescribed benzyl benzoate emulsion application to a patient diagnosed with scabies. The nurse teaches the patient regarding the prescribed treatment. Which of the following instructions is appropriate?

A. 'All your family members should be treated simultaneously with the medication'
B. 'If someone develops symptoms tell him to apply the medicine'
C. 'Do not share towels and linens with other family members'
D. 'Apply the medication as prescribed, otherwise the infection will spread to other family members'

Q24. A patient with contact dermatitis is prescribed topical corticosteroids to be applied twice a day. Which of the following instructions regarding the application of topical corticosteroids is appropriate?

A. 'Apply the medicine on the affected part as a thick coating'
B. 'Stop applying the medicine as soon as symptoms disappear'
C. 'Apply the medicine in long upward strokes in the direction opposite hair growth for better absorption'
D. 'Too frequent and prolonged application of the drug may cause skin atrophy'

Q25. Which of the following factors may be the cause of atopic dermatitis?

A. Contact with allergen
B. Infection by virus
C. Nutritional deficiencies
D. Family history of allergy

Q26. A common site for the lesions associated with atopic dermatitis is:

A. Elbow bends
B. Axilla
C. Groin
D. Buttocks

Q27. Which of the following nursing diagnoses is not appropriate for an young boy suffering from atopic dermatitis?

A. Impaired skin integrity related to skin dryness
B. Alteration in comfort related to pruritus
C. Risk for infection transmission to others
D. Body image disturbance related to unsightly skin lesions

Q28. Physician has prescribed soaks, application of topical corticosteroid followed by the occlusive dressings for a young girl having lesion of atopic dermatitis in the antecubital area. What is the purpose of occlusive dressings in this condition?

A. Promote absorption of topical corticosteroid
B. Promote hydration of the skin by preventing evaporation from hydrated epidermis
C. Promote cooling of the skin
D. All of the above

Q29. Which of the following statements accurately describes intertrigo?

A. Epidermal thickening resulting in elevated plaque with accentuated skin markings
B. Unpigmented skin patches associated with the lack of melanin formation
C. Irritation of opposing skin surfaces caused by the friction
D. Raised, firm, thickened scabs that form at the site of a wound

Q30. A patient attends the hospital clinic with the complain of pruritus on buttocks. On examination, the nurse finds sharply demarcated scaling plaques on both sides in the sacral area, and discolored nails with pits and ridges. The nurse suspects:

A. Contact dermatitis
B. Psoriasis
C. Scabies
D. Candidiasis

Q31. Majority of the household burn occurs from:

A. Defective wiring
B. Unattended cooking
C. Carelessness with cigarettes, bidis, and open flames
D. Improper storage of flammables

Q32. Major cause of the burn injury in the toddlers is from:

A. Contact with scalding liquids
B. Direct contact with flames from an explosion of flammable liquid
C. Clothing ignition while playing with matches
D. All of the above

Q33. The injury that is most likely to result in a full thickness burn is:

A. Sunburn
B. Ionizing radiation
C. Contact with hot objects
D. Electric current

Q34. If a white skinned individual remains exposed for 2 hours to the summer's sun unprotected may get sunburn which is:

A. Superficial partial-thickness burn
B. Deep partial-thickness burn
C. A full thickness burn
D. No real burn, sunburn merely means tanning of skin

Q35. A deep partial-thickness (second degree) burn is characterized by:

A. Injury to the epidermis
B. Injury to the epidermis and varying depth of dermis
C. Damage throughout the dermis and nerve endings
D. Damage to the skin, fat, muscle and bone

Q36. Which of the following characteristics is found in a third-degree full-thickness burn wound?

A. Blanching on pressure
B. Erythema
C. Fluid-filled vesicles
D. Eschar

Q37. During assessment of a patient with partial-thickness burn (second-degree) the nurse is expected to find:

A. Leathery or hard appearance of the skin
B. Exposed thrombosed vessels
C. Red, shiny and wet appearance of the skin
D. Erythema and blanching on pressure

Q38. The severity of burns is assessed by:

A. Estimating the percentage and depth of injured skin
B. Determining the presence of pre-existing diseases
C. Presence of burn in the specific site
D. Using established guides to indicate burn location relative to the total body surface and age of victim

Q39. Immediately following a burn injury, vasoactive substances released from the injured tissue alter capillary permeability. The first consequence of the altered capillary permeability is:

A. Movement of albumin into interstitial space
B. Movement of the potassium into the interstitial fluid
C. Movement of sodium and water into the interstitial space
D. Movement of red blood cells into the interstitial space

Q40. A person received burns to his entire chest, abdomen and left arm. According to the 'rule of nines' the victim has sustained burns to which of the following percentages of his body?

A. 18% **B.** 27%
C. 30% **D.** 36%

Q41. A female patient has been admitted in the burn unit with second and third-degree burn over 50% of the body caused by catching fire in her clothes. It has been 8 hours since admission. During this time which of the following data should have the highest priority for intervention?

A. Restlessness
B. Intense thirst
C. Feeble peripheral pulses
D. Difficulty in talking and hoarseness of voice

Q42. A 35-year-old woman weighing 60 kg is admitted in the burn ward with 50% burn. Using Parkland (Baxter) formula, how much fluid will be replaced during the first 12 hours?

A. 6750 mL **B.** 7500 mL
C. 9000 mL **D.** 10500 mL

Q43. Which of the following intravenous fluid is most appropriate for a patient with second and third-degree burn on 40% of the body during the first 24 hours?

A. Normal saline
B. 5% dextrose
C. Ringer's lactate solution
D. Albumin

Q44. A 50-year-old person weighing 70 kg is receiving fluid resuscitation therapy for sustaining an electrical burn over 25% of his body. In order to evaluate the adequacy of fluid replacement therapy the nurse should assess which of the following parameters?

A. ECG showing sinus rhythm
B. Urine output of 50 mL per hour
C. Urine output of 100 mL per hour
D. Systolic blood pressure 120 mm Hg

Q45. The nurse caring for a patient with 40% full-thickness burn is aware that the patient is at risk of developing which of the following electrolyte disturbances during the emergent phase?

A. Hypernatremia
B. Hyperkalemia
C. Hypomagnesemia
D. Hypochloremia

Q46. A hypermetabolic state observed after a burn injury resulting in protein and lipid catabolism that affects wound healing. In order to maintain a positive nitrogen balance the patient must adhere to which of the following dietary regimens?

A. High protein, low fat, low carbohydrate diet
B. High caloric and high protein diet
C. Small and frequent diet providing at least 2000 calories
D. Low sodium, high potassium and high fiber diet

Q47. Which of the following pain relieving drugs may be ordered for a person with second-degree partial-thickness burns over 20% of body surface area?

A. Acetaminophen
B. Morphine sulfate
C. Ibuprofen
D. Haloperidol

Q48. A 25-year-old young woman is admitted to the burn unit of the hospital with partial and full-thickness burns on her face, chest and arms. On arrival at the burn unit, which of the following will the nurse anticipate as an immediate action?

A. Collecting blood samples for arterial blood gases
B. Administering morphine sulphate IM
C. Inserting indwelling catheter for measuring hourly urine output
D. Assessing body image disturbances of the woman

Q49. Which of the following actions would a nurse take before changing dressings of a patient who has sustained a large partial-thickness burn?

A. Checking vital signs including blood pressure
B. Obtaining a signed consent for this procedure
C. Administering the pain medication as prescribed
D. Arranging music of patient's choice to be played during the procedure for distraction.

Q50. An autograft has been placed on the anterior chest of a 3-year-old child for a partial –thickness scald injury. Which of the following nursing interventions is appropriate?

A. Positioning the child on his abdomen immediately after operation
B. Immobilizing the arms of the child with elbow restraints
C. Applying a pressure dressing around the chest
D. Encouraging early ambulation

Q51. A patient has received an autograft in his left hand for a partial-thickness chemical burn. Postoperatively which of the following nursing interventions is appropriate?

A. Monitor the pulse in the left arm every 4 hours.
B. Change dressing every shift
C. Administer pain medication every 4 hours as prescribed to relieve pain in the donor site
D. Both A and C

Q52. A patient has received an autograft for a third-degree burn on his right arm. Postoperatively the nurse instructs the patient to:

A. Perform range of motion with the affected arm
B. Keep the arm in a dependent position to increase arterial circulation
C. To restrict fluid to prevent fluid accumulation under the graft
D. To protect the grafted site from direct sunlight

Q53. Two weeks after a skin graft a patient questions the nurse regarding the possibility of scarring at the donor site. Which

of the following instructions regarding the care of the donor site by the nurse is most appropriate?

A. Clean the area with soap and water everyday
B. Apply hydrogen peroxide over the area twice a day
C. Apply an antibiotic ointment once a day after cleaning with soap and water
D. Apply moisturizing lotion or cream on the area several times a day

Q54. A patient who has sustained an extensive partial-thicknes burn is undergoing daily hydrotherapy. The main purpose of hydrotherapy is to:

A. Prevent infection
B. Cleanse the wound
C. Restore fluid and electrolyte balance
D. Control elevated body temperature associated with the burn

Q55. When planning care for a person with burns on the upper part of the body involving face and neck, which of the following nursing diagnoses should take the highest priority?

A. Fluid volume deficit
B. Body image disturbances
C. Ineffective airway clearance
D. Risk for infection

Q56. A patient with a partial-thickness burns over 60% body surface area admitted in the burn unit. While planning care the nurse gives priority to which of the following goals of therapy?

A. Providing emotional support to the patient and family members
B. Relieving pain
C. Preventing infection
D. Maintaining the patient's fluid, electrolyte and acid-base balance

Q57. A patient is recovering from an extensive partial-thickness burn of 50% body surface area. While planning care during the acute stage the nurse gives priority to which of the following nursing diagnoses?

A. Fluid volume deficit
B. Risk for infection
C. Body image disturbance
D. Impaired physical mobility

Q58. A patient who is being treated for extensive burn in the burn unit is receiving H_2-receptor antagonist. The nurse explains to the patient that the purpose of administering this drug is to:

A. Aid in digestion
B. Stimulate intestinal motility
C. Facilitate protein absorption
D. Prevent stress ulcer

Q59. A patient has severe burns involving the lower extremities. Which of the following nursing actions would prevent contractures in this patient?

A. Keeping the legs elevated by 2 pillows
B. Applying splints to the patient's legs
C. Keeping the legs separated by placing a pillow in between the two legs
D. Instructing patient to do quadriceps drill

Q60. Hypertrophic scarring is a common complication of burn injury. Hypertrophic scarring can be prevented by:

A. Skin grafting of all burn wounds
B. Massaging the healed area with moisturizing cream several times a day
C. Exposing the healed tissue to direct sunlight
D. Continuous wearing of pressure garments after healing is complete

Q61. To assess the risk of development of pressure ulcer the nurse should use a validated assessment tool. Which of the following assessment tools is used to assess the risk of development of pressure ulcer?

A. Braden scale
B. Glasgow coma scale

C. Pressure sore status tool (PSST)
D. Pressure ulcer scale of healing (PUSH)

Q62. The nurse is assessing a 65-year-old patient for pressure ulcer risk using Braden scale. The numeric score obtained by the patient is 10. The nurse understands that the patient:

A. Is not at risk of developing a pressure ulcer
B. Is at high-risk of developing pressure ulcer
C. Has an existing pressure ulcer
D. Is not at risk at present but requires daily assessment

Q63. A 60-year-old patient with cirrhosis of liver and altered sensorium is assessed to be at the risk for the development of a pressure ulcer. The nurse should instruct the family member caring for the patient to:

A. Reposition the patient at every 2 hours
B. Increase fluid intake to hydrate the skin
C. Encourage patient to take high carbohydrate and high protein diet
D. All of the above

Q64. A 70-year-old lady with hemiplegia is being cared for at home. The public health nurse identifies a 1cm wide and 2 cm long superficial open blister over the patient's sacrum. The nurse would document this as being which of the following stages of pressure ulcer?

A. Stage I
B. Stage II
C. Stage III
D. Stage IV

Q65. Which of the following agents should be used to clean a pressure ulcer?

A. Soap and water
B. Normal saline
C. Hydrogen peroxide
D. Povidone-iodine

Q66. The nurse is providing care for a patient who has a sacral pressure ulcer with a wet to dry dressing. The wet to dry dressing:

A. Keep the wound bed and surrounding skin moist
B. Keep the wound bed moist and the surrounding skin dry
C. Is applied on an infected pressure ulcer
D. Consists of a wet dressing covered by a plastic sheet type dressing

Q67. Which of the following diets promotes wound healing?

A. Low carbohydrate, high protein and high vitamin C
B. Diet containing high carbohydrate, high protein and vitamin C
C. High protein, high vitamin A and C
D. Adequate calorie, protein, vitamin D and E

Q68. Which of the following conditions is a risk factor for the development of skin cancers?

A. Increased melanin content in skin
B. Exposure to systemic arsenicals
C. Young age
D. Persons living away from the equator

Q69. All of the following statements are true about nonmelanoma skin cancers *except:*

A. Nonmelanoma skin cancers are most common form of skin cancers
B. They arises from the dermal layer of skin
C. Common sites are the exposed areas of skin
D. Responsible for permanent disfigurement and disability

Q70. Which of the following types of skin cancer has the ability to metastasize to any organ including the brain and heart?

A. Basal cell carcinoma
B. Squamous cell carcinoma
C. Actinic keratosis
D. Malignant melanoma

ANSWERS AND RATIONALS OF INTEGUMENTARY SYSTEM AND BURNS

1. **B.** The innermost layer of the epidermis is stratum germinativum. The other layers of the epidermis from innermost to outermost and above the stratum germinativum are stratum granulosum, stratum lucidum, and stratum corneum.

2. **C.** The eccrine glands secrete sweat. These glands are widely distributed over the body except in a few areas, e.g. lips. These glands exit the body independently of the hair shaft. The other gland that secretes sweat is apocrine gland. Melanine is secreted by the melanocytes present in the basal layer of epidermis. Sebaceous glands secrete sebum and endocrine glands secrete hormones.

3. **B.** The most important function of the skin is to protect the underlying tissues of the body by serving as a surface barrier to the external environment. It acts as a barrier against mechanical, thermal, chemical, radiant, microorganisms, etc. Absorption of medications, sensory perception and synthesis of vitamin D are the other important functions of the skin but the protection of underlying tissues is the primary function.

4. **D.** Chronic exposure to ultraviolet rays is the major contributor to the wrinkling of skin. Sun damage to the skin is cumulative. Wrinkling of skin is more marked in the sun exposed areas of the body, e.g. face. Heredity, poor nutrition and general ill health all contribute to wrinkling but most important contributor is the exposure to ultraviolet rays.

5. **D.** When a person ages, the rate of wound healing diminishes due to decreased proliferative capacity of the skin. Other changes associated with aging are decreased not increased sweat production, diminished not increased growth of nails and hairs, diminished not increased awareness of pain, touch and temperature.

6. **A.** During physical examination of the skin, the nurse should have a private examination room with good lighting preferably daylight. She should carry out the examination systematically, proceeding from head to toe and perform a general inspection first followed by examination of specific lesion. The nurse determines skin turgor by gently pinching an area of skin under the clavicle and not by inspection. Areas of bruising are inspected and not palpated for possible blanching.

7. **B.** Elevated, sharply defined lesions that are less than 1cm in diameter and filled with serous fluid are called vesicles, e.g. lesions of chickenpox, herpes zoster, etc. Papules are elevated solid lesion less than 1 cm in diameter. Cysts are elevated thick-walled lesions containing fluid or semisolid matter and pustules are elevated superficial lesions filled with purulent fluid.

8. **C.** Firm, edematous and irregularly shaped areas of varying diameter are called wheals, e.g. insect bites, urticaria. Macules are circumscribed flat areas of less than 1 cm diameter with change in color, e.g. petechiae, measles. Papules are elevated solid lesion less than 1 cm in diameter and pustules are elevated superficial lesions filled with purulent fluid.

9. D. Biopsy techniques employed for obtaining skin tissue specimen for histological assessment include punch, incisional, excisional and shave biopsies. Any of the method may be adopted depending upon the site, cosmetic result desired and the type of tissue to be obtained.

10. B. Splinter hemorrhages are vertical linear red or brown streaks in the nail bed result from minor trauma to the nail bed, subacute bacterial endocarditis and trichinosis. Beau's line is a horizontal depression in the nail plate occurs alone or in multiple results from systemic infection or direct injury to the nail root. Clubbing is an increased angle between the nail plate and nail base usually results from long-standing hypoxia. Paronychia refers to inflammation of the skinfold at the nail margin usually due to trauma.

11. D. An effective sunscreen should have a wide range of absorbance. Benzophenones block both UVA and UVB rays. So the sunscreen containing benzophenones as an ingredients would be most effective sunscreen. Parsol blocks only UVA rays. Salicylates and cinnamets block only UVB rays.

12. D. Impetigo is a contagious superficial skin infection caused by beta hemolytic streptococci, staphylococci or combination of both. A severe untreated infection may lead to glomerulonephritis. Treatment consists of warm saline soaks followed by soap and water removal of crusts, topical antibiotics and systemic antibiotics, e.g. penicillin and erythromycin. Topical antibiotics are less effective in healing impetigo so systemic antibiotics are administered.

13. A. Antibacterial agent erythromycin or tetracycline may be administered orally or as a topical agent to treat severe acne. Acne is a common skin disorder of adolescence and is caused by *P.acnes*. Pyrimethamine is an antimalarial agent, miconazole is an antifungal agent and acyclovir is an antiviral agent. These agents do not have an impact on bacterial infections.

14. C. The nurse will teach the patient to apply warm moist compresses to the affected area every 4 hours to promote circulation and relieve pain. Cellulitis is a bacterial infection caused by streptococci and *Staphylococcus aureus*. Treatment includes moist heat application, immobilization and elevation, systemic antibiotics. The patient should rest in bed with the affected leg elevated. Movement, e.g. range of motion exercise is not encouraged. Elastic bandage and use of splints are contraindicated as they may compromise blood supply.

15. B. Gentamicin may cause ototoxicity. So the patient should be taught to report symptoms of loss of hearing, ringing or roaring in ears caused due to damage in ears. Visual problems, hoarseness of voice and tightness of chest are not associated with gentamicin.

16. B. Herpes zoster is a highly contagious viral infection. The organism is transmitted by direct contact with the vesicular fluid and airborne droplets from the respiratory tract of the patient. So the patient should be in a private cabin. Isolation room with negative pressure airflow is not required. Patient with previous history of chickenpox may have immunity against the virus but his visitors will be unnecessarily exposed.

17. B. Herpes zoster occurs due to activation of the varicella zoster virus. The treatment of herpes zoster will include administration of an antiviral agent, e.g. famciclovir. Tetracycline is used in bacterial infection, liquid nitrogen is used in planter warts and miconazole is given in fungal infection.

18. C. Oral famciclovir may cause adverse gastrointestinal effects as diarrhea, nausea and vomiting. It is not associated with hypotension, burning urination and palpitation.

19. A. Infection caused by *Candida albicans* (fungus) also known as moniliasis. Infection by *Candida albicans* presents in the warm moist areas e.g. mouth, vagina and overlapping areas of skin. Moniliasis appears as diffuse papular erythematous rash with pinpoint satellite lesions around edges of affected area. Lesions of tinea corporis appear as annular with well defined margins and erythematous. Scabies are seen as linear patches of grouped vesicles on erythematous base.

20. B. Fungal infection of the foot is termed as tinea pedis. Tinea corporis is the fungal infection of the body, tinea capities is the fungal infection of the scalp and tinea curis is the fungal infection of the inner thigh and inguinal creases.

21. D. Adult lice usually bite the scalp behind the ears and along the back of the neck. Lice may bite any part of the scalp but bites are less common on the top of the head.

22. C. The nurse should isolate patient's bed linen and towel until patient is no longer infectious usually after 24 hours after treatment begins. Handwashing is a good practice to prevent transmission. Scabies mites are not found in feces, so enteric precaution is not necessary. Application of pediculicide to patient's scalp does not treat scabies.

23. A. The patient and all his family members should be treated against scabies by applying benzyle benzoate emulsion simultaneously in order to prevent recurrence and eradicate the disease as scabies can be transmitted from a patient to other family members by direct physical contact and by shared personal items before symptoms manifestation and recurrence.

24. D. The nurse should teach the patient to apply the medicine only once or twice as prescribed. More frequent application does not increase effectiveness, rather increases the chance of side effects. Side effects are more likely when medium or high potency drug is applied for prolonged time. The most common side effect is skin atrophy that presents as thin, shiny skin with increased prominence of blood vessels, telangiectasia, easy bruising and stria. The patient should apply the medicine evenly and sparingly and not as a thick coating should not abruptly stop applying medicines even if symptoms disappear, and apply it in long, downward strokes in the direction of hair growth to prevent irritation of follicle and not against the growth of hair.

25. D. Exact cause of atopic dermatitis is unknown. The condition is associated with a personal or family history of asthma, eczema or food allergies. It is not due to contact with allergen. Contact with allergen causes contact dermatitis. The condition is not caused by infection with bacteria, virus or fungus. Specific nutritional deficiency is also not known as a cause of the problem. In some patients with eczema the ratio of omega-3 to omega-6 fatty acids is found to be lowered. But this factor has not yet been established as a cause of the disease.

26. A. The common site for the lesions associated with atopic dermatitis in adults is the large folds of the extremities. It is mainly found on elbow bends (antecubital area), backs of the knees (popliteal area), neck, eyelids, and the back of the hands and feet. Axilla, groin and buttocks are not the common sites for atopic dermatitis.

27. C. Atopic dermatitis is not due to infection and it is not contagious. So the nursing diagnosis of risk for infection transmission to others is not appropriate. All other nursing diagnosis are appropriate.

28. D. Occlusive dressings if applied immediately after soaking or on wet skin prevent evaporative water loss and correct dryness of the skin caused by the atopic dermatitis. Application of occlusive dressings also promotes topical therapy and cooling of the skin. All these effects give better relief from the distressing symptoms of dryness, itching and scaling.

29. C. Intertrigo is a superficial inflammatory dermatitis that occurs due to irritation of apposing (touching) skin surfaces caused by friction. Inadequate ventilation, heat and moisture build up result in erythema and maceration, itching and burning. Epidermal thickening resulting in elevated plaque with accentuated skin markings is lichenification. Unpigmented skin patches associated with the lack of melanin formation is vitiligo and raised, firm, thickened scabs that form at the site of a wound is keloid.

30. B. Psoriasis, a chronic skin disorder of unknown etiology shows these characteristic skin changes. Psoriatic skin lesions are covered with silvery white scales, symmetrically distributed and commonly occur on the scalp, elbows, knees and sacral regions. Nail dystrophies and pitting occur in about 30 to 50% of patients. In contact dermatitis lesions are itchy, erythematous and edematous and not scaly. Burrows present in lesions of scabies that appear in interdigital webs. Fingernails are not affected in scabies. In candidiasis there is diffuse papular erythematous rash, not scaling plaques.

31. C. Most of the burn injuries occur from the actions of the victims. Majority of the burn injury in the household takes place from the carelessness of the victim with cigarettes, bidis, and open flames from candles, etc. Defective wiring, unattended cooking and improper storage of flammables are also the cause of burn, but their incidence is low.

32. A. Most of the burn injury occurs in toddlers from scalding liquids. Toddlers suffer more scald injuries than any other age group. Scald injuries are frequently the result of mishaps in the performance of daily activities such as bathing and cooking. Overturned teapots, cooking pans spilling hot liquid and oil, hot tap water are the specific source. Other causes of burn injury listed are less frequently seen in toddlers.

33. D. Burn injuries from electrical current may result in full- thickness burn. The extent of injury is influenced by the duration of contact, the intensity of current (voltage), the type of current (direct or alternating), the pathway of the current and the resistance of the tissues as the electrical current passes through the body. Contact of electrical current greater than 40 volts is potentially dangerous. Sunburn and ionizing radiation may cause superficial partial thickness burn and contact with hot objects may cause deep partial-thickness burns.

34. A. A sunburn is a superficial partial-thickness burn. A prolonged exposure to sun's rays can cause a superficial partial-thickness burn which is typically called 'sunburn.' All persons particularly white skinned individuals should be advised to wear protective clothing or sunscreen to protect against such injury. Deep partial-thickness burns are less common in the sun exposed individual who is conscious and able to retreat from the sun's rays. Sunburn is a real injury and should be treated as such.

35. B. A deep partial-thickness (second-degree) is characterized by the injury to epidermis and varying depth of dermis. In this type of burn some skin elements from which epithelial regeneration can occur remain viable. Epidermis is affected in superficial partial-thickness (first-degree) burn. (Third-degree) full-thickness burns are characterized by damage through the dermis and nerve endings. Damage to skin, fat, muscle and bone takes place in (fourth-degree) full-thickness burn.

36. D. In a third-degree, full-thickness burn the skin appears dry and may be black, brown, white or ivory. The denatured skin is called eschar. Fluid-filled vesicles or wet skin (if vesicles have ruptured) are seen in the deep partial-thickness second-degree burn. Erythema and blanching on pressure are seen in the superficial partial-thickness or first-degree burn wound.

37. C. During assessment of a second-degree or partial-thickness burn the nurse is expected to find the burned area as red, shiny and wet or blistered. Other additional assessment findings are severe pain due to nerve injury and mild to moderate edema. Leathery, hard, dry or waxy appearance of the skin with visible thrombosed vessels is seen in full-thickness or third-degree burn wound. Erythema, blanching on pressure, pain and mild swelling and absence of blisters are found in the first-degree partial-thickness burn.

38. D. The severity of burn depends on many factors, e.g. burn size, depth of burn, location of burn injury, age and general health of the victim and mechanism of the injury. To help clinician in determining the injury severity for the burn patient, guidelines are established by individual institution or professional association (like American Burn Association) that take into account all these factors.

39. C. Immediately after a burn injury, vasoactive substances (catecholamine, histamine, leukotrien, kinin and prostaglandins) are released from the injured tissue. These substances along with direct damage to vessels from heat increases capillary permeability allowing movement of water, sodium from the vascular space to the interstitial spaces and other surrounding tissues resulting into intravascular volume depletion, edema and blister formation. With movement of water and sodium into interstitial spaces colloidal osmotic pressure decreases resulting into movement of protein (albumin) from the vascular space to interstitial space. So movement of albumin takes place later and not the first consequence of altered capillary permeability. Potassium that is mostly intracellular move into the intravascular space not interstitial space as injured cells and hemolyzed RBCs release potassium. Increased capillary permeability does not allow RBCs to leave intravascular compartment resulting into increased hematocrit concentration.

40. B. The victim has sustained a burn of total 27% of his body (entire chest and abdomen 18% and left arm 9%). The 'rule of nines' is a quick assessment used to determine the extent of burn based on the body surface area. It does not take into consideration the depth of burn. According to 'rule of nines' an adult's head and neck and each upper extremity are 9%, the anterior chest and abdomen, the entire back and each leg are 18% and the perineum is 1%.

41. D. Difficulty in talking and hoarseness of voice are assessment findings that have the highest priority for intervention at this time. These findings are indicative of inhalation injury that is potentially life-threatening and requires immediate intervention by intubation and mechanical ventilation. Restlessness, intense thirst and feeble peripheral pulses are the signs of hypovolemic shock that occurs due to massive fluid shift and would not take precedence over potential respiratory failure.

42. B. 7500 mL of fluid will be replaced to a woman weighing 60 kg and having 50% BSA burn. Parkland (Baxter) formula is 4 mL × kg body weight × % BSA burned. So the fluid requirement of this woman is 4 × 60 × 50 = 12,000 mL = 12 L in 24 hours. Now –

½ of total in first 8 hours = 6 L or 6,000 mL (750 mL/ hr)

¼ of total in second 8 hours = 3 L or 3,000 mL (375 mL/hr)

¼ of total in third 8 hours = 3 L or 3000 mL (375 mL/hr)

So the required fluid during 12 hours = 6000 + 375 × 4 = 6000 + 1500 +7500 mL. 6,750 ml of fluid is required during first 10 hours, 9,000 mL fluid in first 16 hours and 10,500 mL during the first 20 hours.

43. C. During the first 24 hours the most appropriate fluid to be used is Ringer's lactate solution which is a balanced salt solution. This solution replaces lost sodium and corrects metabolic acidosis, both of which commonly occur after burn injury. According to Parkland formula which is used by most of the institution, Ringer's lactate solution is the only fluid used for first 24 hours after burn injury. Albumin which is a colloid solution is administered during the second 24 hours after burn injury when capillary permeability returns to normal or near normal. A combination of normal saline, 5% dextrose and colloids are used during the first 24 hours of burn injury by a few institutions that use Evans formula. Institutions using Brook formula uses Ringer's lactate solution, colloids and 5% dextrose in combination during the first 24 hours of burn injury.

44. C. Adequacy of fluid replacement is assessed by the various parameters. Urinary output is the most commonly used parameter. Adequate fluid replacement will result in adequate kidney perfusion which will produce urine at least 5 mL/kg of body weight/hour. So an adult with burn injury should have 30-50 mL urine per hour. But in case of an electrical burn an urine output of 75 to 100 mL/hour should be used as an acceptable parameter. The other assessment parameters for adequate fluid replacement are—arterial blood pressure greater than 90 mm Hg (peripheral measurement of blood pressure is often invalid because of vasoconstriction and edema), pulse rate less than 120, respiration 16 to 20 breaths per minute and an alert and oriented sensorium.

45. B. A patient with full-thickness burn injury is at risk of developing hyperkalemia because large amounts of potassium are released from the injured cells and hemolyzed RBCs and move into the extracellular spaces. During the emergent phase patient is at risk of developing hyponatremia not hypernatremia because sodium along with water rapidly shifts from the intravascular spaces to the interstitial spaces and remains there until edema formation ceases. Hypomagnesemia and hypochloremia are not identified in a patient with burn.

46. B. Burn patients should eat by mouth as soon as their condition permits. Dietary intake should be optimum to prevent massive protein and lipid breakdown from hypermetabolic state that exists after burn. Diet should consists of high calories which may be 3 times of normal adult caloric intake and high protein. This kind of diet will promote positive nitrogen balance and help healing. Vitamins would be used to supplement the diet and to aid in tissue repair. Other diets listed are not indicated for the burn patient.

47. B. Morphine sulfate is an opioid analgesic acts on the central nervous system diminishing pain sensation. It is a very potent analgesic. As the patient has sustained a second-degree partial-thickness burn that is very painful, he requires a potent analgesic like morphine sulfate. Acetaminophen and ibuprofen may be helpful in mild to moderate pain and are not effective in relieving pain of burn injury. Haloperidol has antipsychotic and sedative action and is given in combination with morphine to produce sedative effect not to relieve pain.

48. A. Since the woman has sustained a burn of upper part of the body including face, most probably she has sustained inhalation injury of respiratory tract. Hence the nurse should first draw blood for arterial blood gases to establish pulmonary function levels. Administration of morphine is important to relieve pain but intramuscular administration is contraindicated. Morphine is given in intravenous route after fluid replacement is initiated. Inserting indwelling catheter to monitor urine output is very important but it is not a priority over evaluation of blood gas levels. Assessing body image disturbances is a low priority during this stage. It may be important during the rehabilitative phase.

49. C. The nurse will administer pain medication before changing dressings because dressing changes for the burn patient can be very painful. Dressings of burn wound often involves removal of eschar (burned leathery crust that forms over burned tissue and harbors pathogenic microorganism) or debridement. Analgesics preferably narcotics should be administered at least ½ hour before the procedure in order to allow sufficient time for the medication to take effect before beginning dressing. Distraction by music therapy is not an appropriate measure for the relief of pain associated with change of dressings. Checking vital signs prior to dressing change is not required. A signed consent is not necessary for dressing change.

50. B. Immobilizing the arms of the child with elbow restraints is the appropriate nursing intervention in caring a child after skin graft, as this will keep the child's hands away from the grafted site. The child should be positioned on his back (supine) not on abdomen to prevent dislodgment of the graft. Grafted area should be covered with a dressing but pressure should not be applied over grafted area, as it would impede circulation of the wound bed. Child will require bed rest to prevent dislodgment of the graft and not ambulated early.

51. A. Optimum circulation is needed for the survival of the graft, so nurse must check pulse for adequate circulation.

52. D. The patient who has received a skin graft must be instructed to protect the graft site from direct sunlight to prevent burning and sloughing. Patient should not perform range of motion exercises of the affected hand as it may dislodge the graft. He should keep the hand slightly elevated, not keep in a dependent position. Patient should not restrict fluid as optimum hydration and nutrition are important for healing. Blisters (small blebs of serum) if formed under the graft are drained periodically by inserting a small sterile needle into the blister.

53. D. Moisturizing lotion or cream, e.g. lanolin should be applied over the donor site several times a day. Application of moisturizing lotion will keep the area soft and minimize scarring. However, patient should be explained that possibility of scarring could not be predicted so early as scar tissue requires a full year to mature. Soap and hydrogen peroxide are irritant and their use should be avoided. Patient does not require an antibiotic ointment as healing has already taken place.

54. B. The main purpose of hydrotherapy for patients with burns is to cleanse the wounds by removing loose tissue and debris. Hydrotherapy also promotes active range of motion exercises. Proper cleaning minimizes infection but it can not prevent infection. Infection of wound is prevented by topical microbial therapy after cleansing. Fluid and electrolyte replacement is essential in the management of patient with burns and is achieved by intravenous infusion of fluid and electrolytes. However, hydrotherapy if given for a prolonged time may cause hyponatremia (sodium loss through the burn wound to the hypotonic water). So hydrotherapy should always be given for only 30 minutes or less. Hydrotherapy reduces elevated body temperature but this is not the main purpose in the management of burn.

55. C. A patient with burns in the upper part of the body involving face and neck is at high-risk for ineffective airway clearance related to possible upper airway edema, secondary to inhalation of superheated air, smoke or noxious chemicals. So the nursing diagnosis of ineffective airway clearance should receive highest priority. Fluid volume deficit, body image disturbances and risk for infection are all important nursing diagnoses for this patient but not priority.

56. D. The nurse should give priority to maintain the patient's fluid, electrolyte and acid-base balance to avoid potential life-threatening complications, e.g. hypovolemic shock, respiratory failure, cardiac failure and acute renal failure. Providing emotional support, relieving pain and preventing infection are all important goals for this patient but maintenance of fluid, electrolyte and acid-base balance are the most immediate goals.

57. B. The acute phase begins with the mobilization of extracellular fluid and subsequent diuresis. During the acute stage the nurse should give priority to risk for infection. The high-risk of infection is related to loss of the skin barrier, an impaired immune response, the presence of invasive lines and catheters. Care of the patient during the acute phase focusses on the infection control, care of wound,nutritional support, pain management, physical therapy and psychosocial care. Fluid volume deficit is a priority problem in the emergent phase, not in acute phase. Body image disturbance and impaired physical mobility are appropriate nursing diagnoses but do not have higher priority than risk for infection.

58. D. Curling's ulcer occurs in burn patients and is caused by generalized stress response. Prophylactic use of antacids and H_2 receptor antagonist prevents this complication. H_2 receptor antagonists do not aid in digestion, stimulate intestinal motility and facilitate protein absorption.

59. B. In order to prevent contractures in the lower extremities of the patient the nurse should position the legs extended with help of splints. A contracture is an abnormal condition of a joint characterized by flexion and fixation. Because of pain the patient will prefer to assume a flexed position for comfort, which predisposes to contracture formation. So the nurse should properly position the patient's legs extended with the help of splints. Keeping legs elevated or placing pillow in between legs will not prevent contractures. Exercise, e.g. quadriceps drill strengthens muscles but do not prevent contractures. To prevent contractures the patient must perform the range of motion exercises every 4 hours throughout the healing process.

60. D. Hypertrophic scarring can be prevented by wearing pressure garments for 24 hours a day for as long as 1-2 years after burn injury. Pressure can help to keep a scar flat and thus prevents hypertrophic scarring. Skin grafting does not result in hypertrophic scarring but it is not possible to treat all wounds by skin graft. Massaging the healed area with moisturizing cream prevents itching but not hypertrophic scar formation. Exposure to direct sunlight does not prevent hypertrophic scar formation, but causes hyper-pigmentation and sunburn injury. So the patient must be instructed to protect healed burn areas from direct sunlight for a period of 1 year.

61. A. Pressure sore risk assessment is done by Braden scale. 6 factors are considered in the Braden scale, e.g. sensory perception, moisture, activity, mobility, nutrition and friction and shear. Numeric scores are given against each factors. Total scores can range from 6-23. The lower the score on the Braden scale the higher is the risk for development of pressure ulcer. Glasgow coma scale is used for the assessment of level of consciousness. Pressure ulcer scale of healing tool and pressure sore status tool are used for the documentation of healing of already developed pressure ulcer and not to assess the risk of pressure ulcer.

62. B. A score of 10 at Braden scale signifies that the patient is at high-risk of developing a pressure ulcer. Scores on Braden scale can range from 6-23. The lower the score the higher is the patient's predicted risk of developing a pressure ulcer. A score of (6-9), very high-risk; (10-12), high-risk; (13-14) moderate-risk; (15-18), at risk: (19-23), no risk.

63. A. The nurse should instruct the family member caring for the patient to reposition the patient at every 2 hours. Although optimum hydration prevents skin breakdown, this patient with cirrhosis may be on fluid restriction because of edema and ascites. High protein diets although beneficial for healthy skin but patient with cirrhosis and altered sensorium needs protein restricted diet to decrease ammonia level in the blood.

64. B. Stage II pressure ulcers are identified by the skin that is not intact. There is a partial-thickness skin loss involving epidermis, dermis or both. The ulcer is superficial and presents as an abrasion, blister or shallow crater. Stage I pressure ulcer identified as skin that is intact. The ulcer appears as persistent red area (in lightly pigmented skin) or blue or purple area (in darker skin) that does not blanch with external pressure. Stage III pressure ulcers are identified by the full-thickness skin loss involving damage to or necrosis of subcutaneous tissue. The ulcer presents as deep crater. Stage IV pressure ulcers are identified as full-thickness skin loss with extensive destruction, tissue necrosis, or damage to muscle, bone and supporting structures.

65. B. Pressure ulcer should be cleaned with normal saline. Antiseptic lotions should never be applied on wound bed as most of the antiseptic lotions are cytotoxic, i.e. they damage cell especially fibroblasts. Hydrogen peroxide and povidone- iodine are cytotoxic and should not be applied on wound bed. Soap is irritating and should not be used.

66. B. Following cleansing of a pressure ulcer the wound should be covered with a wet-to-dry dressing. Wet-to-dry dressing keep the wound bed moist and the surrounding skin dry. Wet-to-dry dressing is never applied on an infected wound. Dry gauze dressing not a plastic sheet-type dressing covers a wet dressing.

67. B. Malnutrition delays wound healing. A positive nitrogen balance is essential for healing of wound. A diet containing high carbohydrate, high protein and vitamin C promotes wound healing. High carbohydrate prevents protein breakdown and maintains positive nitrogen balance. Other nutrients necessary for the wound healing are vitamin A, K, pyridoxine, riboflavin and thiamin. Vitamin D and E are not necessary for wound healing.

68. B. One of the risk factor for development of skin cancer is exposure to systemic arsenicals, e.g. drinking water with high arsenic concentration. The other risk factors include fair skin individual (having low melanin in skin), middle aged or elderly person, history of chronic sun exposure, persons living near the equator, working outdoors and frequent outdoor recreational activities.

69. B. Nonmelanoma skin cancers arise from the epidermis not dermis. Melanoma skin cancers arise from melanocytes, situated in the deeper layer of the epidermis. The other statements are all true about nonmelanoma skin cancers.

70. D. Malignant melanoma is the most deadly skin cancer. Basal cell carcinoma and squamous cell carcinomas are the nonmelanoma skin cancers. They do not metastasize but causes severe local destruction, permanent disfigurement and disability. Actinic keratosis also known as solar keratosis is a premalignant form of squamous cell carcinoma and a most common form of premalignant skin lesion.